Handbook of Preoperative Assessment and Management

Provided as an Educational
Service by

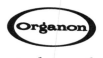

makers of

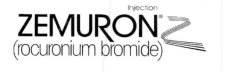

Injection

ZEMURON®
(rocuronium bromide)

Handbook of Preoperative Assessment and Management

Edited by

BobbieJean Sweitzer, M.D.

Assistant Professor of Anesthesia and Critical Care
Harvard Medical School
Assistant Anesthetist
Massachusetts General Hospital
Boston, Massachusetts

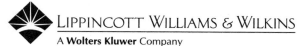

LIPPINCOTT WILLIAMS & WILKINS
A **Wolters Kluwer** Company

Philadelphia · Baltimore · New York · London
Buenos Aires · Hong Kong · Sydney · Tokyo

Acquisitions Editor: R. Craig Percy
Developmental Editor: Sonya L. Seigafuse
Supervising Editor: Mary Ann McLaughlin
Manufacturing Manager: Kevin Watt
Cover Illustrator: Kevin Kall
Production Editor: JoAnn Schambier, Silverchair Science + Communications
Compositor: Silverchair Science + Communications
Printer: RR Donnelley/Crawfordsville

© **2000 by LIPPINCOTT WILLIAMS & WILKINS**
530 Walnut Street
Philadelphia, PA 19106 USA
LWW.com

Printed in the USA

Library of Congress Cataloging-in-Publication Data

Handbook of preoperative assessment and management / edited by
  BobbieJean Sweitzer.
    p. ; cm.
  Includes bibliographical references and index.
  ISBN 0-7817-1633-0
    1. Preoperative care--Handbooks, manuals, etc. I. Sweitzer, BobbieJean.
    [DNLM: 1. Preoperative Care--methods. 2. Risk Assessment--methods.
  WO 179 H236 1999]
  RD49 .H364 1999
  617'.919--dc21
                                                    99-048127
                                                      CIP

Care has been taken to confirm the accuracy of the information presented and to describe generally accepted practices. However, the authors, editors, and publisher are not responsible for errors or omissions or for any consequences from application of the information in this book and make no warranty, expressed or implied, with respect to the currency, completeness, or accuracy of the contents of the publication. Application of this information in a particular situation remains the professional responsibility of the practitioner.
The authors, editors, and publisher have exerted every effort to ensure that drug selection and dosage set forth in this text are in accordance with current recommendations and practice at the time of publication. However, in view of ongoing research, changes in government regulations, and the constant flow of information relating to drug therapy and drug reactions, the reader is urged to check the package insert for each drug for any change in indications and dosage and for added warnings and precautions. This is particularly important when the recommended agent is a new or infrequently employed drug.
Some drugs and medical devices presented in this publication have Food and Drug Administration (FDA) clearance for limited use in restricted research settings. It is the responsibility of health care providers to ascertain the FDA status of each drug or device planned for use in their clinical practice.

10 9 8 7 6 5 4 3 2 1

To Stephen, who motivates and sustains me,
and to Sydney, Sheridan, and Schuler,
who give me much joy and inspire me with their curiosity

Contents

Contributing Authors

Rae M. Allain, M.D.
Assistant in Anesthesia
Department of Anesthesia and Critical Care
Massachusetts General Hospital
55 Fruit Street
Boston, Massachusetts 02114

Jane Ballantyne, M.D.
Assistant Professor of Clinical Anesthesia
Department of Anesthesia and Critical Care
Massachusetts General Hospital
55 Fruit Street
Boston, Massachusetts 02114

Charles Beattie, Ph.D., M.D.
Professor and Chairman
Department of Anesthesiology
Vanderbilt University Medical Center
1313 Twenty-first Avenue S
Nashville, Tennessee 37232

Joshua A. Bloomstone, M.D.
Instructor
Department of Anesthesia and Critical Care
Harvard Medical School
Massachusetts General Hospital
55 Fruit Street
Boston, Massachusetts 02114

Ok Yung Chung, M.D., M.B.A.
Assistant Professor
Department of Anesthesiology
Assistant Medical Director
Vanderbilt Pain Control Center
Vanderbilt University Medical Center
1211 Twenty-first Avenue S
Nashville, Tennessee 37212

Gregory Crosby, M.D.
Associate Professor of Anesthesia
Harvard Medical School
Brigham and Women's Hospital
75 Francis Street
Boston, Massachusetts 02115

Deborah J. Culley, M.D.
Instructor
Department of Anesthesiology
Harvard Medical School
Brigham and Women's Hospital
75 Francis Street
Boston, Massachusetts 02115

Francisco DeLaCruz, M.D.
Resident in Anesthesiology
Massachusetts General Hospital
55 Fruit Street
Boston, Massachusetts 02114

Lynne R. Ferrari, M.D.
Associate Professor of Anesthesia
Harvard Medical School
Medical Director, Perioperative Services
Children's Hospital
300 Longwood Avenue
Boston, Massachusetts 02115

Stephen P. Fischer, M.D.
Associate Professor of Anesthesiology
Stanford University School of Medicine
Medical Director
Preoperative Anesthesia Evaluation Program
Stanford University Medical Center
300 Pasteur Drive, H3580
Stanford, California 94305

Lee A. Fleisher, M.D.
Associate Professor of Anesthesiology
Department of Anesthesiology and Critical Care Medicine
Chief, Division of Perioperative Health Services Research
Johns Hopkins University School of Medicine
600 N Wolfe Street
Baltimore, Maryland 21287

Michael E. Henry, M.D.
Instructor in Psychiatry
Harvard Medical School
Director of Electroconvulsive Therapy
McLean Hospital
115 Mill Street
Belmont, Massachusettes 02478

Michael S. Higgins, M.P.H., M.D.
Assistant Professor of Anesthesiology
Vanderbilt University School of Medicine
Twenty-first and Garland
Nashville, Tennessee 37232

Joseph M. Hughes, M.D., M.B.A.
Instructor in Anesthesia
Department of Anesthesia and Critical Care
Harvard Medical School
Massachusetts General Hospital
55 Fruit Street
Boston, Massachusetts 02114

William E. Hurford, M.D.
Associate Professor of Anesthesia
Department of Anesthesia and Critical Care
Harvard Medical School
Massachusetts General Hospital
55 Fruit Street
Boston, Massachusetts 02114

Mary Kraft, M.D., M.P.A.
Instructor in Anesthesia
Department of Anesthesia and Critical Care
Massachusetts General Hospital
55 Fruit Street
Boston, Massachusetts 02114

Stephanie L. Lee, M.D., Ph.D.
Assistant Professor of Medicine
Tufts University School of Medicine
New England Medical Center
750 Washington Street
Boston, Massachusetts 02111

Ricardo Martinez-Ruiz, M.D.
Assistant Professor
Department of Anesthesiology
University of Puerto Rico School of Medicine
P.O. Box 365067
San Juan, Puerto Rico 00936

James B. Mayfield, M.D.
Instructor
Department of Anesthesia and Critical Care
Harvard Medical School
Massachusetts General Hospital
55 Fruit Street
Boston, Massachusetts 02114

L. Reuven Pasternak, M.D., M.P.H., M.B.A.
Chairman and Associate Professor
Department of Anesthesiology and Critical Care Medicine
Johns Hopkins Bayview Medical Center
4940 Eastern Avenue
Baltimore, Maryland 21224

Robert A. Peterfreund, M.D., Ph.D.
Assistant Professor of Anesthesia
Harvard Medical School
Associate Anesthetist
Department of Anesthesia and Critical Care
Massachusetts General Hospital
55 Fruit Street
Boston, Massachusetts 02114

Donald F. Pierce, Jr., M.D., Ph.D.
Instructor in Anesthesiology
Vanderbilt University Medical Center
1313 Twenty-first Avenue S
Nashville, Tennessee 37232

Zenaide M. N. Quezado, M.D.
Instructor in Anesthesia
Department of Anesthesia and Critical Care
Harvard Medical School
Massachusetts General Hospital
55 Fruit Street
Boston, Massachusetts 02114

Michael F. Roizen, M.D.
Chairman
Department of Anesthesia and Critical Care
Professor of Internal Medicine
University of Chicago Pritzker School of Medicine
5841 S Maryland
Chicago, Illinois 60637

Stanley P. Sady, Ph.D., M.D.
Anesthesia Associates of New Mexico
1720 Louisiana NE, #401
Albuquerque, New Mexico 87110

Devashish Sen, M.D.
Department of Anesthesia and Critical Care
Harvard Medical School
Massachusetts General Hospital
55 Fruit Street
Boston, Massachusetts 02114

Kenneth E. Shepherd, M.D.
Assistant Professor of Clinical Anesthesia
Harvard Medical School
Department of Anesthesia and Critical Care
Massachusetts General Hospital
55 Fruit Street
Boston, Massachusetts 02114

BobbieJean Sweitzer, M.D.
Assistant Professor of Anesthesia and Critical Care
Harvard Medical School
Assistant Anesthetist
Massachusetts General Hospital
32 Fruit Street
Boston, Massachusetts 02114

Jeffrey Uppington, M.B., B.S.
Assistant Professor of Anesthesia
Department of Anesthesia and Critical Care
Harvard Medical School
Massachusetts General Hospital
55 Fruit Street
Boston, Massachusetts 02114

Preface

A number of converging forces have created a need for a practical reference for clinicians interested in performing high-value preoperative assessments. These include growing information about managing risk in the context of various patient and disease characteristics, increased emphasis on systems approaches to simultaneously increase quality and decrease cost, and greater penetration of technology at the front line of patient care. In addition, care has become more distributed, specialized, and discontinuous while production and cost pressures have increased. These trends threaten to multiply gaps in service and challenge safety. In care characterized by multiple handoffs among different disciplines, such as preoperative assessment, it is clear that clinicians today must have ready access to the information they need, when they need it, and in a form that they can use.

This book is the first of its kind to integrate current knowledge about risk, data management systems, pathophysiology, the clinical examination, cost-effective diagnostics, and methods for optimizing patient status preoperatively. Historically, no widely accepted curriculum for preoperative evaluation that encompasses these areas has been available to anesthesia clinicians, specialists, surgeons, or primary care providers. Although valuable information exists, it is often presented in a number of overlapping areas or in a way that makes it difficult for practitioners to synthesize opposing views. Furthermore, a lack of rigorous, controlled studies have prevented professional organizations, health care institutions, and quality-assurance bodies from developing and disseminating standards and guidelines to reduce uninformed, costly, and potentially harmful variance in practices.

Leaders in clinical and academic arenas have suggested it is the right time to lay the foundation for creating a scientific basis for preoperative evaluation. Taking its cue from this vision, this book builds a case for consensus on the assessment and management of surgical patients formulated on an evidence-based perspective and expert opinion.

Many caregivers find preoperative assessment a challenge both clinically and organizationally, yet preoperative preparation and education have been shown to facilitate recovery and reduce postoperative morbidity. Preoperative health status predicts operative outcomes and resource use. We acknowledge that a gap currently exists between best and actual practices. We believe that a reference source is needed to support generation of state-of-the-art preoperative assessment curricula and stimulate research.

By emphasizing pathophysiology of disease states that are particularly relevant to surgery and anesthesia, the pertinent history and physical examination that are required for diagnosis, and focused laboratory tests, we have striven to give the reader the necessary knowledge and tools to adapt our approach to patients in diverse individual practices. With the contemporary emphasis on problem-oriented learning, case studies are provided to enhance relevancy of the material. These can be flexibly adapted for small group, problem-based learning sessions. Unique aspects of the book include chapters on risk assessment, data management, electronic medical records, and development of practice guidelines presented in an effort to streamline the preoperative assessment process.

Our goal is to present a cohesive body of information to assist clinicians taking responsibility for providing a comprehensive, value-added approach to preoperative assessment and management. We challenge future practitioners to develop preoperative evaluation, risk assessment, and best-practice models to meet and exceed the demands of today's health care system and the needs of our patients. The culture change will be no less difficult than the drive to advance scientific practice.

BobbieJean Sweitzer, M.D.

Acknowledgments

I thank the contributors who gave their knowledge and time to bring this work to fruition. In addition, I would like to acknowledge Jennifer Padelford Lofton for her unflagging dedication to the book and manuscript preparation. I am indebted to Sonya Seigafuse and Craig Percy at Lippincott Williams & Wilkins and JoAnn Schambier at Silverchair Science + Communications for their sincere support, advice, and collegiality. I also owe a debt of gratitude to the following reviewers who generously provided their expertise to help ensure a high level of quality across the book:

Michael Bailin, M.D.
Keith Baker, M.D.
George Battit, M.D.
Daniel Carr, M.D.
Charles Coté, M.D.
David Cullen, M.D.
William Denman, M.D.
Peter Dunn, M.D.
Gordon Gibby, M.D.
Douglas Hansell, M.D.
Michael S. Higgins, M.D., M.P.H.
William Kimball, M.D.
Michael Laposata, M.D.
Edward Lowenstein, M.D.
Alex Macario, M.D.
John Marota, M.D.
L. Reuven Pasternak, M.D.
Harvey Rosenbaum, M.D.
James T. Roberts, M.D.
Michael F. Roizen, M.D.
Nina Rubin, M.D.
John Ryan, M.D.
Adam Sapirstein, M.D.
Leslie Shaff, M.D.
Erik Shank, M.D.
Scott Streckenbach, M.D.
Elizabeth Vancott, M.D.
Warren Zapol, M.D.

Risk Assessment and Risk Modification

Charles Beattie, Ok Yung Chung, and Donald F. Pierce, Jr.

This chapter provides a critical appraisal of the current state of preoperative evaluation and risk assessment. Although the discussion encompasses, conceptually, all aspects of perioperative risk, special emphasis is given to cardiac morbidity. The argument is made that, for the most part, enough is now known about the preexisting conditions that lead to untoward outcomes. Attempts to further refine the quantification of risk based on preoperative data will not result in better patient care. The real issue confronting perioperative clinicians at this point is risk reduction.

After its discovery, surgical anesthesia was eagerly embraced by the general public and the medical profession, even as complications associated with its use were noted with concern.[1] From those early times to the present, efforts to improve safety have included the discovery of agents with higher therapeutic indices, creation of accurate and reliable drug delivery devices, and development of sophisticated monitoring modalities. These pharmacologic and technological advances have provided important tools to the modern anesthesiologist. Meanwhile, innovative clinicians and researchers have systematically addressed a broad array of conditions known to be associated with perioperative sequelae. Each problem or potential problem, many of which are reviewed in this book, now has one or more accepted countermeasures. Indeed, one might say that the dominant portion of anesthesia training consists of acquisition of the knowledge and experience to protect patients from the negative effects of surgical procedures and drug toxicity as these interact with preexisting comorbidities. Thus, anesthesiologists are always engaged in risk assessment (Is this patient at risk for particular complications?) and risk modification (What can I do about it?), although it is not customary either to express their activity in that manner or to quantify the risk. For example, practitioners widely accept that the risk of regurgitation during anesthetic induction is greater in patients who have recently eaten. Because regurgitation may lead to aspiration, pneumonia, and death, protection of the airway is mandatory, and many techniques and procedures have been developed to prevent this complication. However, practitioners do not, in general, know actual values either for the risk of regurgitation leading to aspiration or for the reduction of that risk by the special precautions taken. Most anesthesia-related risk can be so described.

HISTORICAL AND CONTEMPORARY APPROACHES TO RISK ASSESSMENT

Preoperative placement of patients into risk categories may have several advantages. These include addressing patient demand for information, containing costs, providing documentation in the event of litigation, and adjusting outcome data (between providers and institutions) for variations in severity of disease. The first attempt to formally assign risk based on preoperative findings was the Physical Status Assessment of the American Society of Anesthesiologists (ASA-PS), published in 1941.[2] The ASA-PS is a five-category scale. This subjective assignment has been shown to stratify patients with reasonable accuracy according to their overall anesthetic risk. More recent and more involved assessment scales or indices have been developed, but the ASA-PS scale has compared favorably with them.[3] The most obvious way of altering the ASA-PS scale to promote realistic morbidity prediction would be to include modifiers reflecting the severity of the surgical case, which would allow the separation of low-risk or superficial surgical procedures from those resulting in extensive tissue trauma or other physiologic perturbations (e.g., vascular clamping). A five-point surgical severity scale was developed at Johns Hopkins University Hospital to differentiate patients for whom evaluations by an anesthesiologist could be deferred until the day of surgery from those for whom a preoperative visit should be scheduled (R. Pasternak, personal communication, 1993). The ASA Task Force on Preoperative Evaluation has modified these surgical risk categories to low, medium, and high.

GOLDMAN STUDY

In 1977, Goldman et al.[4] published outcome data from 1,001 unselected patients older than 40 years undergoing major noncardiac operations. The authors identified preoperative conditions or findings that were associated with increased cardiac morbidity (see Table 3-1). A novel feature of this paper was the quantification of risk as a function of the number of "points" accumulated in a measure known as the *Goldman Cardiac Risk Index* (CRI). Several modifications and competitors for further accuracy have appeared since that time. Jeffery et al.[5] demonstrated that the CRI greatly underestimated risk in abdominal aortic aneurysm (AAA) surgery. Detsky et al.[6] applied the CRI and modified it to include factors not found significant by Goldman (see Table 3-2). Gerson et al.[7] added exercise to the Goldman CRI and improved the predictive value.

Experienced clinicians had known for some time, even before the Goldman study, those significant elements of procedures and comorbidities that create challenging problems. Skinner and Pearce summarized their observations 10 years before development of the Goldman CRI, essentially covering the major relevant risk factors.[8] These included the following:

1. High mortality rate was associated with intraperitoneal and intrathoracic surgery.
2. Patients with healed myocardial infarction had a 14% mortal-

ity; those with an acute myocardial infarction (less than 3 months earlier) had a mortality of 40%.

3. Higher mortality rates were seen if systolic blood pressure was less than 100 mm Hg or diastolic blood pressure was less than 50 mm Hg in patients who went to surgery in shock, despite efforts to stabilize blood pressure.
4. Patients with mitral valvular disease were relatively safe, whereas patients with aortic valve disease did not tolerate major procedures.
5. Patients with chronic pulmonary disease undergoing thoracic or abdominal procedures had a 37% mortality rate.
6. Patients with congestive heart failure (CHF) had increased mortality in proportion to the severity of CHF; mortality was 4% for those with mild CHF versus 67% for those with severe CHF.
7. Patients with electrocardiographic (ECG) abnormalities of atrial fibrillation, atrial flutter, heart block, or bundle branch block had an increased mortality compared with those whose ECGs were normal.
8. Emergency surgery was not well tolerated.

The identification of these specific factors based on clinical experience is remarkable. One might legitimately question whether the various indices and their modifications have contributed to improving patient care and whether the focus should continue to be the discovery of more specific predictive formulas.

The thesis here is that the extensive effort put forth to *quantify* the risk of intraoperative and postoperative cardiac morbidity and mortality, based on preoperative conditions or findings, has been of little practical value either for the practicing clinician or for patients. To illustrate, consider a 71-year-old man presenting for colon resection for carcinoma of the bowel. He has a history of hypertension, controlled with a diuretic; stable angina, controlled with atenolol; and premature atrial contractions on his ECG. The Goldman CRI[4] predicts this patient's risk of postoperative cardiac complications to be 14%.

1. What meaningful information does this number convey to the practitioner or to the patient?
2. Is the prediction independent of the surgical and anesthetic perioperative management the patient is to receive?

Preoperative cardiac risk prediction has become a virtual fetish among a sizable number of investigators who have moved beyond indices based on simple evaluations to study the specificity and sensitivity of testing modalities that are both costly and risky (see Chapter 3). These include exercise stress testing, ambulatory ECG, echocardiography, transesophageal echocardiography, radionucleotide ventriculography, dipyridamole-thallium imaging, and dobutamine stress echocardiography. Chapter 3 reviews studies that have reported positive predictive values and those that have not. The problem with these tests is that they are derivative means of determining the state of coronary flow and myocardial function under various conditions. Predictors of cardiac risk are actually measures of the degree of cardiac disease. They are useful for that purpose. They are related to perioperative morbidity only through the effectiveness or infectiveness of perioperative management to ameliorate the complex physiologic changes and maintain homeostasis in the face of the underlying disease.

Risk assessment without risk modification is an exercise in sophistry. Missing from virtually all risk assessment studies is information about the details of patient management. The reader is left ignorant regarding such issues as preoperative and postoperative administration of medications (including cardiovascular drugs); principles of anesthetic induction, maintenance, and emergence; definitions of hemodynamic extremes; the physiologic and pharmacologic interventions intended to control hemodynamics; postoperative pain management; and other treatments through discharge. These essential aspects of patient care are not addressed. They vary among institutions and individuals or groups within institutions with potentially serious variations in outcome.

The rush to assign risk without systematic work to determine what to do about it has resulted in virtual chaos. A survey of cardiovascular anesthesiologists showed a broad range of testing for all vascular procedures, devoid of consensus.[9] Not only does disagreement exist as to who should be tested, even less agreement is found on what should be done with the results of testing. At the time of this publication, many of the institutions with the highest testing rates had no provisions for altering care based on the results. Interestingly, cardiologists and surgeons were responsible for most of the test ordering.

The above issues have been extensively reviewed by a task force of the American College of Cardiology (ACC) and the American Heart Association (AHA). The culmination of this review was a publication entitled *Guidelines for Perioperative Cardiovascular Evaluation for Noncardiac Surgery.*[10] Much of this document addresses the risk of vascular surgery, because patients undergoing such surgery have the highest probability of coronary artery disease (CAD). Both preoperative findings or "predictors" and surgical procedures are stratified by levels of severity.

Aortic surgery and lower-extremity bypass grafting are high-risk procedures, whereas carotid endarterectomy is considered to be of intermediate risk. As an example, consider a 65-year-old man presenting for elective infrarenal AAA repair. He has premature atrial contractions and inferior lead Q waves on his ECG. He is taking medication for hypertension and walks 1 mile daily. This patient has intermediate clinical predictors, good exercise tolerance, and is to undergo a high-risk surgical procedure. Based on the algorithm, he should undergo further noninvasive testing procedures, leading to coronary revascularization if indicated before AAA surgery. Note the importance of exercise tolerance in this algorithm, which is not based on well-established investigations but rather derives from the experience of "domain experts" on the task force. When these guidelines are applied, approximately 50% of major vascular surgery patients undergo noninvasive testing.[11] If the results of such testing are negative, the recommendation is to proceed with the vascular procedure. If testing is positive, angiography is recommended, with some patients receiving coronary revascularization before vascular surgery.

Although the guidelines[10] serve to organize the preoperative approach to patients at risk, they do not guide actual medical management.

DECISION ANALYSIS

Two publications have specifically introduced the concept of cumulative risk and have emphasized institutional variability in mortality rates as a major factor in determining the advisability of preoperative testing.[12,13] They complement and underpin development of the ACC/AHA guidelines.[10] The question is whether to proceed directly to major vascular surgery (AAA) with a patient who has risk factors for CAD or rather to recommend a noninvasive test that may lead to angiography and coronary revascularization. Three presumptions influence this approach: (a) patients undergoing AAA repair who have been successfully revascularized have a low mortality,[14] (b) perioperative clinicians are skilled in the special needs of AAA surgery, and (c) all tests and procedures are associated with risk and the cumulative effects are of concern.

In a decision analysis, each step in the process is assigned a probability for one of two potential outcomes. The pathway with the highest probability of a good outcome may be identified, so that essentially the appropriate decision is reached as to whether to conduct a test before surgery or to proceed directly to surgery. As an example of the application of this methodology, consider the question of whether to perform dipyridamole thallium imaging for patients requiring AAA repair. The decision analysis variables for AAA repair with their assumed values are shown below:

1. MBase—baseline perioperative mortality of AAA repair in patients *without* CAD (0.5%).
2. MCAD—perioperative mortality of AAA repair in patients *with* CAD (9.5%).
3. MCABG—perioperative mortality of AAA repair in patients with prior coronary artery bypass grafting (CABG) (0.5%).
4. MRevasc—perioperative mortality of patients with AAA undergoing coronary revascularization (6.4%).
5. MAngio—perioperative mortality of patients with AAA undergoing coronary angiography (0.1%).

Also relevant are the prior probability of CAD in the AAA population (36%) and the sensitivity (86%) and specificity (74%) of dipyridamole thallium imaging.

Revisiting the case of the 65-year-old man presenting for AAA repair, the results of a two-way sensitivity analysis holding constant all of the above variables except MRevasc and MCAD show that, for a given MRevasc of 7.9%, the institution should proceed to AAA repair without further testing if the MCAD is less than 9.5%. Conversely, the institution should *precede* AAA repair with testing (leading to angiography, then CABG, as indicated) if the MCAD is greater than 9.5%. The appeal of this approach is that, at each step, it emphasizes the local risks, which, in turn, are dependent on perioperative management and therefore presumably modifiable. The decision to test could change if practitioners decrease the associated mortality. Note that the MBase is based on data from only a few institutions. A review of AAA mortality throughout New York State[15] showed rates of 5.8% to 10.4% depending on the volume of operations performed by the surgeon and the institution. These data blend MBase with MCAD and suggest that MBase is probably greater than 0.5%.

RISK MODIFICATION

For inexplicable reasons, most perioperative risk studies have been designed and conducted by cardiologists and internists who view the perioperative period as a "black box." Patients go into this box and most of them emerge relatively unscathed. As inhabitants of the black box, anesthesiologists, surgeons, intensivists, and others may have the ability to modify risk and propose meaningful assessments, plans, and alternatives.

Efforts to reduce risk and improve care include continuous reassessment of the methods and techniques of anesthetic practice. The introduction of the laryngeal mask airway and large studies comparing regional and general anesthesia[16,17] are examples of ongoing work that results in improvements. Serious morbidity and mortality due solely to anesthesia may possibly have reached an irreducible minimum. Major improvements in outcome may be realized only by restructuring the processes of care[18] and by leveraging the expertise of specially trained professionals.

Two important elements have affected risk assessment: the role of perioperative management in patient outcome and the importance of the surgical stress response on postoperative recovery, morbidity, and length of hospitalization.[19,20]

Several observations support the rational presumption that the patient's medical and anesthetic management throughout the perioperative period is relevant to outcome. The New York State review of major vascular surgery showed wide variations in morbidity and mortality among institutions, with the best results coming from centers that perform the largest numbers of surgeries, especially for the more complex procedures.[15] Superficially, the finding is thought to reflect surgeon performance; however, it is measuring the entire process, including preoperative preparation, anesthetic management, and postoperative care, involving a host of personnel. Surgical skill, although obviously important, may not be the major factor. A study of outcomes at Veterans Administration hospitals throughout the country has shown marked differences between the worst and best performances.[21] This institutional variation in risk implies that medical decisions and procedures are of critical importance. Moreover, clinical trials with standardized care before, during, and after surgery have shown lower morbidity rates than those of uncontrolled series.[16,22,23]

Preoperative Preparation

Risk modification begins with careful preoperative preparations that include, but are by no means limited to, a variety of day-of-surgery maneuvers known or presumed to reduce morbidity. These range from administration of antacids and drugs to increase gastric motility for patients at risk of aspiration to administration of cardiovascular medications for patients with heart disease. Many patients do not receive their medications on the day of surgery because of patient misunderstanding or improper instructions. This omission could influence intraoperative and postoperative stability and possibly lead to morbidity, yet clinical data sets do not include such information. Advancing risk assessment and quality improvement processes require the identification of relevant data and their inclusion in relational databases for analysis. This is important to test the validity and efficiency of current protocols as well as new proposals to modify risk.

Certain interventional preoperative preparations, such as pulmonary artery catheterization, undertaken to optimize specific physiologic parameters may be warranted.[24,25] Anesthesiologists and others have developed progressive sophistication in the measurement, interpretation, and manipulation of physiologic parameters. These practitioners control cardiac loading conditions; myocardial oxygen supply and demand; brain, kidney, and splanchnic perfusion; acid-base status; electrolyte levels; oxygen-carrying capacity; and body temperature throughout complex and prolonged surgical procedures. These skills may vary substantially among groups as well as among individuals within them.

Advanced management is likely to improve outcomes, but this improvement has been difficult to establish because of problems in standardizing care and designing investigations with appropriate control groups. The utility of aggressive management of cardiovascular and pulmonary physiology, guided by pulmonary artery catheterization data, repeatedly has been questioned in intensive care units (ICUs) and is under national debate.[26] Less dissension exists regarding the use of intraoperative pulmonary artery catheterization, except when it is used *routinely* without regard to patient characteristics. Some studies have found improvement in surgical outcome and morbidity when pulmonary artery catheterization has been used.[24,25]

Whether or not pulmonary artery catheterization is used, intraoperative care can and should be modified for patients with known CAD or myocardial systolic or diastolic dysfunction. Careful surveillance for myocardial ischemia, using monitors with ST segment analysis, permits immediate correction of the contributing conditions with vasodilators, vasoconstrictors, negative chronotropic agents, inotropic drugs, volume expansion, and other therapies. The anesthetic technique may be altered to enhance cardiac performance.

Anesthetic Technique

Beyond obtundation of conciousness and the production of a quiescent surgical field (the classic goals of general anesthesia), investigations have demonstrated that anesthetic techniques differ in their ability to block or attenuate the surgical stress response. These neurohumoral phenomena are mediated by noxious stimuli through neural pathways and by direct tissue injury. The unchecked stress response leads to hyperdynamic cardiovascular activity, hypercoagulability, delayed wound healing, and suppressed immune function.[19,27-29] Mounting evidence that stress can suppress immune function may have profound implications for perioperative care.[20] Intense stress-ablative techniques may be beneficial for oncologic surgery, for example. Conceivably, recurrence of primary and metastatic lesions could be influenced by control of surgical stress.[30] These untoward sequelae may be prevented by careful anesthetic management using regional anesthesia alone and in combination with general anesthesia or by balanced anesthesia using narcotics.[19,20,31]

Preemptive analgesia (preincisional ablation of noxious stimuli) and blunting of the stress response has been demonstrated to result in reduced pain several weeks after surgery.[32] Additionally, or alternatively, the end-organ response may be treated. β-Blockers given preoperatively and continued during and after surgery have been shown to increase survival rates several months after surgery.[33] One study showed better graft patency and more blunted catecholamines and procoagulant response in patients undergoing lower-extremity vascular bypass grafting when regional anesthesia was used than when general anesthesia was used.[16,29]

Postoperative Issues

Patient management in the hours to days after surgery influences outcome. The physiologic phenomena of emergence from general anesthesia are complex, characterized by a return of sympathetic tone, reflex responsiveness, and the central processing of noxious impulses from the surgical site or sites. Bronchospasm, atelectasis, cardiovascular disturbances, hypertension, tachycardia, hypotension, and arrhythmias may lead to morbidity. Heart rate generally increases postoperatively, and myocardial ischemia and infarctions follow the same pattern.[34,35] Fluid management is complex as the patient may continue to "third-space," requiring large volumes for several hours after surgery, while mobilization of fluid occurs over the succeeding days.

Pain management after surgery is a topic of growing interest. Epidural analgesia is likely to result in better pain control, earlier mobilization, improved bowel motility with earlier feeding and better stress response attenuation, with the potential benefits as noted above.[19]

The organization of people and processes are vital components of optimal perioperative care, but this complicated issue is rarely identified or accounted for in risk assessment and outcome studies. Data show that morbidity after high-risk surgery is affected by the intensity and quality of care.[36] Length of stay, need for reintubations, acute renal failure, cardiac arrest, and return to the ICU were markedly different under different models of ICU care. The practice of twice-daily rounds by ICU physicians and the holding of morbidity and mortality conferences were associated with the best results. Financial and professional territorial concerns in specific institutions frequently inhibit the development of programs that optimize patient outcomes.

We have tried to demonstrate that preoperative risk assessment based on aggregate data has limited meaning to both patients or physicians. The question is, given a patient with a disease or physiologic conditions known to be associated with perioperative morbidity, what level of clinical expertise, interspecialty collaboration, and system management can be applied to optimize care and reduce or eliminate untoward events?

Bodenheimer has written, "what question should the clinician consider? It should not be 'who among the population with, or at risk for, coronary disease needs further evaluation before noncardiac surgery?', rather it should be 'why do patients experience adverse events and how might these events be prevented . . . ?"[37] Improved clinical outcomes are more likely to result from preventing excess oxygen demand after surgery than from deciding which tests optimally predict adverse events.

TOWARD A NEW PARADIGM

How does risk modification proceed? Three important elements are proposed: (a) creation of a standard language or terminology to characterize algorithms of care developed to address known risk factors, (b) formation of procedure-specific protocols that promote standardization of care, and (c) availability of a clinical information system with carefully chosen data elements.

Precaution Protocols

As previously noted and discussed throughout this book, many effective techniques have been devised by clinicians and researchers to address conditions that lead to morbidity. A graded series of interventions, scaled in proportion to the likelihood of the presence of disease, the severity of the outcome, and the significance of the surgical procedure, presumably lessen the probability of adverse outcomes. We propose that these interventions be formally grouped into three levels of intensity (I = lowest, II = intermediate, III = highest) and labeled as **precaution protocols**. The management of patients at risk for cardiac ischemia would fall under *Cardiac Ischemia Precautions, Level I, II, or III*. First local groups, and later multicenter panels, would determine the elements of cardiac ischemia precautions for each level. As an example, Tables 1-1 through 1-3 are proposed as starting points. Note that the recommendations either repeat or become more stringent as the level of precaution increases. A detailed algorithm can be developed for each level. Surgical intensity is categorized into three risk levels (low, medium, high) (Table 1-4). Table 1-5 shows the care matrix that results from incorporation of surgery-specific risk and precaution criteria. A patient requiring bowel surgery who had stable CAD would be treated with Cardiac Ischemia Precautions, Level II.

Other examples of precaution lists include (a) Cardiac Failure Precautions, (b) Bronchospastic Precautions, (c) Aspiration Precautions, (d) Allergic Precautions, (e) Difficult Airway Precautions, (f) Arrhythmia Precautions, (g) Endocrine Precautions, and (h) Hypertension Precautions.

Table 1-1. Cardiac Ischemia Precautions, Level I

On day of surgery, administration of all cardiovascular medications.

Intraoperative ST segment surveillance on "diagnostic" mode with accurate lead placement.

Perioperative hemodynamic management to avoid extremes of blood pressure and heart rate (±20% of baseline), including during induction, emergence, and institution of regional blockade.

Maintenance of hematocrit ≥30% and normal oxygenation.

Adequate postoperative pain management.

Reestablishment of preoperative cardiac medications.

Table 1-2. Cardiac Ischemia Precautions, Level II

On day of surgery, administration of all cardiovascular medications.

Continuous intraoperative ST segment analysis.

Careful control of hemodynamics with avoidance of high or low
    excursions, especially during induction and intubation, emergence,
    and institution of regional blockade. Invasive arterial pressure
    monitoring may be required. Central venous pressure monitoring
    (blood loss, fluid shifts) may be required. Nitroglycerin, β-blockers,
    and calcium channel antagonists must be readily available.

Maintenance of hematocrit ≥30% and supplemental oxygen delivery.

Maintenance of body temperature >35°C.

Adequate postoperative pain management (patient-controlled
    analgesia or epidural analgesia) and hemodynamic control.

Reinstitution of preoperative cardiac medications.

Table 1-3. Cardiac Ischemia Precautions, Level III

On day of surgery, administration of all cardiovascular medications.

Continuous intraoperative ST segment analysis.

Strict hemodynamic control requiring invasive arterial monitoring,
    possible pulmonary artery catheterization, and/or transesophageal
    echocardiography. Maintenance of heart rate below 85 beats/min.
    Vasodilators, vasoconstrictors, β-blockers, and calcium channel
    blockers must be immediately available.

Strict maintenance of body temperature >35°C.

Assurance of adequate oxygenation (hematocrit ≥30%, supplemental
    oxygen delivery, adequate cardiac output).

Maximum effort to ablate perioperative stress response, including
    minimization of pain. Neuraxial blockade techniques may be
    indicated.

Reinstitution of preoperative cardiac medications.

Table 1-4. Surgery-specific risk classifications

Low risk
    Nonvascular extremity surgery of moderate duration (<3 hours)
    Cataract resection
    Dermatologic operations
    Short, superficial procedures amenable to local anesthesia
Intermediate risk
    Most orthopedic procedures
    Urologic procedures
    Carotid surgery
    Kidney transplant
    Uncomplicated bowel resection
High risk
    Long or complicated procedures of the abdomen, thorax, head,
        and neck
    Aortic and lower extremity vascular surgery
    Transplants (other than kidney)

Table 1-5. Appropriate cardiac ischemia precaution level as a function of surgical risk and severity of heart disease

Surgery-specific risk classification	Risk factors for CAD, PVD, HTN, age >60 yr, smoking, DM	Known CAD, MI >6 mo, stable angina	Severe CAD, MI <6 mo, unstable angina, CHF
Low	—	Level I	Level II
Intermediate	Level I	Level II	Level III
High	Level II	Level III	Level III

CAD, coronary artery disease; CHF, congestive heart failure; DM, diabetes mellitus; HTN, hypertension; MI, myocardial infarction; PVD, peripheral vascular disease.

Features of precaution lists include the following:

1. Outline processes of care
2. Facilitate communication between anesthesiologists and consultants (i.e., no more "avoid hypoxia and hypotension"; rather, "suggest Cardiac Ischemia Precautions, Level II")
3. Standardize therapy to allow comparisons for outcomes research and utilization review
4. Amenable to change as new studies define important variables to control or advantageous therapeutic modalities are developed

Importantly, the precaution list facilitates communication between anesthesiologists and others within an institution and among groups in different institutions.

Procedure-Specific Protocol

Although the creation of clinical pathways has swept through much of medicine, anesthesiologists have been particularly resistant to their implementation. This resistance is partly because the choice of anesthesia is personal, subjective (reflective of the culture of the training program), and laden with idiosyncrasies. After training is completed, styles of practice may progressively solidify unless the environment is challenging and stimulating. Many anesthesiologists feel that standardization of anesthetic care and perioperative medical management is impossible and undesirable. The authors' experience, however, is that intraoperative and postoperative care can be standardized, usually with demonstrably good outcomes.[22]

The Perioperative Ischemia Randomized Anesthesia Trial (PIRAT), a 4-year trial of regional anesthesia and epidural analgesia versus general anesthesia and patient-controlled intravenous analgesia in patients undergoing lower-extremity vascular bypass grafting, was designed and conducted with specific clinical algorithms that guided preoperative, intraoperative, and postoperative management. Seven anesthesiologists, two surgeons, five intensivists, and three acute pain specialists agreed on details of induction, maintenance, emergence, weaning, pain control, and anticoagulation for the procedure and for the first 24 hours after surgery. Blood pressure limits (based on preoperative baseline blood pressure) and heart rate limits (40 to 85 beats per minute) were defined. Treatments of excursions in blood pressure and heart rate, fluid administration, and analgesia adjustments were standardized. The rate of myocardial ischemia, detected by continuous Holter monitoring, was lower in patients treated under the protocol than in observational patients given nonstandardized treatment.[16] The rate of myocardial infarction during hospitalization was much lower in the PIRAT study (4%) than in another study (13%).[11] This example demonstrates the benefits of standardized care. The definition of 85 beats per minute as the upper limit of acceptable heart rate was probably a factor in reducing ischemia. The ICU group reported that, based on this study, the surgical and anesthesia house staff began redefining their treatment thresholds for tachycardia for nonstudy patients with CAD (T. Buchman, personal communication, 1989).

Defining **procedure-specific protocols** may have advantages as well. Cardiac, vascular, neurosurgical, trauma, and other surgical subspecialty procedures involve complex physiologic perturbations such as vascular clamping or other circulatory compromise, unclamping and reperfusion, hypercoagulability and hypocoagulability, brain swelling, blood loss, and fluid shifts. Techniques have evolved to prevent or lessen sequelae related to these phenomena, but their details vary among practitioners and controversies are common. Through standardization of procedure-specific protocols, baseline outcomes can be established that allow comparative evaluation of alternative methodologies.

After creation of the precaution protocols and procedure-specific protocols, the anesthesia care plan could be summarized as follows:

> 65-year-old man for elective AAA repair with stable
>   CAD, a history of reflux, hypertension, and good exercise
>   tolerance
> Plan: AAA Procedure-Specific Protocol
> Aspiration Precautions, Level I
> Arrhythmia Precautions, Level I
> Hypertension Precautions, Level I
> Myocardial Ischemia Precautions, Level III

SUMMARY

The best opportunity to positively influence perioperative patient care and outcomes does not lie in further refinements of predictive models of preoperative risk. Rather, the time has come to evaluate our management processes, discover the proximate causes of morbidity, and alter the delivery of care, thereby reducing morbidity and mortality. The task is complex, but the potential benefits are significant. A plan of action is listed below.

1. Local consensus groups create details of precaution lists based on experience and review of the literature. Medical and surgical collaboration is necessary.
2. Local groups of anesthesiologists and surgeons create procedure-specific protocols. Other important collaborators include postanesthesia care unit and ICU nurses, and intensive care and acute pain specialists.

3. Preoperative, intraoperative, and postoperative data collection mechanisms are developed.
4. Baseline outcomes are established for comparison with national standards.
5. Apparent antecedents of common morbidities are identified.
6. Revision of precaution lists and procedure-specific protocols continues.
7. Modification of perioperative care to improve outcomes continues.

Future efforts should determine why events occur and which surveillance and treatment modalities need revision to prevent adverse outcomes.

REFERENCES

1. Codman EA. A study in hospital efficiency. Boston: Thomas Todd Co, 1916.
2. Saklad M. Grading of patients for surgical procedures. *Anesthesiology* 1941;2:281–284.
3. Waters J, Wilkinson C, Golmon M, et al. Evaluation of cardiac risk in noncardiac surgical patients. *Anesthesiology* 1981;55: A343.
4. Goldman L, Caldera DL, Nussbaum SR, et al. Multifactorial index of cardiac risk in noncardiac surgical procedures. *N Engl J Med* 1977;297:845–850.
5. Jeffrey CC, Kunsman J, Cullen DJ, et al. A prospective evaluation of cardiac risk index. *Anesthesiology* 1983;58:462–464.
6. Detsky AS, Abrams HB, Forbath N, et al. Cardiac assessment for patients undergoing noncardiac surgery, a multifactorial clinical risk index. *Arch Intern Med* 1986;146:2131–2134.
7. Gerson MC, Hurst JM, Hertzberg VS, et al. Cardiac prognosis in noncardiac geriatric surgery. *Ann Intern Med* 1985;103:832–837.
8. Skinner JF, Pearce ML. Surgical risk in the cardiac patient. *J Chronic Dis* 1964;17:57–72.
9. Fleisher LA, Beattie C. Current practice in the preoperative evaluation of patients undergoing major vascular surgery: a survey of cardiovascular anesthesiologists. *J Cardiothorac Vasc Anesth* 1993;7:650–654.
10. Eagle KA, Brundage BH, Chaitman BR, et al. Guidelines for perioperative cardiovascular evaluation for noncardiac surgery. Report of the American College of Cardiology/American Heart Association Task Force on Practice Guidelines (Committee on perioperative cardiovascular evaluation for noncardiac surgery). *J Am Coll Cardiol* 1996;27:910–948.
11. L'Italien GJ, Cambria RP, Cutler BS, et al. Comparative early and late cardiac morbidity among patients requiring different vascular surgery procedures. *J Vasc Surg* 1995;21:935–944.
12. Fleisher LA, Skolnick ED, Holroyd KJ, et al. Coronary artery revascularization before abdominal aortic aneurysm surgery: a decision analytic approach. *Anesth Analg* 1994;79:661–669.
13. Mason JJ, Owens DK, Harris RA, et al. The role of coronary angiography and coronary revascularization before noncardiac vascular surgery. *JAMA* 1995;273:1919–1925.
14. Foster ED, Davis KB, Carpenter JA, et al. Risk of noncardiac operation in patients with defined coronary disease: the Coronary Artery Surgery Study (CASS) registry experience. *Ann Thorac Surg* 1986;41:42–50.
15. Hannan EL, Kilburn H, O'Donnell JF, et al. A longitudinal analysis of the relationship between in-hospital mortality in New York

State and the volume of abdominal aortic aneurysm surgeries performed. *Health Serv Res* 1992;27:517–542.

16. Christopherson R, Beattie C, Frank SM, et al. Perioperative morbidity in patients randomized to epidural or general anesthesia for lower extremity vascular surgery. Perioperative Ischemia Randomized Anesthesia Trials Study Group. *Anesthesiology* 1993;79:422–434.

17. Bode RH Jr, Lewis KP, Zarich SW, et al. Cardiac outcome after peripheral vascular surgery: comparison of general and regional anesthesia. *Anesthesiology* 1996;84:3–13.

18. Hammermeister KE, Shroyer AL, Sethi GK, Grover FL. Why it is important to demonstrate linkages between outcomes of care and processes and structures of care. *Med Care* 1995;33:OS5–OS16.

19. Liu S, Carpenter RL, Neal JM. Epidural anesthesia and analgesia: their role in postoperative outcome. *Anesthesiology* 1995;82:1474–1506.

20. Kehlet H. Multimodal approach to control postoperative pathophysiology and rehabilitation. *Br J Anaesth* 1997;78:606–617.

21. Khuri SF, Daley J, Henderson W, et al. The National Veterans Administration surgical risk study: risk adjustment for the comparative assessment of the quality of surgical care. *J Am Coll Surg* 1995;180:519–531.

22. Beattie C, Roizen MF, Downing JW. Cardiac outcomes after regional or general anesthesia: do we know the question? *Anesthesiology* 1996;85:1207–1208.

23. L'Italien GJ, Paul SD, Hendel RC, et al. Development and validation of a Bayesian model for perioperative cardiac risk assessment in a cohort of 1,081 vascular surgical candidates. *J Am Coll Cardiol* 1996;27:779–786.

24. Berlauk JF, Abrams JH, Gilmour IJ, et al. Preoperative optimization of cardiovascular hemodynamics improves outcome in peripheral vascular surgery: a prospective, randomized clinical trial. *Ann Surg* 1991;214:289–297.

25. Shah KB, Kleinman BS, Hafez S. Re-evaluation of perioperative myocardial infarction in patients with prior myocardial infarction undergoing noncardiac operations. *Anesth Analg* 1990;71:231–235.

26. Pulmonary Artery Catheterization and Clinical Outcomes Workshop. Sponsored by National Heart, Lung, and Blood Institute; National Institutes of Health; Center for Devices and Radiological Health; and Food and Drug Administration, September 1997; Bethesda, Maryland.

27. Breslow MJ, Parker SD, Frank SM, et al. Determinants of catecholamine and cortisol responses to lower extremity revascularization. *Anesthesiology* 1993;79:1202–1209.

28. Tuman K, McCarthy R, March R, et al. Effects of epidural anesthesia and analgesia on coagulation and outcome after major vascular surgery. *Anesth Analg* 1991;73:696–704.

29. Rosenfeld BA, Beattie C, Christopherson R, et al. The effects of different anesthetic regimens on fibrinolysis and the development of postoperative arterial thrombosis. *Anesthesiology* 1993;79:435–443.

30. Andersen BL, Farrar WB, Golden-Kreutz D, et al. Stress and immune responses after surgical treatment for regional breast cancer. *J Natl Cancer Inst* 1998;90:30–36.

31. Mangano DT, Siliciano D, Hollenberg M, et al. Postoperative myocardial ischemia. *Anesthesiology* 1992;76:342–353.

32. Gottschalk A, Smith DS, Jobes DR, et al. Preemptive epidural analgesia and recovery from radical prostatectomy. *JAMA* 1998;279:1076–1082.

33. Mangano DT, Layug EL, Wallace A, et al. Effect of atenolol on mortality and cardiovascular morbidity after noncardiac surgery. *N Engl J Med* 1996;335:1713–1720.

34. Badner NH, Knill RL, Brown JE, et al. Myocardial infarction after noncardiac surgery. *Anesthesiology* 1998;88:572–578.
35. Landesberg G, Luria MH, Cotev S, et al. Importance of long-duration postoperative ST-segment depression in cardiac morbidity after vascular surgery. *Lancet* 1993;341:715–719.
36. Pronovost P, Jenckes M, Dorman T, et al. Impact of ICU organization and staffing on outcomes after abdominal aortic surgery. *Crit Care Med* 1998;26:A38.
37. Bodenheimer MM. Noncardiac surgery in the cardiac patient: what is the question? *Ann Intern Med* 1996;124:763–766.

Preoperative Testing

Michael F. Roizen

Preoperative laboratory tests are intended to help an anesthesiologist optimize care for a patient's specific medical conditions. Selection of tests preoperatively is an adjunct to the primary purpose of preoperative evaluation: to facilitate return of the patient to normal function as soon as possible after surgery. More than 80% of surgeries rely on same-day admission or outpatient care. Many of these patients are not seen by an anesthesiologist before the day of surgery. Test results are sometimes considered substitutes for the lost interaction between anesthesiologist and patient. Batteries of tests, however, are not a substitute for history taking, physical examination of a patient, and exchange of medically related information between physician and patient. This chapter examines the theoretical and statistical bases for testing, describes specific preoperative tests, and presents a strategy for preoperative testing.

IDENTIFICATION OF PATIENT FACTORS THAT INCREASE THE RISK OF ANESTHESIA

To assess the individual patient's anesthetic risk, the anesthesiologist must be familiar with patient factors that increase perioperative risk. These risk factors must be addressed preoperatively so that therapeutic intervention can be planned to reduce risk.

Major surgery places a tremendous stress on the human organism. The body has an elaborate defense mechanism that alerts it to and helps it escape from trauma. The job of the anesthesiologist is *not* simply to put the patient to sleep and to awaken the patient when surgery is over, but also to maintain homeostasis during the stress of surgery and to provide pain relief to blunt the effects of the stress response. To do this, the anesthesiologist must interfere with the stress response induced by pain, anticipate periods when the stress response will not be present, and manage both common and rare problems presented by the patient's underlying medical conditions.

Although the stress of surgery is not consciously perceived, it evokes a complex physiologic response. Much of this response is intended to allow the body to escape trauma. For example, blood flow is diverted from the kidney and liver and is supplied to the heart and head. Blood pressure rises. Thus, the system that is most needed to be in a good state of health, the cardiovascular system, has first priority.[1-3] Elaborate and simple tests and history taking processes have evolved to evaluate the cardiovascular system, especially in aged patients or patients with comorbid disease[4] (see Chapters 3 and 4).

DETECTION OF DISEASE: HISTORY, PHYSICAL EXAMINATION, AND CHART REVIEW VERSUS LABORATORY TESTS

The primary problem with ordering batteries of laboratory tests is that laboratory tests are not very good screening devices for disease. In addition, the subsequent "extra" tests that physicians order as a follow-up to supposedly abnormal results are costly. More important, however, is the fact that unindicated tests often represent additional risk to the patient, increase medicolegal risk to the physician, and result in inefficient use of operating rooms in outpatient centers and hospitals.

In the perioperative management of a patient, the anesthesiologist may alter the care of the patient based on preoperative laboratory test results. If a preoperative test suggests a change in the care of an individual that leads to improvement in the health of the patient or avoidance of a potential problem, then that test has been beneficial to the patient. *Other preoperative tests, the results of which are normal or merely borderline abnormal, may only distract the physician.* The results of these tests create no benefit but merely inconvenience—or worse, harm through distraction. Finally, if a preoperative test suggests a change in the care of an individual that causes the health of the patient to suffer or a problem to arise, then that test decreases the overall quality of medical care and is harmful to the patient. One not uncommon example is a case in which abnormal results on a chest radiograph (CXR), obtained for a 40-year-old man solely because he is scheduled for surgery, lead to a computed tomographic needle biopsy that produces normal results but is complicated by a pneumothorax. This sequence of events shows how a "benign" test can result in harm. Thus, testing can have an unfavorable risk-benefit ratio.

On the whole, not much benefit appears to arise from unindicated routine laboratory testing. Leonard et al.[5] reported that biochemical screening tests had no significant value in the preoperative screening of pediatric patients expected to be hospitalized for less than 1 week. When Korvin et al.[6] reviewed biochemical tests given routinely to 1,000 patients on hospital admission, they found that none of the tests produced a new diagnosis that was unequivocally beneficial to the patient. In an ambitious, controlled trial of multiphasic screening of 1,500 patients, Olsen et al.[7] found no difference in morbidity between control groups and groups subjected to screening tests. Durbridge et al.[8] compared results for 1,500 patients randomly assigned to undergo or not undergo screening tests on hospital admission. With respect to length of hospital stay and patient outcome, no benefit resulted from the 8,363 extra tests performed for the group undergoing screening tests. Narr et al.[9] found that more than 3,000 patients who were categorized as class I or II according to the classification of the American Society of Anesthesiologists (ASA) failed to benefit from laboratory testing.

Many studies have compared the yield from indicated (warranted based on history or risk group) versus unindicated (unwarranted) preoperative testing.[9-21] Few unindicated tests have yielded beneficial changes in perioperative care; at most, only 16 patients of more than 16,000 who had unindicated preoperative tests benefited from such testing. Furthermore, this figure represents the most optimistic interpretation; four patients in a study conducted by Kaplan et al.[10] received no benefit, and for at least another seven patients in a study by O'Connor and Drasner,[15] the benefit of treating asymptomatic anemia before non–blood loss surgery was not clear.

Although laboratory tests can aid in ensuring that a patient's preoperative condition is optimal once a disease is suspected or diagnosed, such tests have several shortcomings as screening devices for the discovery of unknown disease. First, they frequently fail to uncover pathologic conditions and are inefficient in screening for asymptomatic diseases. Second, they discover abnormalities the identification of which does not necessarily lead to improved patient care or outcome. Finally, most abnormalities discovered on preoperative screening, or even on admission screening for nonsurgical purposes, are not recorded appropriately (other than on the laboratory report) or pursued appropriately.

The detection of abnormalities does not justify testing because most abnormalities in asymptomatic patients do not reflect the presence of disease. For tests reported as continuous results, the distribution of results in a population of patients is Gaussian (i.e., normal). The values defining "abnormal" are set arbitrarily, so that test results above the 97.5 percentile or below the 2.5 percentile of values obtained from healthy individuals are said to be abnormal. Test results between these two extremes are "within the reference range." Therefore, 5% of test results from patients without disease are "outside the hospital reference range." If one were to order 100 hemoglobin determinations for a sample of healthy patients, 5% of the results would be expected to be "abnormal." Ordering multiple preoperative tests increases the chances of at least one abnormal result.

Assuming that the results of tests are independent of one another, the more tests ordered, the higher the likelihood of an abnormal result. For example, if two tests are ordered for a patient without disease, the chance of both being normal is 0.95×0.95, or 0.90. For 20 tests, the chance that all will be normal is only 36%. The chance that at least one result will be abnormal is 64%. Thus, if one chooses to use more than 13 tests to screen patients before surgery, one should expect at least one abnormal result.

Testing for acquired immunodeficiency syndrome (AIDS) provides another example. More than 92% of the population at low risk of human immunodeficiency virus (HIV) infection who have positive (abnormal) results on two enzyme-linked immunosorbent assays and one Western blot test in reality do not have HIV infection. Therefore, the fact that the benefit from nonselective testing is so low or that so few abnormal results arising from unwarranted tests are acted on is not surprising. Even for the very elderly, a patient group at high risk of morbidity and mortality during surgery, the ultimate benefit of routine laboratory screening is doubtful. Domoto et al.[22] examined the yield and benefit of a battery of 19 screening laboratory tests performed routinely in 70 functionally intact elderly patients (average age, 82.6 years) who resided at a chronic care facility. The 70 patients underwent 3,905 screening tests. "New abnormal" results occurred in 5 of the 19 screening tests. Most of these new abnormalities were only minimally outside the normal range. Only four discoveries (0.1% of all tests ordered) led to a change in patient management, none of which changes, Domoto et al. concluded, benefited any patient in any important way.

Wolf-Klein et al.[23] retrospectively studied the results of annual laboratory screening of a population of 500 institutionalized and ambulatory elderly patients (average age, 80 years). From the 15,000 tests performed, 756 new abnormalities were discovered, 690 of which were ignored. Sixty-six of the new abnormalities were evaluated; the result was 20 new diagnoses, 12 of which led to treatment. Two patients of the 500 ultimately may have benefited from eradication of asymptomatic bacteriuria (although eradication of this condition has not been shown to improve the quality of life or to extend life).[24]

Studies show that the history and physical examination are the best ways to screen for disease. Delahunt and Turnbull[25] evaluated 803 patients who were assessed preoperatively for varicose vein stripping or inguinal herniorrhaphy. A total of 1,972 tests produced only 63 abnormalities not indicated by history or physical findings. Furthermore, in no instance did the discovery of these abnormalities influence patient management. Another study retrospectively evaluated 690 admissions for elective pediatric surgical procedures.[26] The history and physical examination indicated the probability of abnormalities in all 12 patients for whom an abnormality was detected by laboratory testing. Clinical diagnosis, and not laboratory testing, was the apparent basis for any change in operative plans. Bates et al. found that at least 40% of repeat tests in a large teaching hospital were redundant.[27] At the Mayo Clinic, Narr et al.[28] found that no harm resulted from omitting all laboratory testing in a group of ASA class I patients whose median age was 21.4 years. The sample size of this study was sufficiently large to permit the conclusion that testing is more likely to cause harm than to provide benefit to ASA class I patients. Whether ASA class I patients older than 40 years would benefit from testing is unclear.

Patients who benefit from testing have risk factors, symptoms, or other history that calls forth testing. In our own study of patients who were symptomatic or only had risk factors for disease, 606 (5.8%) of 10,419 test results were significantly abnormal (J. L. Apfelbaum et al., unpublished data). Of these, the results of 124 tests (1.2%) affected care. Among the patients whose care was changed, six patients suffered harm (6 of 10,419, or 0.06%), whereas 91 patients (91 of 10,419, or 0.9%) benefited from the change in care. By contrast, for asymptomatic patients who had no risk factors for disease, only 121 (1.1%) of the 10,899 tests results were significantly abnormal. Of these, results of 13 tests (13 of 10,899, or 0.01%) affected care. During the study, every change in care that benefited or harmed a patient stemmed from a single test result. Therefore, the 13 care-affecting tests represented 13 care-affected patients. Of these 13 patients, five asymptomatic patients (5 of 10,899, or 0.05%) were harmed, whereas only one of the patients (1 in 10,899 tests results, or 0.009%) benefited from a change in care. Neither harm nor benefit was thought to result from the other seven changes in care.

In summary, the studies cited point to the lack of benefit from routine laboratory testing as a method of assessing patients preoperatively. Many of these laboratory tests have been shown to be superfluous to patient management. History and physical examination are considered the most effective ways of screening for disease. Laboratory tests can be used to screen for disease when the patient has appropriate risk factors and when such tests have proved effective. The better use of such tests, however, is to confirm clinical diagnoses or to optimize the patient's condition before surgery.

PATIENT RISK

Unnecessary testing may lead physicians to pursue and treat borderline and false-positive laboratory abnormalities. This observation does not imply that all standard screening tests should be discontinued. Some are beneficial, such as the mammogram for all women 50 years or older, the test for occult blood in stool for all people 40 years or older, and the Papanicolaou (Pap) smear for sexually active women.[29,30] However, few studies have examined whether increased testing and the follow-up on false-positive test results adversely affect patients. In one study addressing this issue, Roizen et al.[31] retrospectively examined the adverse effects of chest radiography on patients. For 606 patients, 386 additional CXRs were ordered without indication of need. Among those 386 patients, the discovery of only one abnormality (an elevated hemidiaphragm probably caused by phrenic nerve palsy) may have resulted in improved care for that patient. On the other hand, the existence of three lung shadows on CXR led to three sets of invasive tests, including one thoracotomy, but no discovery of disease. These procedures caused considerable morbidity, including one pneumothorax and four months of disability, for those three patients.

Tape and Mushlin[32] found a similar result when examining the benefits and risks of CXRs obtained preoperatively in Rochester, New York. Of 341 patients admitted for vascular surgery, nine had radiographic findings that led to clinical action. Specifically, three patients (two with congestive heart failure and one with pulmonary fibrosis) may have benefited from the findings. However, all three patients were known by history to have the disease shown on CXR. In addition, six patients were subjected to a potentially detrimental clinical intervention. Two had a false diagnosis of tuberculosis, with subsequent therapy for one patient; two others had false diagnosis of nodules; and the last two had falsely normal CXRs readings. All the beneficial effects attributed to preoperative CXRs accrued to patients who had an obvious clinical history of pulmonary or cardiac disease.

Orkin[33] has further explained the basis of the risk of testing asymptomatic patients. Testing of asymptomatic patients is more risky than beneficial to patient health. Specifically, for 1 in every 2,000 preoperative tests (1 in 300 patients), the test results led to patient harm because of the pursuit of abnormalities indicated by those tests; for 1 in 10,000 tests (1 in 1,746 patients), the tests led to benefit (J. L. Apfelbaum et al., unpublished data).

In another study, Turnbull and Buck[12] examined the charts of 2,570 patients undergoing cholecystectomy to determine the value of preoperative tests. With four possible exceptions, history and physical examinations successfully indicated the need for all tests that ultimately benefited the patients. Again, whether those four

Table 2-1. Risk of potassium supplementation

	Route of administration			
	Oral	Intravenous	Oral and intravenous	All routes
Number of patients	1,910	2,192	819	921
Deaths	3 (0.2%)	3 (0.15%)	1 (0.1%)	7 (0.14%)
Life-threatening reaction or death	6 (0.3%)	7 (0.35%)	14 (1.7%)	28 (0.57%)
Hyperkalemia	74 (3.9%)	34 (1.6%)	71 (8.7%)	179 (3.6%)
Other side effects	53 (2.8%)	18 (0.8%)	33 (4.0%)	283 (5.7%)

One in 200 patients given potassium supplementation dies or has a life-threatening reaction.
Data from Lawson DH. Adverse reactions to potassium chloride. *QJM* 1974; 43:433–440; Lawson DH, Hutcheon AW, Jick H. Life threatening drug reactions amongst medical in-patients. *Scott Med J* 1979;24:127–130.

patients actually experienced any benefit as a result of the preoperative tests is doubtful. Among them was one patient who had emphysema detected only by CXR. This patient had preoperative physiotherapy without subsequent postoperative complication. Two patients had unsuspected hypokalemia (potassium levels of 3.2 and 3.4 mEq per L) and received treatment before operation. Current data in the literature indicate that no harm occurs to patients undergoing surgery with this degree of hypokalemia and that severe harm may be caused by treating such patients with oral or intravenous administration of potassium (Table 2-1).[34,35] The fourth patient possibly benefiting from preoperative testing had an asymptomatic hemoglobin concentration of 9.9 g per dL and was given a blood transfusion before cholecystectomy. Because cholecystectomy is not normally associated with major blood loss, one might conclude that this patient also received no benefit from preoperative laboratory testing and its pursuit but was exposed to the risk of transfusion. Thus, it is not clear that any patient in this study benefited from preoperative screening tests without indication for need by history or physical examination.

In another study, only two patients at most (who had eradication of asymptomatic bacteriuria) benefited from the 9,720 screening tests that were obtained.[36] At least one patient was seriously harmed from pursuit and treatment of abnormalities on screening tests. This patient developed atrial fibrillation and congestive heart failure after institution of thyroid therapy for borderline low levels on thyroxine and free thyroxine index tests. Whether these investigators examined other patients for potential harm arising from the pursuit and treatment of abnormalities on screening tests is unclear.

Screening mammography has been evaluated in a real-life practice setting to determine benefits and risks. Although yearly screening was determined to be beneficial, more than 20% of women without disease were subjected to a breast biopsy. Calculations were that more than 49% of women without disease would have been subjected to a breast biopsy had they obtained a yearly mammogram and clinical breast examination. Thus, even when benefit exceeds risk, substantial risk attaches to routine testing.[37]

Even sophisticated laboratory tests have not been better in controlled trials than the history and physical examination in estimating the risk from a diagnosis. This lack of benefit from laboratory testing has applied to diagnoses as relatively amenable to laboratory diagnosis as the differential diagnosis of systolic murmurs,[38] assessment of nutritional status,[39] and evaluation of cardiac and gastrointestinal disease.[40]

MEDICOLEGAL LIABILITY

Extra testing—testing not warranted by findings on a medical history—does not provide medicolegal protection against liability. Studies show that 30% to 95% of all unexpected abnormalities found on preoperative laboratory tests are not noted on the chart before surgery. This lack of notation occurs not only at university medical centers but at community hospitals as well. Moreover, the failure to pursue an abnormality appropriately poses a greater risk of medicolegal liability than does failure to detect that abnormality.[41] In this way, extra testing increases the medicolegal risk to physicians.

OPERATING ROOM SCHEDULES

According to hospital administrators in the United States, surgeons say they order preoperative tests to satisfy anesthesiologists. Surgeons find it easier just to order all the tests and let the anesthesiologist sort them out. Surgeons also believe that ordering batteries of tests is more efficient than having an anesthesiologist, who sees the patient the night before or the day of surgery, obtain the tests on an emergency basis. This line of reasoning overlooks the fact that abnormalities arising from tests performed in battery fashion usually are not discovered until the night before or the day of surgery, if at all. The discovery of abnormal results on the day of surgery delays the operating room schedule or postpones scheduled cases as effort and time are wasted to obtain consultant review of false-positive or slightly abnormal results. Data show cost reductions and other benefits from delegating test selection to anesthesiologists.[42,43]

LOW PREDICTIVE VALUE OF AN "ABNORMAL" LABORATORY TEST RESULT

Of prime importance in preoperative evaluation is knowing the percentage of abnormal laboratory test values that truly indicates disease. If the anesthetic management of a patient is altered because of a test abnormality, that abnormality should indicate a condition that (a) poses a significant risk of preoperative morbidity that can be lessened by preoperative treatment, (b) cannot be discovered through history taking and physical examination, and (c) is sufficiently prevalent in the population to justify the risk of performing the follow-up test. To be cost efficient, the test should be sufficiently sensitive (yield a positive result when disease is present) and specific (yield a negative result in the absence of disease).[44] What a clinician wants to know is what a positive or negative test result means for an individual patient. The positive or negative predictive values depend on the probability of disease in the pretest population. For example, assume that patients with pneumonia would have the notation "pneumonia" (or some significant abnormality) written as the diagnosis on their CXR reports. Assume also that the specificity of a test (the rate of negative findings when the patient is healthy) is 98.3%. That is, 983 of 1,000 people who actually do not have pneumonia have a comment such as "without evidence of pneumonia" or "normal" written on their CXR reports. Third, assume that 0.5% of the asymptomatic population younger than age 40 years who are about to undergo routine elective surgery has pneumonia. Given the preceding assumptions, what is the likelihood that a person whose CXR report reads "pneumonia" actually has pneumonia?

If 100,000 asymptomatic persons are tested and 0.5% are assumed to be diseased, then 500 people have undetected pneumonia. If the sensitivity of the CXR for pneumonia is assumed to be 75%, 375 of these people would have abnormal CXRs. Then, if specificity is assumed to be 98.3%, 97,809 of the 99,500 healthy people would have normal results on CXR. This means that 1,691 (1.7%) would have abnormal radiographic results. Thus, of 2,066 patients having a diagnosis of pneumonia based on CXR, 1,691 (82%) would have CXR results that are falsely positive. Therefore, it is entirely possible that 82% of the CXR reports indicating "infiltrate compatible with pneumonia" in otherwise asymptomatic persons would actually be describing totally healthy people. Expressed in another way, when the above assumptions are applied, the likelihood that an asymptomatic person would actually have pneumonia when the CXR report contains that notation (the positive predictive value of a positive test in this group) is only 18%.

Assume that the CXR in the under-40 population has a sensitivity of 75% and a specificity of 95% (these values are better than the best reported in the literature for readings referenced by a single radiologist). Assume also that the prevalence of disease detectable by the test is 0.5% and that the benefit from true positive results is 20 in 100 (better than the best in the literature). For the asymptomatic under-40 population, the result would be harmful to three individuals and beneficial to only 0.8 individuals per 1,000 CXRs. Similar analyses are possible for other tests and situations.

Two other important concepts related to the reported benefits and risks of screening tests deserve consideration: lead-time and length-time biases.[45] These two factors, which can indicate an apparent benefit of testing when none exists, have been discussed in detail elsewhere.[46]

Before one concludes that no tests should be ordered preoperatively, one should remember that detection of subclinical conditions in high-risk groups and optimization of therapy for clinical conditions can result in fewer perioperative morbidities, fewer changes in perioperative plans, and improved discussions of informed risk with the patient and others.

Table 2-2. Types of surgical procedures

Class A, minimally invasive
  Little potential to disrupt normal physiology
  Rarely associated with morbidity related to the anesthetic
  Rarely require blood administration, invasive monitoring, or post-operative management in a critical care setting
  Examples: cataract extraction, diagnostic arthroscopy, postpartum tubal ligation
Class B, moderately invasive
  Modest potential to disrupt normal physiology
  May require blood administration, invasive monitoring, or post-operative management in a critical care setting
  Examples: carotid endarterectomy, abdominal hysterectomy, laparoscopic cholecystectomy
Class C, highly invasive
  Typically produce significant disruption of normal physiology
  Almost always require blood administration, invasive monitoring, and postoperative management in a critical care setting
  Examples: total hip replacement, open aortic aneurysm resection, aortic valve replacement, posterior fossa craniotomy for aneurysm

SURGICAL PROCEDURES AND LABORATORY TEST ABNORMALITIES IN ASYMPTOMATIC POPULATIONS

Does surgical procedure influence laboratory test selection? A decade ago the answer to that question was no. Now the answer is yes. Some operations have such low rates of associated morbidity and mortality (diagnostic knee arthroscopy or cataract extraction, for example) that, unless a test represents routine preventive care for a particular patient, testing is not warranted.

Surgical procedures can be divided into three categories (Table 2-2). The first type, call it class A, is minimally invasive, results in little tissue trauma, and is associated with minimal blood loss. The opinion of the author is that no routine laboratory testing is indicated for healthy patients before class A procedures. Some laboratory tests may be required for a particular subset of patients to optimize their medical status before surgery. The next two types of procedures, class B and class C, are progressively more risky and invasive. They may require that the anesthesiologist optimize the condition of less-threatening medical processes in the perioperative period and therefore often require more preoperative laboratory tests.

Chest Radiographs

What abnormalities on CXR would influence management of anesthesia? Certainly, it may be important to know about the existence of tracheal deviation or compression; mediastinal masses; pulmonary nodules; a solitary lung mass; aortic aneurysm; pulmonary edema; pneumonia; atelectasis; new fractures of the vertebrae, ribs, and clavicles; dextrocardia; or cardiomegaly before proceeding to anesthesia and surgery. A CXR, however, probably would not detect the degree of chronic lung disease requiring a change in anesthetic technique any better than would the history or physical examination. Abnormalities are rare in the asymptomatic individual. In fact, the risks associated with CXR probably exceed their possible benefit if the patient is asymptomatic and younger than 75 years. This analysis is predicated on maximizing benefit to all patients as a group, as one cannot say which individual patient will benefit and which will be harmed. Thus, no CXR is indicated for an asymptomatic patient younger than 75 years old who is free of risk factors for lung disease. This statement may also be true of patients older than 75 years.

Electrocardiograms

The incidence of electrocardiogram (ECG) abnormalities has been determined by studies of patients (J. Hsu et al., unpublished data)[12,13,47] and epidemiologic surveys of healthy people.[48] The abnormalities on ECG that have the potential to alter management of anesthesia are as follows: atrial flutter or fibrillation; first-, second-, and third-degree atrioventricular block; changes in ST segments suggesting myocardial ischemia or recent pulmonary embolism; premature ventricular and atrial contractions; left or right ventricular hypertrophy; short PR interval; Wolff-Parkinson-White syndrome; myocardial infarction; prolonged QT segment; and tall, peaked T waves. What is the incidence of finding these abnormalities on the 12-lead preoperative screening ECG but not on a standard monitor lead 1 or an MCL_5 lead applied immediately before induction of anesthesia in the operating room?

Before answering that question, we must apply some qualifiers. First, few of the studies on the incidence of ECG abnormalities[12,13,49] excluded patients with histories or physical examinations indicating cardiac problems. Second, the studies do not distinguish those findings evident on monitoring leads from findings evident on only 6-lead or 12-lead ECGs.

Abnormalities on ECG are relatively common and increase exponentially with age. Averaging all of the data indicates that the incidence of abnormal preoperative ECG results would exceed 10% at 40 years of age and would be 25% by 60 years of age. These estimates pool abnormalities for both genders. Clearly, those studies that looked for abnormalities on ECG after first ensuring that the patient was asymptomatic (McKee and Scott,[11] Yipintsoi et al.[49] and Blery et al.[50]) found a much lower incidence of significant abnormalities. McKee and Scott found no abnormalities significant to perioperative care for 160 individuals who had no cardiac symptoms and were younger than 60 years, and only two abnormalities for 163 patients older than 60 years. Moorman et al.[47] found only 1 of 275 asymptomatic patients 45 years or younger who had abnormalities on preoperative ECGs. In the study by Blery et al., only 0.6% of 2,256 patients younger than 40 who had no cardiac or pulmonary symptoms had an abnormality on preoperative ECG. Our group found no abnormalities on ECG that were significant to, or altered, perioperative care among 510 patients judged to be asymptomatic on the basis of results from a video questionnaire.[51]

How useful is it to repeat an ECG if the patient has had an ECG within the past 2 years? Rabkin and Horne[52] addressed this question. New abnormalities on a subsequent ECG occur with significant frequency—25% to 50% as frequently as all abnormalities occurring on the previous ECG. Thus, one would be justified in obtaining screening ECGs before elective surgery for all patients older than 40 years, even those who have recently had an ECG, if it is older than 2 months or was abnormal.

Some physicians have questioned even that conclusion. Goldberger and O'Konski[53] believe that the most important potential benefit of the preoperative ECG is detection of a previously unrecognized myocardial infarction. This risk increases with age. However, even for the highest risk group, men 75 years or older, the estimated incidence of unrecognized Q wave myocardial infarction within the preceding 6 months is relatively small (less than 0.5%). Goldberger and O'Konski concluded that the risk of obtaining a preoperative ECG and subsequent reactions probably exceeds its benefit if patients are asymptomatic, do not have important risk factors for coronary artery disease, and are younger than 45 (men) or younger than 55 (women). If the benefit-risk analysis described in the section on CXRs is applied, then ECGs are indicated for asymptomatic men 40 years or older and for asymptomatic women 50 years or older who are scheduled to undergo procedures in class B or class C.

Hemoglobin Levels, Hematocrit, and White Blood Cell Counts

Wasserman and Gilbert[54] found that, of 28 patients with uncontrolled polycythemia (hemoglobin level higher than 16 g per dL) who underwent major surgery, 22 (79%) had complications and ten (36%) died. This group was compared with 53 patients who had controlled polycythemia (hemoglobin level less than 16 g per dL) and major surgery; of this group, 15 (28%) had complications and three (5%) died. For both groups, most of the complications were related to polycythemia (e.g., hemorrhage or thrombosis). Admittedly, the study of Wasserman and Gilbert had deficiencies. It was a retrospective study, and no time frame was given. "Minor" surgery was excluded. Also, the study did not explain why polycythemia was controlled preoperatively for some patients but not for others. Nevertheless, knowledge and pretreatment of polycythemia decreased perioperative morbidity and mortality. Data from another study confirm that polycythemia is an independent risk factor for cardiovascular mortality.[55]

No such evidence exists for normovolemic anemia. Rothstein[56] concluded that a hemoglobin level of 9 g per dL is adequate for patients older than 3 months, but the level should exceed 10 g per dL for younger patients. As emphasized by Roy et al.,[17] the age of the patient at the time of discovery of anemia often points to its cause. Anemia in the neonatal period is often attributable to recent blood loss, isoimmunization, congenital hemolytic anemia, or congenital infection. Anemia first detected 3 to 6 months after birth suggests a congenital disorder of hemoglobin synthesis or structure. Thus, assays of hemoglobin concentration in the first 6 months may represent the first opportunity for analysis. This use of the perioperative period for screening (or case finding) necessitates a proactive procedure for referring the patient and parents for counseling and treatment.

The point—that preoperative evaluations and documentation of data from the history are often not complete—was reiterated by Hackmann et al.[16] in their study of the prevalence of anemia. Several patients whose anemia was not properly suspected had conditions (Hirschsprung's disease, pyloric stenosis, or history of anemia accompanying juvenile rheumatoid arthritis) that should have alerted the anesthesiologist. These investigators also emphasize the importance of obtaining a thorough history.

Should asymptomatic anemia be treated before non–blood loss surgery, as O'Connor and Drasner[15] and others have done? Does this practice produce more benefit than harm? Does iron therapy at this early age contribute to late ischemic heart disease? Is the function of preoperative testing to spot chronic conditions? Although these questions have no definite answers, the author agrees with O'Connor and Drasner that these practices are indicated if one sets up the preoperative assessment to function in that role. Under such conditions, anesthesiologists would constitute second-opinion consultants to the primary care physician. An important requirement is that the preoperative assessment be performed sufficiently early (at least 1 week before surgery) and be vested with enough authority so that surgery can be postponed in a timely enough fashion to avoid any decrease in operating room efficiency.

If the preoperative assessment is not performed in advance or is not vested with sufficient authority, perhaps asymptomatic anemia before non–blood loss surgery should not be treated preoperatively. These impressions are confirmed by studies showing that humans survive anesthesia and class A–type surgery with hemoglobin levels higher than 80 g per L.[57,58] No data confirm the hypothesis that preoperative treatment of moderate or mild normovolemic anemia in such patients decreases perioperative morbidity or mortality.

Similarly, no data exist regarding the possible harm from an abnormal white blood cell (WBC) count found preoperatively. Therefore, the following ranges of surgically acceptable values are arbitrary: for hematocrit, 29% to 57% for men and 27% to 54% for women; for WBC count, 2,400 to 16,000 per mm^3 for both men and women. When values fall outside these ranges, a medical evaluation should be sought before instituting anesthesia or surgery.[59]

How many healthy patients have this degree of abnormality in hematocrit or WBC count? No such patient was found among the 223 of 2,010 patients judged healthy by history (i.e., history indicated no need for tests) in two different studies.[10,51] If 10% of all abnormalities are assumed to be outside the surgically acceptable range, and if the benefit-risk analysis described in the section on CXRs is applied, then the conclusion is that preoperative hematocrit or hemoglobin levels and red cell antigen screening should be performed for all surgical patients older than 64 years who are undergoing class B or class C procedures involving possible blood loss of more than 2 units per 70 kg of body weight.[60] Taking a WBC count appears to be justified rarely, if ever, for asymptomatic patients.

Blood Chemistries, Urinalysis, and Clotting Studies

What blood chemistries would have to be abnormal, and how abnormal would they have to be, to justify changing one's perioperative management? Abnormal hepatic or renal function might change the choice and dose of anesthetic or adjuvant drugs. Approximately 1 in 700 supposedly healthy patients actually harbors hepatitis, and 1 in 3 of those patients becomes jaundiced.[61] However, our group found no asymptomatic patient who denied exposure to hepatitis who then became jaundiced after uneventful surgery[51] (M. F. Roizen, unpublished data for more than 11,500 patients in a prospective study; J. Hsu et al., unpublished data). These data suggest that either the screening history suffices or the incidence of asymptomatic hepatitis is decreasing.

Unexpected abnormalities are reported for 2% to 10% of patients screened, and these abnormalities lead to many additional tests that usually (in approximately 80% of cases) have no significance for the patient. In fact, as described above, if 20 chemistry tests were ordered for a healthy individual, a 64% chance would exist that results from at least one test would be abnormal. Unexpected abnormalities that are significant arise in 2% to 5% of patients studied. Of these abnormalities, approximately 70% are related to blood glucose[62] and blood urea nitrogen (BUN) levels. The screen for diabetes may soon shift from determination of random blood glucose to determination of hemoglobin A_{1C}. The 9 to 20 additional tests on the screening simultaneous multichannel analysis of 12 to 20 variables lead to very few important discoveries affecting anesthesia. In fact, the false-positive rate is so high (i.e., 96.5% for calcium testing) that the value representing cost versus benefit for most of these tests (even when the tests are free) is negative, as is the value representing benefit versus risk. Berwick[63] clarified the difficulty of screening using data from screening at health fairs. More than 75% of the abnormalities for 76,519 patients were not even outside the range that caused the laboratories to notify the patient or physician of an abnormal value, let alone in a range judged significant to the patient's health.

If a screening test for hepatitis is desired (because the incidence of hepatitis is 0.14% or because one wishes to avoid the potential legal problems of postanesthetic jaundice), then a determination of serum glutamic-oxaloacetic transaminase or its successor aspartate aminotransferase, is warranted. BUN and glucose (or hemoglobin A_{1C}) level determination is indicated only for individuals older than 65 years. In fact, if the data from our group regarding asymptomatic liver disease can be generalized, no blood chemistry tests are warranted for healthy patients younger than 65 years. Furthermore, the availability of antibody testing for hepatitis C infection should diminish the medicolegal risk posed by postanesthetic jaundice.[64]

Abnormalities are commonly found on urinalysis. The quality of urinalysis results obtained by the dipstick technique has been variable at best.[65] In addition, these abnormal results usually do not lead to beneficial changes in management. Most of the results that do lead to beneficial changes could have been obtained by history or determination of BUN and glucose (or hemoglobin A_{1C}) levels, tests that are already recommended for all patients older than 65 years. Thus, urinalysis, although initially inexpensive, becomes an expensive test to justify on a benefit-cost or benefit-risk basis.

Although partial thromboplastin time and prothrombin time are useful tests with which to screen patients who have a history of bleeding, their value as screening tests for asymptomatic patients has never been shown.[9,10,12,14,66–69] Virtually no asymptomatic patient in the literature has had unequivocal benefit from clotting function studies performed preoperatively. Most patients show symptoms or have a medication history suggesting the possible need for clotting function tests. Suchman and Mushlin[69] and Macpherson[70] reviewed the data and concluded that preoperative clotting function testing for asymptomatic patients who have no risk factors for coagulopathy is incapable of predicting perioperative bleeding. No information is gained from either an abnormal or a normal result on clotting studies in low-risk patients. Figure 2-1 presents an algorithm that can be used to segregate high-risk and low-risk patients.

One situation deserves special comment: that in which the patient is taking aspirin or aspirin-containing compounds. Aspirin use at 3 to 10 mg per kg of body weight per day does not seem to pose a risk of bleeding. Data are not available, however, for situations in which 300 mg or more is administered within 12 hours of surgery. Because the pharmacokinetics of aspirin change when more than 2 g per 70 kg is consumed per day, a patient should be evaluated if he or she has not discontinued aspirin consumption sufficiently early to ensure that there will be no appreciable level of acetylsalicylic acid in the blood for 24 hours before surgery. This is the period that acetylsalicylic acid would have to be absent for the generation of the approximately 50,000 new platelets per mm^3 needed for normal platelet aggregation. The patient should also be evaluated if surgical hemostasis cannot be ensured or if a regional procedure into a closed space is planned.

TESTS FOR HUMAN IMMUNODEFICIENCY VIRUS, PREGNANCY, HEMOGLOBINOPATHIES, AND MALIGNANT HYPERTHERMIA

Tests for HIV infection and pregnancy, and screening for hemoglobinopathy and malignant hyperthermia (MH) raise ethical questions that may require close attention to institutional policy and the immediate availability of counseling services. Moreover, all of these tests have risks. The physician may therefore decide to limit testing only to populations at risk (e.g., for pregnancy testing, only to female patients who believe they may be pregnant).

Testing of asymptomatic patients for AIDS is not likely to be the most effective means of uncovering the disease. Of the more than 700,000 people in the United States who have had AIDS, fewer than 200 have not been gay, had sex with a prostitute, engaged in other at-risk sexual behavior, used intravenously administered drugs or shared needles, had a needlestick, been cared for by a family member with AIDS, or received a blood transfusion after 1979. One program screening for HIV in asymptomatic individuals was able to produce an "acceptably low false-positive rate" by diagnosing HIV infection only after one sample of blood produced positive results on three different tests, and after the second sample of blood had been used for verification.[71] Thus, for pregnancy, hemoglobinopathies, and HIV infection, the

Coagulation Tests

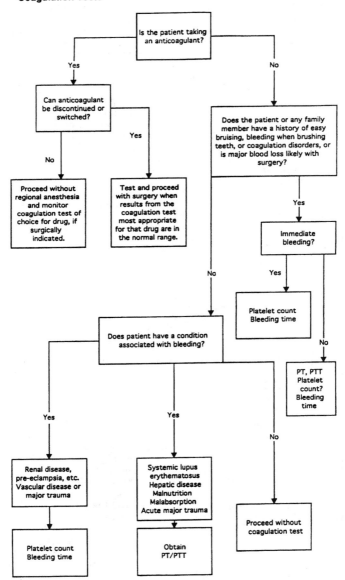

Fig. 2-1. Algorithm for determining whether coagulopathy or coagulation tests are needed. (PT, prothrombin time; PTT, partial thromboplastin time.) (Modified with permission from Roizen MF. Preoperative evaluation. In: Miller RD, ed. *Anesthesia*, vol 1, 5th ed. New York: Churchill Livingstone, 2000:824–883.)

history is still the best tool for identifying those who should be tested or those who are at risk for the condition.

In the past, no screening test existed for malignant hyperthermia other than a personal or family history of the condition. Although several tests may be available in the future, none, including genetic testing, is now available. It is still too early to predict the usefulness of screening tests for susceptibility to malignant hyperthermia or even for other genetic diseases (e.g., diabetes). Some screening tests have not been reliable enough to use for any but at-risk individuals (e.g., children with a history of myopathies who are undergoing surgery for strabismus; patients with a family history of problems with anesthesia; or patients with a history of abnormal red appearance, thermoregulation, and reactions to minor stresses).

Tests for Magnesium Deficiency and Albumin Level

Magnesium (Mg) deficiency represents a special situation. Putatively, it is much more common than other ion deficiencies, and Mg treatment has been advocated as extremely beneficial.[72] Because no data appear to link preoperative treatment of Mg deficiency with benefit, however, screening with tests appears superfluous. Hypomagnesemia is a prevalent laboratory finding in hospitalized patients (11% to 16%). The total serum level of Mg represents the protein-bound (physiologically inactive) Mg, as well as the ionized (physiologically active) Mg. Total serum Mg constitutes less than 1% of total body Mg, and no constant ratio exists between the two values.

Fanning et al.[73] showed that intravenous Mg given over 4 days after coronary artery bypass grafting decreased the incidence and severity of atrial fibrillation. Specifically, 14 patients in the control group had 42 episodes of atrial fibrillation; two of these required cardioversion. By contrast, seven patients in the Mg-treated group had 12 episodes of atrial fibrillation, and none required cardioversion. In a similar study, intraoperative administration of Mg after coronary artery bypass grafting decreased the frequency of postoperative ventricular arrhythmias; 8 of 50 (16%) in the Mg-treated group experienced arrhythmia versus 17 of 50 (34%) in the placebo-treated group ($P < .04$).[74]

Some investigators believe that serum Mg should be measured routinely in hospitalized patients because of the high prevalence of hypomagnesemia coupled with the difficulty of diagnosing hypomagnesemia.[72] One investigator argued that common sense dictates that nonessential surgery be deferred until Mg depletion has been corrected, again with no data to support such an assertion.[75] The benefit of decreased frequency of cardiac dysrhythmias with Mg administration after cardiac surgery[73,74] occurred with or without preoperative hypomagnesemia. If one is going to use Mg empirically, one probably should have a measure of renal function and should monitor Mg levels (or reflexes in the awake patient), but no data indicate that such levels should be routinely obtained preoperatively.

In the National Veterans Affairs Surgical Risk Study,[76] albumin level was an important predictor of perioperative morbidity and mortality in every surgical specialty. Changes in albumin level after enteral nutrition predicted perioperative outcome in malnourished or otherwise very sick patients. Perhaps this laboratory test should be added to those recommended for patients undergoing surgical class C procedures and for patients older than 85 years old undergoing class B procedures.

CONCLUSION

No laboratory tests are indicated in any patient of any age undergoing a minimally invasive class A procedure. A few tests may be indicated for patients undergoing a class B procedure, but the lack of data forces the individual practitioner to use clinical judgment for test selection. The tests shown in Table 2-3 are indicated for class C procedures. For class C procedures for asymptomatic males and females, regardless of age, a hematocrit and a blood typing and screening for unexpected antibodies is recommended. For an asymptomatic woman with pregnancy status in doubt, a pregnancy test is suggested. An ECG is recommended for men 40 years and older and for women 50 years and older. For individuals 65 years and older, an albumin test, a test for diabetes (glucose or hemoglobin A_{1C}), and a test of renal function (BUN) are recommended. Selecting these and only these tests will maximize benefit and minimize risk to patients and may reduce costs.

Table 2-3. Simplified strategy for preoperative testing for class B and C procedures

Group/preoperative condition	Hgb M	Hgb F	WBC	PT/PTT	PLT, BT	Elect	Creat/BUN	Blood glucose or Hgb A$_{1C}$	SGOT/Alk PTAse	Radiograph	ECG	Pregnancy test	Albumin	T/S
Neonates	X	X												
Physiologic age ≥75 yr	X	X					X	X		X	X		X	X
Class C procedure	X	X					X	X			X		X	X
Cardiovascular disease							X				X			
Pulmonary disease										X	X			
Malignancy	X	X	—[a]							X				
Radiation therapy			X							X	X			
Hepatic disease				X					X					
Exposure to hepatitis									X					
Renal disease	X	X				X	X							
Bleeding disorder				X	X						X			
Diabetes						X	X	X						
Smoking ≥20 pack/yr	X	X								X				

continued

Table 2-3. *Continued*

Group/preoperative condition	Hgb M	Hgb F	WBC	PT/ PTT	PLT, BT	Elect	Creat/ BUN	Blood glucose or Hgb A$_{1C}$	SGOT/Alk PTAse	Radiograph	ECG	Pregnancy test	Albumin	T/S
Possible pregnancy												X		
Use of diuretics						X	X							
Use of digoxin						X	X				X			
Steroid use						X		X						
Anticoagulant use	X	X		X		X	X							
CNS disease			X			X	X	X			X			

X indicates that test should be performed.

BT, bleeding time; CNS, central nervous system; Creat/BUN, creatinine and blood urea nitrogen level; ECG, electrocardiogram; Elect, levels of electrolytes (i.e., sodium, potassium, chloride, carbon dioxide); F, female; Hgb, hemoglobin level; Hgb A$_{1C}$, hemoglobin A$_{1C}$; M, male; PLT, platelet count; PT, prothrombin time; PTT, partial thromboplastin time; SGOT/Alk PTAse, serum glutamic-oxaloacetic transaminase and alkaline phosphatase; T/S, blood typing and screening for unexpected antibodies; WBC, white blood cell count.

Note: For minimally invasive class A procedures (cataracts, diagnostic arthroscopy), no tests are indicated. Not all diseases are included in this table. The physician's own judgment is needed regarding patients with diseases not listed.

For moderately invasive class B procedures (in which blood loss or hemodynamic changes are rare), use clinical judgment in test selection.

Highly invasive class C procedures typically disrupt normal physiology. These procedures commonly require blood administration, invasive monitoring, or postoperative management in a critical care setting; examples are total hip replacement, open aortic aneurysm resection, aortic valve replacement, and posterior fossa craniotomy for aneurysm.

^{a}Obtain for leukemias only.

Modified from Roizen MF. Preoperative evaluation. In: Miller RD, ed. *Anesthesia*, vol 1, 5th ed. New York: Churchill Livingstone, 2000;824–883.

REFERENCES

1. Goldman L, Caldera DL, Nussbaum SR, et al. Multifactorial index of cardiac risk in noncardiac surgical procedures. *N Engl J Med* 1977;297:845–850.
2. Duncan PG, Cohen MM, Tweed WA, et al. The Canadian four-centre study of anaesthetic outcomes. III. Are anaesthetic complications predictable in day surgical practice? *Can J Anaesth* 1992;39:440–448.
3. Pedersen T, Eliasen K, Henriksen E. A prospective study of mortality associated with anaesthesia and surgery: risk indicators of mortality in hospital. *Acta Anaesthesiol Scand* 1990;34:176–182.
4. Older P, Hall A. The role of cardiopulmonary exercise testing for preoperative evaluation of the elderly. In Wasserman K, ed. *Exercise gas exchange in heart disease*. Armonk, NY: Futura Publishers, 1996:287–297.
5. Leonard JV, Clayton BE, Colley JRT. Use of biochemical profile in Children's Hospital: results of two controlled trials. *BMJ* 1975;2:662–665.
6. Korvin CC, Pearce RH, Stanley J. Admissions screening: clinical benefits. *Ann Intern Med* 1975;83:197–203.
7. Olsen DM, Kane RL, Proctor PH. A controlled trial of multiphasic screening. *N Engl J Med* 1976;294:925–930.
8. Durbridge TC, Edwards F, Edwards RG, Atkinson M. Evaluation of benefits of screening tests done immediately on admission to hospital. *Clin Chem* 1976;22:968–71.
9. Narr BJ, Hansen TR, Warner MA. Preoperative laboratory screening in healthy Mayo patients: cost-effective elimination of tests and unchanged outcomes. *Mayo Clin Proc* 1991;66:155–159.
10. Kaplan EB, Sheiner LB, Boeckmann AJ, et al. The usefulness of preoperative laboratory screening. *JAMA* 1985;253:3576–3581.
11. McKee RF, Scott EM. The value of routine preoperative investigations. *Ann R Coll Surg Engl* 1987;69:160–162.
12. Turnbull JM, Buck C. The value of preoperative screening investigations in otherwise healthy individuals. *Arch Intern Med* 1987;147:1101–1105.
13. Johnson H Jr, Knee-Ioli S, Butler TA, et al. Are routine preoperative laboratory screening tests necessary to evaluate ambulatory surgical patients? *Surgery* 1988;104:639–645.
14. Muskett AD, McGreevy JM. Rational preoperative evaluation. *Postgrad Med J* 1986;62:925–928.
15. O'Connor ME, Drasner K. Preoperative laboratory testing of children undergoing elective surgery. *Anesth Analg* 1990;70:176–180.
16. Hackmann T, Seward DJ, Sheps SB. Anemia in pediatric day-surgery patients: prevalence and detection. *Anesthesiology* 1991; 75:27–31.
17. Roy WL, Lerman J, McIntyre BG. Is preoperative haemoglobin testing justified in children undergoing minor elective surgery? *Can J Anaesth* 1991;38:700–703.
18. Nigam A, Ahmed K, Drake-Lee AB. The value of preoperative estimation of haemoglobin in children undergoing tonsillectomy. *Clin Otolaryngol* 1990;15:549–551.
19. Baron MJ, Gunter J, White P. Is the pediatric preoperative hematocrit determination necessary? *South Med J* 1992;85:1187–1189.
20. Rohrer MJ, Michelotti MC, Nahrwold DL. A prospective evaluation of the efficacy of preoperative coagulation testing. *Ann Surg* 1988;208:554–557.

21. Lawrence VA, Kroenke K. The unproven utility of preoperative urinalysis. Clinical use. *Arch Intern Med* 1988;148:1370–1373.
22. Domoto K, Ben R, Wei JY, et al. Yield of routine annual laboratory screening in the institutionalized elderly. *Am J Public Health* 1985;75:243–245.
23. Wolf-Klein GP, Holt T, Silverstone FA, et al. Efficacy of routine annual studies in the care of elderly patients. *J Am Geriatr Soc* 1985;33:325–329.
24. Boscia JA, Kobasa WD, Knight RA, et al. Therapy vs no therapy for bacteriuria in elderly ambulatory nonhospitalized women. *JAMA* 1987;257:1067–1071.
25. Delahunt B, Turnbull PRG. How cost-effective are routine preoperative investigations? *N Z Med J* 1980;92:431–432.
26. Rosselló PJ, Ramos Cruz A, Mayol PM. Routine laboratory tests for elective surgery in pediatric patients: are they necessary? *Bol Asoc Med P R* 1982;72:614–623.
27. Bates DW, Boyle DL, Rittenberg E, et al. What proportion of common diagnostic tests appear redundant? *Am J Med* 1998;104:361–368.
28. Narr BJ, Warner ME, Schroeder DR, Warner MA. Outcomes of patients with no laboratory assessment before anesthesia and a surgical procedure. *Mayo Clin Proc* 1997;72:505–509.
29. Sox HC Jr, ed. *Common diagnostic tests: use and interpretation*, 2nd ed. Philadelphia: American College of Physicians, 1990.
30. Hayward RSA, Steinberg EP, Ford DE, et al. Preventive care guidelines: 1991. *Ann Intern Med* 1991;114:758–783.
31. Roizen MF, Kaplan EB, Schreider BD, et al. The relative roles of the history and physical examination, and laboratory testing in preoperative evaluation for outpatient surgery: the "Starling" curve in preoperative laboratory testing. *Anesthesiol Clin North Am* 1987;5:15–34.
32. Tape TG, Mushlin AI. How useful are routine chest x-rays of preoperative patients at risk for postoperative chest disease? *J Gen Intern Med* 1988;3:15–20.
33. Orkin FK. Practice standards: the Midas touch or the emperor's new clothes? *Anesthesiology* 1989;70:567–571.
34. Lawson DH. Adverse reactions to potassium chloride. *QJM* 1974;43:433–440.
35. Lawson DH, Hutcheon AW, Jick H. Life threatening drug reactions amongst medical in-patients. *Scott Med J* 1979;24:127–130.
36. Levinstein MR, Ouslander JG, Rubenstein LZ, Forsythe SB. Yield of routine annual laboratory tests in a skilled nursing home population. *JAMA* 1987;258:1909–1915.
37. Elmore JG, Barton MB, Moceri VM, et al. Ten-year risk of false positive screening mammograms and clinical breast examinations. *N Engl J Med* 338:1998;1089–1096.
38. Lembo NJ, Dell'Italia LJ, Crawford MH, O'Rourke RA. Bedside diagnosis of systolic murmurs. *N Engl J Med* 1988;318:1572–1578.
39. Baker JP, Detsky AS, Wesson DE, et al. Nutritional assessment. A comparison of clinical judgment and objective measurements. *N Engl J Med* 1982;306:969–972.
40. Mitchell TL, Tornelli JL, Fisher TD, et al. Yield of the screening review of systems: a study on a general medical service. *J Gen Intern Med* 1992;7:393–397.
41. Robertson WM. *Medical malpractice: a preventive approach*. Seattle: University of Washington Press, 1985.

42. Pollard JB, Zboray AL, Mazze RI. Economic benefits attributed to opening a preoperative evaluation clinic for outpatients. *Anesth Analg* 1996;83:407–410.
43. Vogt AW, Henson LC. Unindicated preoperative testing: ASA physical status and financial implications. *J Clin Anesth* 1997;9: 437–441.
44. Pauker SG, Kopelman RI. Interpreting hoofbeats: can Bayes help clear the haze? *N Engl J Med* 1992;327:1009–1013.
45. Black WC, Welch HG. Advances in diagnostic imaging and overestimations of disease prevalence and the benefits of therapy. *N Engl J Med* 1993;328:1237–1243.
46. Roizen MF. Preoperative evaluation. In: Miller RD, ed. *Anesthesia*, vol 1, 5th ed. New York: Churchill Livingstone, 2000:824–883.
47. Moorman JR, Hlatky MA, Eddy DM, et al. The yield of the routine admission electrocardiogram. A study in a general medical service. *Ann Intern Med* 1985;103:590–595.
48. Brill PW, Ewing ML, Dunn AA. The value (?) of routine chest radiography in children and adolescents. *Pediatrics* 1973;52: 125–127.
49. Yipintsoi T, Vasinanukorn P, Sanguanchua P. Is routine preoperative electrocardiogram necessary? *J Med Assoc Thai* 1989;72: 16–20.
50. Blery C, Szatan M, Fourgeaux B, et al. Evaluation of a protocol for selective ordering of preoperative tests. *Lancet* 1986;1: 139–141.
51. Apfelbaum J, Robinson D, Murray WJ, et al. An automated method to validate preoperative test selection: first results of a multicenter study, abstracted. *Anesthesiology* 1989;71:A928.
52. Rabkin SW, Horne JM. Preoperative electrocardiography: effect of new abnormalities on clinical decisions. *Can Med Assoc J* 1983;128:146–147.
53. Goldberger AL, O'Konski M. Utility of the routine electrocardiogram before surgery and on general hospital admission. Critical review and new guidelines. *Ann Intern Med* 1986;105:552–557.
54. Wasserman LR, Gilbert HS. Surgical bleeding in polycythemia vera. *Ann N Y Acad Sci* 1964;115:122–126.
55. Erikssen G, Thaulow E, Sandvik L, et al. Hematocrit: a predictor of cardiovascular mortality? *J Intern Med* 1993;234:493–499.
56. Rothstein P. What hemoglobin level is adequate in pediatric anesthesia? *Anesthesiol Update* 1978;1:2–3.
57. Weiskopf RB, Viele MK, Feiner J, et al. Human cardiovascular and metabolic response to acute, severe isovolemic anemia. *JAMA* 1998;279:217–221.
58. Carson JL, Duff A, Berlin J, et al. Perioperative blood transfusion and postoperative mortality. *JAMA* 1998;279:199–205.
59. Kowalyshyn TJ, Prager D, Young J. A review of the present status of preoperative hemoglobin requirements. *Anesth Analg* 1972; 51:75–79.
60. Moore SB, Reisner RK, Offord KP. Morning admission for a same-day surgical procedure: resolution of a blood bank problem. *Mayo Clin Proc* 1989;64:406–408.
61. Wataneeyawech M, Kelly KA Jr. Hepatic diseases unsuspected before surgery. *N Y State J Med* 1975;75:1278–1281.
62. Singer DE, Samet JH, Coley CM, Nathan DM. Screening for diabetes mellitus. *Ann Intern Med* 1988;109:639–649.
63. Berwick DM. Screening in health fairs. A critical review of benefits, risks, and costs. *JAMA* 1985;254:1492–1498.

64. Alter MJ. Non-A, non-B hepatitis: sorting through a diagnosis of exclusion. *Ann Intern Med* 1989;110:583–585.

65. Challand GS. Is ward biochemical testing cheap and easy? *Intensive Care World* 1987;4:9–11.

66. Baranetsky NG, Weinstein P. Partial thromboplastin time for screening. *Ann Intern Med* 1979;91:498–499.

67. Macpherson DS, Snow R, Lofgren RP. Preoperative screening: value of previous tests. *Ann Intern Med* 1990;113:969–973.

68. Eisenberg JM, Clarke JR, Sussman SA. Prothrombin and partial thromboplastin times as preoperative screening tests. *Arch Surg* 1982;117:48–51.

69. Suchman AL, Mushlin AI. How well does the activated partial thromboplastin time predict postoperative hemorrhage? *JAMA* 1986;256:750–753.

70. Macpherson DS. Preoperative laboratory testing: should any tests be "routine" before surgery? *Med Clin North Am* 1993;77:289–308.

71. Burke DS, Brundage JF, Redfield RR, et al. Measurement of the false positive rate in a screening program for human immunodeficiency virus infections. *N Engl J Med* 1988;319:961–964.

72. Wong ET, Rude RK, Singer FR, Shaw ST Jr. A high prevalence of hypomagnesemia and hypermagnesemia in hospitalized patients. *Am J Clin Pathol* 1983;79:348–352.

73. Fanning WJ, Thomas CS Jr, Roach A, et al. Prophylaxis in atrial fibrillation with magnesium sulfate after coronary bypass grafting. *Ann Thorac Surg* 1991;52:529–533.

74. England MR, Gordon G, Salem M, Chernow B. Magnesium administration and dysrhythmias after cardiac surgery. A placebo-controlled, double-blind, randomized trial. *JAMA* 1992;268:2395–2402.

75. Gambling DR, Birmingham CL, Jenkins LC. Magnesium and the anaesthetist. *Can J Anaesth* 1988;35:644–654.

76. Khuri SF, Daley J, Henderson W, et al. Risk adjustment of the postoperative mortality rate for the comparative assessment of the quality of surgical care: results of the National Veterans Affairs Surgical Risk Study. *J Am Coll Surg* 1997;185:315–327.

Ischemic Heart Disease

Lee A. Fleisher

The high-risk patient presenting for noncardiac surgery represents a diagnostic dilemma with respect to the appropriate degree of preoperative evaluation. In patients with known cardiovascular disease, information on the extent of disease, ventricular function, and stability of disease may be beneficial in directing perioperative management. Many patients, particularly those undergoing major vascular surgery, may be asymptomatic, and no prior or recent evaluations may have been performed; however, the probability of extensive coronary artery disease (CAD) may be high.

Based on the above-noted basic premises, numerous investigators have advocated the use of preoperative evaluation and perioperative interventions as a means of reducing complications for high-risk patients undergoing major surgical procedures. Several authors have questioned the need for such an approach in the modern era, however. Reviews of articles reporting outcome after major noncardiac surgery demonstrate a decrease in the incidence of perioperative fatal and nonfatal myocardial infarction (MI). The question remains whether this decrease in complication rate is a function of improved preoperative evaluation or perioperative management. Compounding this clinical controversy are issues related to medical economics. Increasing emphasis is being given to reducing perioperative cost by reducing preoperative testing. Therefore, the value of preoperative testing has come under great scrutiny. This review examines the value of preoperative testing resulting in perioperative and long-term interventions that improve a patient's health. It focuses on two recent sets of guidelines from the American College of Cardiology/American Heart Association (ACC/AHA) and the American College of Physicians (ACP) that have identified clinical risk stratification and appropriate use of diagnostic testing. Both a short-term (perioperative) and long-term perspective are taken in the discussion because the answer may change based on the perspective used.

ROLE OF THE CONSULTANT

As is discussed throughout this chapter, the evaluation of the patient with known cardiovascular disease or risk factors for cardiovascular disease requires an understanding of the extent and stability of the disease and ventricular function. If the anesthesiologist has sufficient information regarding these factors, then no further consultation is required. Frequently, a simple phone call to the primary physician suffices. If the information is not easily obtainable from the patient or the medical record, then a formal consultation may be required. The focus of the consultation

39

should be to ask *specific* questions regarding the cardiovascular status that are important to perioperative management. Such an approach is advocated in the ACC/AHA guidelines.

RISK INDICES

In 1977, Goldman et al. published their landmark article that studied 1,001 patients undergoing noncardiac surgical procedures, excluding transurethral resection of the prostate. The authors excluded the latter surgery because of their impression that it carried a low morbidity rate when performed under spinal anesthesia. They identified six risk factors and gave each factor a certain number of points (Goldman Cardiac Risk Index, or CRI) (Table 3-1). An MI and S_3 gallop were identified as the most sig-

Table 3-1. Computation of the Cardiac Risk Index

Criteria	Point value
History	
(a) Age >70 yr	5
(b) MI in previous 6 mo	10
Physical examination	
(a) S_3 gallop or JVD	11
(b) Important AS	3
Electrocardiogram	
(a) Rhythm other than sinus or PACs on last preoperative ECG	7
(b) >5 PVCs/min documented at any time before operation	7
General status	
Po_2 <60 or Pco_2 >50 mm Hg; K <3.0 or HCO_3 <20 mEq/L; BUN >50 or Cr >3.0 mg/dL; abnormal SGOT; signs of chronic liver disease or patient bedridden from noncardiac causes	3
Operation	
(a) Intraperitoneal, intrathoracic, or aortic operation	3
(b) Emergency operation	4
Total possible points	**53**

AS, aortic stenosis; BUN, blood urea nitrogen, Cr, creatinine; ECG, electrocardiogram; HCO_3, bicarbonate; JVD, jugular vein distention; K, potassium; MI, myocardial infarction; PACs, premature atrial contractions; Po_2, partial pressure of oxygen; Pco_2, partial pressure of carbon dioxide; PVCs, premature ventricular contractions; SGOT, serum glutamic oxalacetic transaminase.

Class	Point range	Percent cardiac complication
I	0–5	1
II	6–12	7
III	13–25	14
IV	>26	78

Reprinted with permission from Goldman L, Caldera DL, Nussbaum SR, et al. Multifactorial index of cardiac risk in noncardiac surgical procedures. *N Engl J Med* 1977;297:845–850.

nificant risk factors. Based on the total number of points for each patient, patients were placed into one of four classes. The patient's class could then be compared with the rates of morbidity and mortality in the original cohort.

The CRI was subsequently validated using another cohort of patients; however, it has not been found to be predictive for patients undergoing major vascular surgery. Multiple studies have demonstrated that major vascular surgery is associated with a higher rate of morbidity and mortality than is nonvascular surgery. To rectify this problem, Detsky et al. proposed a modification of the CRI that incorporated additional factors for vascular patients (Table 3-2). Importantly, the Detsky modification of the Goldman CRI is used as the starting point for the ACP guidelines.

Although both of these indices were useful when initially proposed, perioperative care has changed significantly in the intervening years. Goldman class III and IV patients continue to represent a high-risk cohort; however, further stratification of the low-risk group is required. In addition, assigning an absolute number or class of risk does not provide the anesthesiologist with the information necessary to modify care. For this reason, the use of risk indices has limited value for management in the perioperative period. In contrast, the preoperative evaluation should focus on the identification of the extent and stability of the patient's cardiovascular disease and the ventricular reserve with stress.

Table 3-2. Modified Cardiac Risk Index of Detsky et al.

Variables	Points
Angina	
Class IV[a]	20
Class III[b]	10
Unstable angina <3 mo	10
Suspected critical aortic stenosis	20
Myocardial infarction	
<6 mo	10
>6 mo	5
Alveolar pulmonary edema	
<1 wk	10
Ever	5
Emergency surgery	10
Sinus plus atrial premature beats or rhythm other than sinus on preop ECG	5
>5 PVCs at any time before surgery	5
Poor general medical status	5
Age >70 yr	5

ECG, electrocardiogram; preop, preoperative; PVCs, premature ventricular contractions.
[a]"Inability to carry on any physical activity without discomfort, anginal syndrome *may* be present at rest."
[b]"Marked limitation of ordinary physical activity." Walking one to two blocks on the level or climbing one flight of stairs in normal conditions and at normal pace.
Reprinted with permission from Detsky A, Abrams H, McLaughlin J, et al. Predicting cardiac complications in patients undergoing non-cardiac surgery. *J Gen Intern Med* 1986;1:211–219.

Clinical Evaluation for Coronary Artery Disease

In evaluating the patient, a critical first step is to identify the presence of unstable symptoms. Frequently, the preoperative evaluation represents an opportunity to evaluate patients who rarely access the health care system otherwise and are not currently being treated for cardiovascular disease. This is particularly true for patients scheduled for vascular surgical procedures, in whom coexisting diabetes mellitus or change in lifestyle may mask cardiac symptoms.

In patients with symptomatic CAD, the preoperative evaluation may lead to the recognition of a change in the frequency or pattern of anginal symptoms. The presence of unstable angina has been associated with a high perioperative risk of MI. The perioperative period is associated with a hypercoagulable state and surges in levels of endogenous catecholamines, both of which may exacerbate the underlying process in unstable angina, increasing the risk of acute MI. The anesthesiologist can influence both a patient's short-term and long-term health by referring patients with unstable angina for further medical or coronary interventions.

Patients with stable angina represent a continuum from those who experience mild angina with extreme exertion to those who experience dyspnea with angina after walking up a few stairs. The patient who manifests angina only after strenuous exercise and does not demonstrate signs of left ventricular dysfunction would not be a candidate for changes in management. In contrast, a patient with dyspnea on mild exertion would be at high risk for developing perioperative ventricular dysfunction, myocardial ischemia, and possible MI. These patients have an extremely high probability of having extensive CAD, and additional monitoring or cardiovascular testing should be contemplated, depending on the surgical procedure and institutional factors.

In virtually all studies, the presence of active congestive heart failure preoperatively has been associated with an increased incidence of perioperative cardiac morbidity. Stabilization of ventricular function and treatment for pulmonary congestion is prudent before elective surgery (see Chapter 4). Also, determining the cause of the left heart failure is important. Congestive symptoms may be due to nonischemic cardiomyopathy or mitral or aortic valvular insufficiency or stenosis (see Chapter 4). Because the type of perioperative monitoring and treatments would be different, clarifying the cause of cardiac congestion is important.

Most patients with a prior MI have CAD, although a small group of patients may sustain an MI from a nonatherosclerotic mechanism. Traditionally, risk assessment for noncardiac surgery was based on the time interval between the MI and surgery. Multiple studies have demonstrated an increased incidence of reinfarction if the MI was within 6 months of surgery. With improvements in perioperative care, this difference has decreased.

The importance of the intervening time interval may no longer be valid, however, in the current era of thrombolytics, percutaneous transluminal coronary angioplasty (PTCA), and risk stratification after an acute MI. Although many patients with an MI may continue to have myocardium at risk for subsequent ischemia and infarction, other patients may have their critical coronary stenosis either totally occluded or widely patent. For example, the use of PTCA is associated with a lower incidence of death or reinfarction within 6 months than is traditional medical therapy or the use of thrombolytics. Therefore, patients should be evaluated from the perspective of their risk for ongoing ischemia. The ACC/AHA Task Force on Perioperative Evaluation of the Cardiac Patient Undergoing Noncardiac Surgery has advocated (without any objective evidence) that patients who have had an MI within 30 days be classified as the group at highest risk, whereas for those whose MI occurred longer ago than that period, risk stratification is based on the presentation of disease and exercise tolerance.

Patients at Risk for Coronary Artery Disease

For those patients without overt symptoms or history, the probability of CAD varies with the type and number of atherosclerotic risk factors present. Peripheral vascular disease has been shown to be associated with CAD in multiple studies. Hertzer et al. examined 1,000 consecutive patients scheduled for major vascular surgery and found that approximately 60% of patients had at least one coronary artery with a critical stenosis. Therefore, the patient with peripheral vascular disease should be evaluated further for evidence of CAD.

Patients with diabetes mellitus have a higher probability of CAD than do nondiabetic patients. Such patients have a high incidence of both silent MI and myocardial ischemia. Eagle et al. demonstrated that diabetes mellitus is an independent risk factor for perioperative cardiac morbidity. In attempting to determine the degree of this increased probability, the length of the disease and other associated end-organ dysfunction should be taken into account. Autonomic neuropathy has been found to be the best predictor of silent CAD. Because these patients are at very high risk for a silent MI, an electrocardiogram (ECG) should be evaluated for the presence of Q waves.

Hypertension also has been associated with an increased incidence of silent myocardial ischemia and infarction. Those hypertensive patients with left ventricular hypertrophy who are undergoing noncardiac surgery are at a higher perioperative risk than nonhypertensive patients. Investigators have suggested that the presence of a strain pattern on ECG suggests a chronic ischemic state. Therefore, these patients should be considered to have an increased probability of CAD and cardiovascular morbidity, and further evaluation is warranted if this is a new finding. The implications of an elevated preoperative blood pressure are discussed in Chapter 4.

Several other risk factors suggest an increased probability of CAD. These include the atherosclerotic processes associated with tobacco use and hypercholesterolemia. Although these risk factors increase the probability of developing CAD, they have not been shown to increase perioperative risk. When an attempt is made to determine the overall probability of disease, the number and severity of the risk factors are important.

Physical Examination of the Patient with Cardiovascular Disease

A complete physical examination is necessary. Auscultation of the heart can reveal a previously undiagnosed murmur or additional heart sounds. An S_3 gallop is associated with congestive heart failure. Frequently, a murmur is detected the day of surgery, and the value of further testing must be balanced against the disadvantages of delaying the procedure. The nature of the murmur and concomitant symptoms can provide important information regarding the underlying pathophysiology (see Chapter 4). Auscultation of the lungs should include evaluation for findings of congestive heart failure, in addition to pulmonary disease. Although wheezing may reflect bronchospastic disease, it may also signify congestive heart failure. Crackles or rales may also signify significant congestive heart failure. In addition to signs of left heart failure, patients at risk for cardiovascular disease should be evaluated for signs of right heart failure, such as hepatomegaly and jugular venous distension.

Blood pressure and heart rate should be determined in both supine and standing positions to assess intravascular volume or autonomic dysfunction. In vascular surgery patients, blood pressure should be obtained in both arms. because significant differences have been observed. Careful cardiac auscultation should be performed to detect clinically important findings. The pulmonary examination and evaluation for lower extremity edema can help determine clinical volume status. Peripheral arterial pulses may suggest valvular disease or the presence of atherosclerotic disease.

Decision to Perform Further Cardiovascular Testing

In addition to helping to determine the need for preoperative cardiovascular testing, risk factors are also important in the interpretation of any noninvasive test. Eagle et al. evaluated the implications of the prior probability of disease based on clinical criteria in determining the value of preoperative testing. Patients without clinical risk factors (angina, Q waves, ventricular ectopic activity requiring treatment, diabetes mellitus, age older than 70 years) had only a 3% incidence of perioperative morbidity, and noninvasive testing could not further stratify risk. Similarly, patients with three or more risk factors had a 50% morbidity, and noninvasive testing did not further discriminate risk. Preoperative dipyridamole-thallium imaging, however, was useful in the group at moderate risk (one or two risk factors). This concept, whereby the probability of a disease outcome after testing is held to be a function of the probability of disease before testing, is an application of Bayes' theorem. It helps to explain differences in predictive values reported between consecutive and selective patient series.

Paul et al. evaluated the ability of these clinical risk factors to predict angiographic severity of CAD in patients undergoing vascular surgery. Using the cohort of patients at the Cleveland Clinic who underwent angiography, they demonstrated that critical three-vessel or left main disease was present in only 5% of low-risk patients (no risk factors) but was found in 43% of high-risk patients (more than two risk factors). The authors developed a clinical predictive rule whereby the absence of angina, prior MI, or history of congestive heart failure is associated with a 94% predictive value of being free of critical coronary disease.

Two studies illustrate the reduced value of noninvasive testing when consecutively treated surgical patients are studied. Mangano et al. studied 60 consecutively treated patients undergoing vascular surgery and reported that dipyridamole-thallium imaging had a positive predictive value of 27% for adverse cardiac events, a negative predictive value of 82%, and no net discriminative ability. Baron et al. studied the largest consecutive population of patients (457) undergoing abdominal aortic surgery and also were unable to demonstrate an association between thallium redistribution and perioperative cardiac morbidity. Both studies illustrate the low positive predictive value of testing and significant incidence of morbidity in patients with negative test results when consecutively treated patients are studied.

L'Italien et al. constructed a Bayesian model that incorporated clinical risk factors and the results of dipyridamole-thallium imaging. The pretest (baseline) probability of an event can be calculated similarly to Goldman's CRI, whereby risk factors are associated with certain numerical weights that can be added to determine overall risk. The results of dipyridamole-thallium imaging can then be used to modify the risk and determine the posttest probability of an event. In this manner, risk factors can be used to determine if the test results will raise the probability of morbidity above some threshold for action. Poldermans also demonstrated that risk factors were an important determinant of the value of preoperative testing in patients undergoing dobutamine stress echocardiography.

The additive value of diagnostic testing was best illustrated by Vanzetto et al. They followed a cohort of consecutively treated abdominal aortic surgery patients and performed dipyridamole-thallium imaging in patients with two or more clinical or electrocardiographic risk factors. Importantly, the results of the test were not made available to the clinicians. Major cardiac events occurred in 23% of patients with reversible defects and in 1% of patients without reversible defects. Results of thallium single photon emission computed tomography in clinically high-risk patients demonstrated significantly greater prognostic value for cardiac events than that provided by clinical variables alone.

GUIDELINES FOR PREOPERATIVE TESTING FOR CORONARY ARTERY DISEASE

Multiple algorithms have been published regarding the use of preoperative cardiovascular testing before noncardiac surgery; however, no studies have been performed to evaluate their validity. The ACC/AHA has published Guidelines on Perioperative Cardiovascular Evaluation for Noncardiac Surgery and has proposed an algorithm based on expert opinion and accumulating evidence. The guidelines integrate clinical risk factors, exercise capacity, and the surgical procedure in the decision process.

As described with regard to anginal pattern, exercise tolerance is one of the strongest determinants of perioperative risk and the need for invasive monitoring. McPhail et al. demonstrated that patients undergoing major vascular surgery who could exercise to 85% of their peak maximal heart rate were at a lower risk for cardiac morbidity than were those who were unable to reach the target heart rate, even in the presence of a positive stress test. An excellent exercise tolerance, even in patients with stable angina, suggests that the myocardium can be stressed without becoming dysfunctional. If a patient can walk a mile without becoming short of breath, the probability of extensive CAD is small. Alternatively, if patients develop dyspnea associated with chest pain during minimal exertion, the probability of extensive CAD is higher. A greater degree of CAD has been associated with a higher perioperative risk. In addition, patients with signs of left ventricular dysfunction are at risk for developing hypotension with ischemia, and therefore may benefit from more extensive monitoring or coronary revascularization. Exercising all patients to obtain a formal assessment would not be cost effective, and several scales exist that are based on activities of daily living. One such scale has been proposed in the guidelines (Table 3-3).

The surgical procedure itself has a significant impact on perioperative risks and the amount of preoperative information required to safely perform anesthesia. For surgical procedures that are not associated with significant stress or a high incidence of perioperative myocardial ischemia or morbidity, the costs of the evaluation are often greater than any perceived benefits from the new information. For example, cataract surgery is associated with minimal stress and exceedingly low morbidity and mortality rates, even after a recent MI. Similarly, outpatient procedures have been shown to be associated with a low incidence of morbidity and mortality, although this may change with the increasing complexity of procedures being performed in the outpatient setting. In such patients, perioperative management is rarely changed by the cardiovascular status unless the patient demonstrates unstable angina or overt congestive heart failure. In contrast, the patient undergoing a procedure associated with significant stress and a high incidence of morbidity and mortality can frequently benefit from a more extensive preoperative evaluation. For example, vascular disease is associated with a high risk of morbidity, and the ischemic potential and incidence of periop-

Table 3-3. Estimated energy requirement for various activities

1 MET	Can you take care of yourself?
	Eat, dress, or use the toilet?
	Walk indoors around the house?
	Walk a block or two on level ground at 2–3 mph or 3.2–4.8 km/h?
	Do light work around the house like dusting or washing dishes?
4 METs	Climb a flight of stairs or walk up a hill? Walk on level ground at 4 mph or 6.4 km/h? Run a short distance?
	Do heavy work around the house like scrubbing floors or lifting or moving heavy furniture?
	Participate in moderate recreational activities like golf, bowling, dancing, doubles tennis, or throwing a baseball or football?
>10 METs	Participate in strenuous sports like swimming, singles tennis, football, basketball, or skiing?

MET, metabolic equivalent.
Adapted from the Duke Activity Status Index and American Heart Association Exercise Standards. Reprinted with permission from Eagle K, Brundage B, Chaitman B, et al. Guidelines for perioperative cardiovascular evaluation of the noncardiac surgery. A report of the American College of Cardiology/American Heart Association Task Force on Assessment of Diagnostic and Therapeutic Cardiovascular Procedures. *Circulation* 1996;93:1278–1317.

erative cardiac morbidity increases with the level of aortic cross clamp in patients undergoing aortic reconstruction. Because further determination of cardiac status may alter perioperative care (i.e., coronary artery revascularization or invasive monitoring) the benefit of further evaluation and treatment can be greater than the associated costs or risks. Finally, intraabdominal, orthopedic, and intrathoracic procedures are associated with an intermediate risk. In this group, the duration of surgery and extent of fluid shifts may modify the need for further evaluation. Using data from long-term follow-up of the Coronary Artery Surgery Study (CASS), the guidelines have suggested three classifications of surgical risk (Table 3-4).

The algorithm to determine the need for testing proposed by the ACC/AHA is shown in Fig. 3-1. First, the clinician must evaluate the urgency of the surgery and the appropriateness of a formal preoperative assessment. Next, the clinician must determine if the patient has undergone a previous revascularization procedure or coronary evaluation. Those patients with unstable coronary syndromes should be identified, and appropriate treatment instituted. Finally, the decision to institute further testing depends on the interaction of the clinical risk factors (Table 3-5), surgery-specific risk, and functional capacity (see Table 3-3). For patients at intermediate clinical risk, both the exercise tolerance and the extent of the surgery are taken into account in determining the need for further testing. Importantly, no preoperative cardiovascular testing should be performed if the results will not change perioperative management.

Table 3-4. Cardiac risk stratification[a] for noncardiac surgical procedures

High (reported cardiac risk often >5%)
    Emergent major operations, particularly in the elderly
    Aortic and other major vascular procedures
    Peripheral vascular procedures
    Anticipated prolonged surgical procedures associated with large
        fluid shifts and/or blood loss
Intermediate (reported cardiac risk generally <5%)
    Carotid endarterectomy
    Head and neck surgery
    Intraperitoneal and intrathoracic surgery
    Orthopedic surgery
    Prostate surgery
Low[b] (reported cardiac risk generally <1%)
    Endoscopic procedures
    Superficial procedure
    Cataract surgery
    Breast surgery

[a]Combined incidence of cardiac death and nonfatal myocardial infarction.
[b]Do not generally require further preoperative cardiac testing.
Reprinted with permission from Eagle K, Brundage B, Chaitman B, et al. Guidelines for perioperative cardiovascular evaluation of the noncardiac surgery. A report of the American College of Cardiology/American Heart Association Task Force on Assessment of Diagnostic and Therapeutic Cardiovascular Procedures. *Circulation* 1996;93:1278–1317.

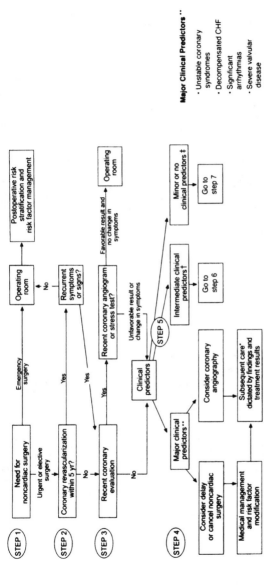

Major Clinical Predictors **

· Unstable coronary syndromes
· Decompensated CHF
· Significant arrhythmias
· Severe valvular disease

Fig. 3-1. The American College of Cardiology/American Heart Association Task Force on Perioperative Evaluation of Cardiac Patients Undergoing Noncardiac Surgery has proposed an algorithm for decisions regarding the need for further evaluation. This represents one of multiple algorithms proposed in the literature. The algorithm is based on expert opinion and incorporates six steps. First, the clinician must evaluate the urgency of the surgery and the appropriateness of a formal preoperative assessment. Next, he or she must determine whether the patient has had a previous revascularization procedure or coronary evaluation. Those patients with unstable coronary syndromes should be identified, and appropriate treatment should be instituted. The decision to perform further testing depends on the interaction of the clinical risk factors, surgery-specific risk, and functional capacity. *Subsequent care may include cancellation or delay of surgery, coronary revascularization followed by noncardiac surgery, or intensified care. (*continued*)

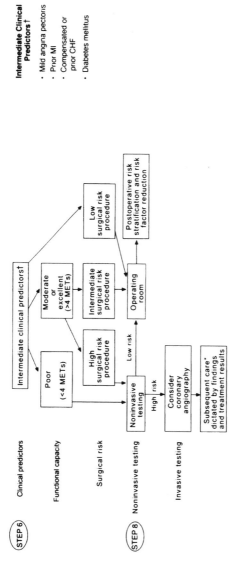

Intermediate Clinical Predictors†

· Mild angina pectoris
· Prior MI
· Compensated or prior CHF
· Diabetes mellitus

Fig. 3-1 *continued.* (CHF, congestive heart failure; ECG, electrocardiogram; MET, metabolic equivalent; MI, myocardial infarction.) (Adapted with permission from Eagle K, Brundage B, Chaitman B, et al. Guidelines for perioperative cardiovascular evaluation of the noncardiac surgery. A report of the American College of Cardiology/American Heart Association Task Force on Assessment of Diagnostic and Therapeutic Cardiovascular Procedures. *Circulation* 1996;93:1278–1317.)

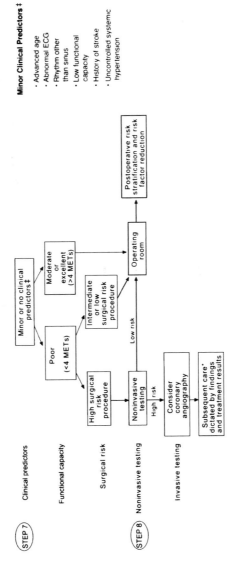

Fig. 3-1 continued.

Table 3-5. Clinical predictors of increased perioperative cardiovascular risk (myocardial infarction, congestive heart failure, death)

Major

Unstable coronary syndromes

    Recent myocardial infarction[a] with evidence of important ischemic risk with clinical symptoms or noninvasive study

Unstable or severe[b] angina (Canadian class III or IV)[c]

Decompensated congestive heart failure

Significant arrhythmias

    High-grade atrioventricular block

    Symptomatic ventricular arrhythmias in the presence of underlying heart disease

    Supraventricular arrhythmias with uncontrolled ventricular rate

Severe valvular disease

Intermediate

Mild angina pectoris (Canadian class I or II)[c]

Prior myocardial infarction by history or pathologic Q waves

Compensated or prior congestive heart failure

Diabetes mellitus

Minor

Advanced age

Abnormal electrocardiogram (left ventricular hypertrophy, left bundle branch block, ST-T abnormalities)

Rhythm other than sinus (e.g., atrial fibrillation)

Low functional capacity (e.g., inability to climb one flight of stairs with a bag of groceries)

History of stroke

Uncontrolled systemic hypertension

---

[a]The American College of Cardiology National Database Library defines recent myocardial infarction as occurring >7 days but ≤ 1 month (30 days) previously.
[b]May include stable angina in patients who are unusually sedentary.
[c]Grading of Angina of Effort by the Canadian Cardiovascular Society:

   I. "Ordinary physical activity [e.g., walking and climbing stairs] does not cause . . . angina." Angina with strenuous or rapid or prolonged exertion at work or recreation.
  II. "Slight limitation of ordinary activity [before onset of angina]." Walking or climbing stairs rapidly, walking uphill, walking or stair climbing after meals, or in cold, or in wind, or under emotional stress, or only during the few hours after awakening. Walking more than 2 blocks on the level and climbing more than one flight of ordinary stairs at a normal pace and in normal conditions.
 III. "Marked limitation of ordinary physical activity [before onset of angina]." Walking one to two blocks on the level and climbing one flight of stairs in normal conditions and a normal pace.
 IV. "Inability to carry on any physical activity without discomfort—anginal syndrome *may* be present at rest."

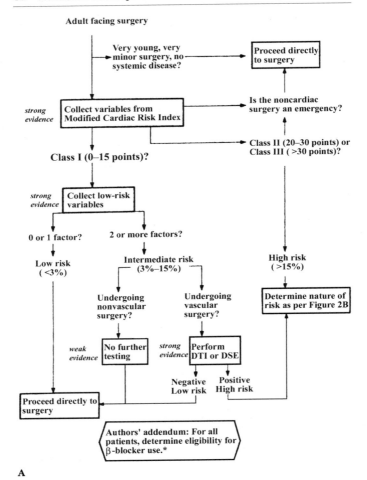

A

Fig. 3-2. The American College of Physicians guidelines for assessing and managing the perioperative risk from coronary artery disease associated with major noncardiac surgery. The commentary in italics indicates the strength of evidence to support each decision process in the algorithm. An evidence-based analysis of the literature accompanied the algorithm in a paper by Palda and Detsky.[2] A: Initially, patients are assessed using the Detsky modification of the Cardiac Risk Index to determine if they fall into class I (low risk), class II, or class III (high risk). If they are class I, information on clinical predictors such as those identified by Eagle is collected to determine if clinical risk is low or high. Only those patients who are positive for several clinical predictors are then determined to be at intermediate perioperative risk. Those patients who have an intermediate risk and are undergoing vascular surgery should be considered for noninvasive imaging with dipyridamole-thallium imaging or dobutamine stress echocardiography. No further testing is suggested in those patients undergoing nonvascular surgery. *This recommendation is to incorporate the perioperative atenolol protocol advocated by Mangano et al.[2]

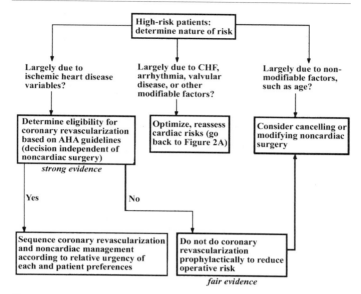

B

Fig. 3-2 *continued.* **B: If the noninvasive testing is positive or the patient is at high clinical risk according to the Detsky index, then determining the nature of the risk is important. If the risk is due largely to ischemic heart disease, then one must determine if the patient would be eligible for coronary revascularization based on American Heart Association (AHA) guidelines, independent of noncardiac surgery. If the risk is due to nonischemic causes, then the ideal choice is to optimize and reassess. Finally, if the risk is due to largely nonmodifiable factors, then either canceling or modifying the noncardiac surgery should be considered. (CHF, congestive heart failure; DSE, dobutamine stress echocardiography; DTI, dipyridamole thallium imaging.) (Reprinted with permission from Palda VA, Detsky AS. Perioperative assessment and management of risk from coronary artery disease.** *Ann Intern Med* **1997;127:313–328.)**

The ACP guidelines attempt to apply an evidence-based approach (Fig. 3-2) The initial decision point is the assessment of risk using the Detsky modification of the Cardiac Risk Index. If the patient is categorized as class II or class III, the patient is considered high risk. If the patient is categorized as class I, the presence of other clinical factors identified by Eagle et al. or Vanzetto et al. are used to further stratify risk. Those who have multiple markers for cardiovascular disease according to these risk indices and are undergoing major vascular surgery are considered appropriate for further diagnostic testing by either dipyridamole-thallium imaging or dobutamine stress echocardiography. The ACP Guidelines suggest that insufficient evidence exists to recommend diagnostic testing for patients undergoing nonvascular surgery.

Many similarities and differences can be noted in the two guidelines. Both apply a Bayesian approach to risk stratification, with the degree of clinical risk defining the appropriateness of further diagnostic testing. The ACC/AHA guidelines use exercise tolerance to stratify risk, whereas the ACP guidelines state that insufficient information exists to justify such an approach. Importantly, the *absence* of evidence does not equal the presence of evidence demonstrating lack of efficacy or harm. The lack of endorsement by the ACP of the use of exercise tolerance and testing for nonvascular procedures is based on an absence of data; however, the ACC/AHA committee felt that sufficient expert opinion existed to endorse such an approach.

TESTING TO CONFIRM THE DIAGNOSIS AND DETERMINE THE EXTENT OF CORONARY ARTERY DISEASE

Multiple noninvasive diagnostic tests have been proposed to evaluate the extent of CAD before noncardiac surgery (Table 3-6). The exercise ECG has been the traditional method of evaluating individuals for the presence of CAD. It represents the least invasive and most cost-effective method of detecting ischemia, with a reasonable sensitivity (68% to 81%) and specificity (66% to 77%) in identifying CAD. The goal of the test is to provoke ischemia through exercise by causing an increase in myocardial oxygen demand relative to myocardial oxygen supply. Electrocardiographic signs of myocardial ischemia and clinical signs of left ventricular dysfunction are considered positive. As outlined above, however, patients with a good exercise tolerance rarely benefit from further testing. Therefore, information regarding maximal heart rate, exercise level, and blood pressure during the test must be provided.

A significant number of high-risk patients are either unable to exercise or have contraindications to exercise. In surgical patients, this phenomenon is most evident in those patients with claudication or an abdominal aortic aneurysm who are undergoing vascular surgery, both of which groups have a high rate of perioperative cardiac morbidity. Therefore, pharmacologic stress testing has become popular, particularly as a preoperative test for vascular surgery patients.

Pharmacologic stress tests for the detection of CAD can be divided into two categories: (a) those that result in coronary

Table 3-6. Sensitivity and specificity of various diagnostic tests for detecting coronary artery disease

Test	Sensitivity (%)	Specificity (%)
Exercise electrocardiography	81	66
Exercise thallium imaging		
Qualitative planar	84	87
Quantitative planar	89	89
Single photon emission computed tomography	94	82
Dipyridamole-thallium imaging	85	90
Stress echocardiography	80–90	80–90
Stress radionuclide angiography	70–80	70–80

artery vasodilatation, and (b) those that increase myocardial oxygen demand. Examples of coronary vasodilators are dipyridamole and adenosine. Dipyridamole works by blocking adenosine reuptake and increasing adenosine concentration in the coronary vessels. Adenosine is a direct coronary vasodilator. After infusion of the vasodilator, flow is preferentially distributed to areas distal to normal coronary arteries, with minimal flow to areas distal to a coronary stenosis. A radioisotope such as thallium chloride Tl 201 or technetium Tc 99m sestamibi is then injected. Normal myocardium shows up on initial imaging, whereas areas of myocardial necrosis or areas distal to a significant coronary stenosis demonstrate a defect. After a delay of several hours, or after infusion of a second dose of technetium Tc 99m sestamibi, the myocardium is again imaged. Those initial defects that remain as defects are consistent with old scar, whereas those defects that demonstrate normal activity on subsequent imaging are consistent with areas at risk for myocardial ischemia. Several authors have shown that the presence of a redistribution defect on dipyridamole-thallium imaging or technetium imaging in patients undergoing peripheral vascular surgery is predictive of postoperative cardiac events (Fig. 3-3). This work has been extended to include patients undergoing nonvascular surgery.

To increase the predictive value of the test, several strategies have been suggested. The redistribution defect can be quantitated, with larger areas of defect being associated with increased risk. In addition, both increased lung uptake and left ventricular cavity dilatation have been shown to be markers of ventricular dysfunction with ischemia. Fleisher et al. demonstrated that the delineation of low-risk and high-risk thallium scans (the latter showing larger area of defect, increased lung uptake, and left ventricular cavity dilatation) markedly improved the test's predictive value. They demonstrated that only patients with high-risk thallium scans were at increased risk for perioperative morbidity and long-term mortality. Therefore, the consultant must provide greater detail regarding the test result than simply a yes or no answer.

The ambulatory ECG (AECG, or Holter monitoring) provides a means of continuously monitoring the ECG for significant ST segment changes during the preoperative period. A positive test is one in which a significant ST segment depression or elevation of at least

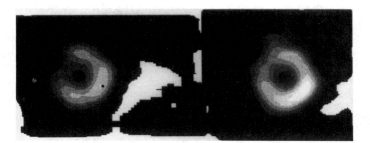

Fig. 3-3. Example of dipyridamole-thallium imaging showing both a stress image (*left*)and a rest image (*right*). A defect is seen on the initial stress image that fills in on the subsequent rest imaging. The presence of a reversible defect has been associated with an increased incidence of perioperative cardiac morbidity.

1 minute's duration is present. Raby demonstrated that the presence of silent ischemia is a strong predictor of outcome, whereas its absence was associated with a good outcome in 99% of patients. Other investigators have demonstrated the value of AECG monitoring, although the negative predictive values have not been as high as originally reported. Fleisher et al. demonstrated a similar predictive value of dipyridamole-thallium imaging and AECG monitoring; however, the quantity of silent ischemia could not be used to identify those patients at greatest risk who might benefit from further testing and coronary revascularization. Preoperative AECG monitoring is rarely used for screening at the current time.

Stress echocardiography has received attention as a preoperative test. Patients are given an infusion of dobutamine to increase both heart rate and inotropy. If heart rate cannot be raised to more than 85% of the age-predicted maximum, then atropine is given. The ECG is monitored continuously for ST segment changes. The echocardiogram is also monitored at discrete time points for the appearance of new or worsened regional wall-motion abnormalities, the presence of which is considered to indicate a positive test. These represent areas at risk for myocardial ischemia. The advantage of this test is that it is a dynamic assessment of the ability to provoke myocardial ischemia in response to increased heart rate, similar to that which might be observed during the perioperative period. As with dipyridamole-thallium imaging, dobutamine stress echocardiography can be further quantified. The presence of wall-motion abnormalities at low heart rate is the best predictor of increased perioperative risk, with large areas of defect being of secondary importance.

The question remains regarding the choice of diagnostic tests for a given patient. Several groups have published metaanalyses of preoperative diagnostic tests. Mantha et al. demonstrated good predictive values for AECG monitoring, radionuclide angiography, dipyridamole-thallium imaging, and dobutamine stress echocardiography. Shaw et al. also demonstrated good predictive values of dipyridamole-thallium imaging and dobutamine stress echocardiography. Although both studies demonstrated the superior predictive value of dobutamine stress echocardiography, significant overlap of the confidence intervals with the values for other tests was noted. The most important determinant with respect to the choice of preoperative testing, however, is the expertise at the local institution.

PERIOPERATIVE INTERVENTIONS TO REDUCE RISK

No randomized trials have evaluated how information is used from the preoperative evaluation, and few randomized trials have addressed the efficacy of different interventions to reduce morbidity during the perioperative period. Modification of perioperative care based on the preoperative evaluation can take the form of medical and coronary interventions performed preoperatively, changes in anesthetic technique, aggressive treatment of hemodynamic perturbations, and utilization of expensive resources such as treatment in the intensive care unit (ICU), ST segment telemetry, or invasive monitoring. Based on the accumulated data, no one anesthetic technique appears to be best; however, information from the preoperative evaluation is taken into account in designing an anesthetic plan.

Although insufficient evidence exists to determine the value of postoperative ICU care or invasive monitoring for the patient with active cardiac disease, these are routinely used for high-risk patients undergoing extensive surgery. The evidence, however, suggests that more intensive monitoring is not needed *in the absence* of active cardiovascular disease (i.e., negative history or negative results on a noninvasive test). Therefore, screening can be used to define the population of patients who would not benefit from intensive monitoring. In an era of rationing of expensive medical resources, the costs of screening may be easily offset by the savings from lower utilization of postoperative resources, such as not placing the patient in the ICU. In addition, identification of very high risk patients (e.g., those with extensive CAD or left ventricular dysfunction) would allow for rational utilization of these intensive resources for extended periods.

Coronary Revascularization

Finally, the preoperative evaluation may occasionally identify a patient who would benefit from coronary revascularization. Several investigators have proposed coronary revascularization before noncardiac surgery as a means of reducing perioperative risk. Preoperative screening may identify patients who have severe CAD. No randomized trials have been performed to address this issue, and such a trial would require a very large sample size and would have multiple confounding issues. Several large cohort studies, however, have suggested that, in patients who survive coronary artery bypass grafting, the risk of subsequent noncardiac surgery is low. Although few data exist to support the notion of coronary revascularization solely for the purpose of improving perioperative outcome, for specific patient subsets, long-term survival may be enhanced by revascularization. Rihal et al., using the CASS database, found that coronary artery bypass grafting significantly improved survival in those patients with both peripheral vascular disease and triple-vessel CAD, especially the group with depressed ventricular function. No benefit was observed in patients with only single-vessel or double-vessel disease.

The value of percutaneous transluminal coronary angioplasty (PTCA) is less well established. In several series, a low incidence of cardiovascular complications was observed in patients undergoing "prophylactic" PTCA before vascular surgery, but determining the expected complication rate in a comparison group with single-vessel or double-vessel disease is difficult. For those perioperative MIs that result from plaque rupture and coronary thrombosis in noncritical lesions, as seen in the ambulatory setting, PTCA theoretically has minimal benefit. Administrative data provides evidence that patients who have undergone PTCA more than 90 days before surgery are at reduced risk, whereas PTCA less than 90 days before has no beneficial effect. Therefore, the current evidence does not support the use of PTCA beyond established indications for nonoperative patients.

Risks versus Benefits of Coronary Revascularization

An alternative approach to determining the optimal strategy for medical care in the absence of clinical trials is construction of a decision analysis. Two decision analyses have been published on the issue of cardiovascular testing before major vascular surgery. Both assumed that patients with significant CAD would undergo coronary artery bypass grafting before noncardiac surgery. Both models found that the optimal decision was sensitive to local morbidity and mortality rates within the clinically observed range. These models suggest that preoperative testing for the purpose of coronary revascularization is not the optimal strategy if perioperative morbidity and mortality are low.

Importantly, the primary cost of preoperative testing and revascularization (both in dollars and in morbidity) is the revascularization procedure itself. Therefore, the indications for revascularization, and thus the frequency of its use, have a significant impact on the model. Second, potential long-term benefits of coronary artery bypass grafting in this population were not included in the analysis, which possibly biased against the revascularization arm. If long-term survival is included in the models, then coronary revascularization may lead to improved overall outcome and be a cost-effective intervention. The patient's age should be included in the equation, however. For example, an 80-year-old diabetic patient with significant comorbid diseases may gain few additional life-years and may actually experience a decrease in the quality of the final years from undergoing coronary artery bypass grafting. In contrast, a 55-year-old man with an abdominal aortic aneurysm who is found to have occult left main disease would experience a substantial increase in both the length and quality of his life from preoperative cardiovascular testing and coronary artery bypass grafting. Therefore, appropriately identified patients with diffuse disease or a significant left main stenosis amenable to surgery with an acceptable risk should undergo coronary artery bypass grafting before noncardiac surgery. In this instance, the procedure is justified based on long-term benefit, and performing it before noncardiac surgery reduces the risk of a fatal or nonfatal perioperative MI.

Pharmacologic Interventions

β-Blockers

In the early 1960s and 1970s, concern existed that continued use of β-blockers during the perioperative period would be detrimental. Several studies in the late 1970s indicated that β-blocker therapy could be safely continued preoperatively and often resulted in a reduction in the incidence of myocardial ischemia. These studies, and the concern for β-blocker withdrawal–induced tachycardia, hypertension, and myocardial ischemia, led to recommendations to continue β-blocker therapy preoperatively. Until recently, the evidence to support the continued use of β-blockers was poor and was based on case-controlled studies or surrogate end points. The effect of the use of atenolol was examined in a randomized, placebo-controlled study of patients either with or at risk for CAD who were undergoing noncardiac surgery. The majority of these patients (66%) had a history of hypertension. Six died during the hospitalization (four in the atenolol group and two in the placebo group), three from noncardiac causes. Treatment with atenolol during the hospitalization was associated with a reduction in mortality and cardiac complications that was noted for the 2-year follow-up period of the study. The effect was particularly prominent in the first 6 months postoperatively. Based on the findings of this trial, the ACP guidelines advocate the perioperative use of atenolol in all high-risk patients. However, the study was small, was fraught with multiple confounding factors (uneven distribution of comorbidities and pre-operative and long-term use of β-blockade), and may not be able to be generalized into routine clinical practice. Importantly, those patients who are on β-blockers should continue on β-blockers.

Despite these concerns, some basic conclusions can be drawn from the literature. The use of β-blockers should not be discontinued before noncardiac surgery. Although the relationship between acute perioperative administration of β-blockers and short-term and long-term outcome has not been definitively established, the periopera-tive use of β-blockers appears to be well tolerated and may lower the incidence of cardiac events in some high-risk patients.

Nitroglycerin

Nitroglycerin has been a mainstay of antiischemic therapy, but its value during the perioperative period is controversial. Two random-ized clinical trials have focused on high-risk noncardiac surgery patients. Coriat et al. studied a cohort of patients undergoing carotid endarterectomy using a high-dose narcotic technique. They demon-strated a significantly reduced incidence of myocardial ischemia with administration of 1.0 μg per kg per minute of nitroglycerin compared with 0.5 μg per kg per minute; however, no patients sus-tained a perioperative MI. Dodds et al. compared nitroglycerin at 1.0 μg per kg per minute to placebo using a balanced anesthetic tech-nique in high-risk patients undergoing a diverse group of noncardiac surgeries and demonstrated no difference in perioperative myocar-dial ischemia or infarction. Many of the effects of nitroglycerin are mimicked by anesthetic agents, which minimizes the potential bene-ficial effects of nitroglycerin and potentially leads to more profound hypotension. Therefore, the evidence does not support the routine prophylactic use of this agent.

Alpha$_2$-Adrenergic Agonists

A great deal of attention has been given to the use of alpha$_2$-adr-energic agonists as adjuvants to anesthetic management. Ellis et al. randomly assigned high-risk noncardiac surgery patients to receive either clonidine or a placebo and demonstrated a significantly decreased incidence of intraoperative but not postoperative ischemia with clonidine. Stuhmeier et al. randomly assigned elective vascular surgery patients to receive either an alpha$_2$-adrenergic agonist or a placebo and demonstrated a significantly reduced incidence of perio-perative myocardial ischemia with fewer nonfatal MIs in the group receiving the alpha$_2$-adrenergic agonist. Clonidine may be useful for the management of postoperative hypertension because it is avail-able for oral and transdermal use. Clonidine stimulates central alpha$_2$ receptors and thereby decreases sympathetic outflow to the vasculature, producing vasodilation and lowering blood pressure. It is particularly appropriate for the patient taking clonidine preopera-tively to continue this drug to avoid the clonidine withdrawal syn-drome. Abrupt cessation of clonidine administration can lead to a withdrawal syndrome characterized by rebound hyperactivity of the central autonomic and sympathetic nervous systems. Patients can present with symptoms similar to those of a pheochromocytoma or severe hypertension with marked agitation. Levels of noradrenaline, adrenaline, and total and free 3-methoxy-4-hydrophenylglycol, indices of sympathetic hyperactivity, are found to be very high. Clonidine should not be used in patients with high-grade conduction disturbances.

Perioperative administration of mivazerol, an intravenous alpha$_2$-adrenergic agonist, was associated with a significantly reduced incidence of myocardial ischemia with no difference in cardiac events. A large-scale trial of mivazerol is currently being analyzed, the results of which should provide important data for management of high-risk patients.

Calcium Channel Antagonists

The calcium channel blockers may be useful in the management of postoperative hypertension. These agents lower blood pressure by reducing afterload but may produce reflex tachycardia; this is particularly true of the dihydropyridine compounds such as nifedipine. However, a large-scale nonrandomized trial involving cardiac surgery patients has been unable to demonstrate any difference in outcome related to the use of these agents.

Intraaortic Balloon Counterpulsation

In patients with unstable angina or severe CAD, placement of an intraaortic balloon counterpulsation device has been used before induction of anesthesia in patients considered at high risk for noncardiac surgical procedures. In several small case series, perioperative morbidity and mortality were low. Because the use of an intraaortic balloon counterpulsation is associated with risks and requires additional knowledge, the individual physician must determine if the benefits outweigh these risks.

CASE STUDY

A 62-year-old white man presents for a total hip replacement. Past medical history shows diabetes mellitus and use of insulin. An ECG demonstrates Q waves in II, III, and aVF leads. Hemoglobin level is 10 g per dL.

This patient is undergoing an intermediate-risk procedure and is at a moderate level of cardiac risk by clinical history. He has previously sustained a silent MI based on ECG changes. He has diabetes mellitus, which may account for the lack of symptoms and increase the probability that he is experiencing silent myocardial ischemia at the current time.

Traditionally, great concern has been shown about performing elective surgery within 6 months of an MI. In this patient, the interval between the silent MI and the current elective surgery is unknown. If a previous ECG is available for comparison, then it may be possible to determine a rough estimate for the time interval between the infarction and the current surgery. If a previous

ECG is not available, then the exact time interval remains unknown. The ACC/AHA Task Force eliminated this arbitrary 6-month time interval and suggested that elective surgery is associated with prohibitive risk only during the initial 4 to 6 weeks. The fact that the MI was silent does not eliminate the increased probability of cardiac risk. If the patient is otherwise asymptomatic, without signs of congestive heart failure or ongoing ischemia on ECG, then placing this patient at intermediate clinical risk based on a more remote MI and history of diabetes mellitus would be reasonable.

In this patient at moderate clinical risk undergoing an intermediate-risk procedure, exercise tolerance is the critical factor in determining the need for further evaluation. If the patient has a good exercise tolerance (greater than four metabolic equivalents or ability to carry a bag of groceries up two flights of stairs), then no further evaluation is necessary. In patients scheduled for joint surgery, exercise tolerance is usually limited by the underlying disease. In this author's opinion, the question is whether the patient has had good exercise tolerance within the previous 1 year. If the patient was able to walk up stairs or around the mall within that 1-year period, then no further testing is necessary. If the patient has had poor exercise tolerance for longer than 1 year, then the question is whether perioperative management would be modified by the results of a test. If coronary revascularization would be considered to improve long-term survival, then preoperative testing is indicated. In this totally asymptomatic patient, severe triple-vessel disease, which is an indication for coronary revascularization, is unlikely to be found. If alternative methods of monitoring are considered, such as the use of a pulmonary artery catheter or ICU resources, then testing might be used to determine if use of such resources would be beneficial.

In summary, preoperative evaluation in this patient should focus on the identification of symptoms and signs of angina or ventricular dysfunction. If the patient demonstrates significant CAD, then preoperative testing is indicated if the patient has poor exercise tolerance. Otherwise, the optimal outcome will be obtained by proceeding to the operating room with an understanding that perioperative management should be directed at minimizing hemodynamic disturbances, particularly tachycardia; avoiding hypothermia; maintaining a hemoglobin level of 10 g per dL; and optimizing postoperative pain relief.

REFERENCES

1. Eagle K, Brundage B, Chaitman B, et al. Guidelines for perioperative cardiovascular evaluation of the noncardiac surgery. A report of the American College of Cardiology/American Heart Association Task Force on Assessment of Diagnostic and Therapeutic Cardiovascular Procedures. *Circulation* 1996;93:1278–1317.
2. Palda VA, Detsky AS. Perioperative assessment and management of risk from coronary artery disease. *Ann Intern Med* 1997;127:313–328.
3. Goldman L, Caldera DL, Nussbaum SR, et al. Multifactorial index of cardiac risk in noncardiac surgical procedures. *N Engl J Med* 1977;297:845–850.
4. Detsky A, Abrams H, McLaughlin J, et al. Predicting cardiac complications in patients undergoing non-cardiac surgery. *J Gen Intern Med* 1986;1:211–219.

5. Rao TL, Jacobs KH, El-Etr AA. Reinfarction following anesthesia in patients with myocardial infarction. *Anesthesiology* 1983;59:499–505.
6. Shah KB, Kleinman BS, Sami H, et al. Reevaluation of perioperative myocardial infarction in patients with prior myocardial infarction undergoing noncardiac operations. *Anesth Analg* 1990;71:231–235.
7. Shah KB, Kleinman BS, Rao T, et al. Angina and other risk factors in patients with cardiac diseases undergoing noncardiac operations. *Anesth Analg* 1990;70:240–247.
8. Mangano DT. Perioperative cardiac morbidity. *Anesthesiology* 1990;72:153–184.
9. Hollenberg M, Mangano DT, Browner WS, London MJ. Predictors of postoperative myocardial ischemia in patients undergoing noncardiac surgery. The Study of Perioperative Ischemia Research Group. *JAMA* 1992;268:205–209.
10. Goldman L, Caldera DL. Risks of general anesthesia and elective operation in the hypertensive patient. *Anesthesiology* 1979;50:285–292.
11. Eagle KA, Coley CM, Newell JB, et al. Combining clinical and thallium data optimizes preoperative assessment of cardiac risk before major vascular surgery. *Ann Intern Med* 1989;110:859–866.
12. Boucher CA, Brewster DC, Darling RC, et al. Determination of cardiac risk by dipyridamole-thallium imaging before peripheral vascular surgery. *N Engl J Med* 1985;312:389–394.
13. Baron JF, Mundler O, Bertrand M, et al. Dipyridamole-thallium scintigraphy and gated radionuclide angiography to assess cardiac risk before abdominal aortic surgery. *N Engl J Med* 1994;330:663–669.
14. Vanzetto G, Machecourt J, Blendea D, et al. Additive value of thallium single-photon emission computed tomography myocardial imaging for prediction of perioperative events in clinically selected high cardiac risk patients having abdominal aortic surgery. *Am J Cardiol* 1996;77:143–148.
15. Poldermans D, Arnese M, Fioretti PM, et al. Improved cardiac risk stratification in major vascular surgery with dobutamine-atropine stress echocardiography. *J Am Coll Cardiol* 1995;26:648–653.
16. Halm EA, Browner WS, Tubau JF, et al. Echocardiography for assessing cardiac risk in patients having noncardiac surgery. Study of Perioperative Ischemia Research Group. *Ann Intern Med* 1996;125:433–441.
17. Eagle KA, Rihal CS, Mickel MC, et al. Cardiac risk of noncardiac surgery: influence of coronary disease and type of surgery in 3368 operations. CASS Investigators and University of Michigan Heart Care Program. Coronary Artery Surgery Study. *Circulation* 1997;96:1882–1887.
18. Huber KC, Evans MA, Bresnahan JF, et al. Outcome of noncardiac operations in patients with severe coronary artery disease successfully treated preoperatively with coronary angioplasty. *Mayo Clin Proc* 1992;67:15–21.
19. Fleisher LA, Eagle KA. Screening for cardiac disease in patients having noncardiac surgery. *Ann Intern Med* 1996;124:767–772.
20. Fleisher LA, Skolnick ED, Holroyd KJ, Lehmann HP. Coronary artery revascularization before abdominal aortic aneurysm surgery: a decision analytic approach. *Anesth Analg* 1994;79:661–669.
21. Mangano DT, Layug EL, Wallace A, Tateo I. Effect of atenolol on mortality and cardiovascular morbidity after noncardiac surgery. Multicenter Study of Perioperative Ischemia Research Group. *N Engl J Med* 1996;335:1713–1720.
22. Stuhmeier KD, Mainzer B, Cierpka J, et al. Small, oral dose of clonidine reduces the incidence of intraoperative myocardial ischemia in patients having vascular surgery. *Anesthesiology* 1996;85:706–712.
23. Grotz RL, Yeston NS. Intra-aortic balloon counterpulsation in high-risk patients undergoing noncardiac surgery. *Surgery* 1989;106:1–5.

Nonischemic Cardiac Disease

Devashish Sen, BobbieJean Sweitzer, and Lee A. Fleisher

Preoperative evaluation identifies patients who might need further assessment or treatment of comorbid conditions. A significant number of patients undergoing surgery have cardiac disease. In some patients, cardiac conditions are discovered during preoperative evaluation and treatment can be lifesaving. In many instances, preoperative evaluation leads to a modification of the anesthetic plan to optimize postoperative outcomes. This chapter provides a comprehensive review of the pathophysiology and anesthetic implications of **hypertension, congestive heart failure, valvular heart disease, rhythm disturbances**, presence of a **pacemaker** or **implantable cardioverter defibrillator, carotid bruits,** and the **transplanted heart,** and examines **perioperative management of drug therapy**. This chapter excludes ischemic heart disease, which is covered in Chapter 3. An approach to pertinent history taking, physical examination, and diagnostic algorithms is presented. The description includes methods to assess risk and to diagnose and treat cardiac diseases in the perioperative period.

HYPERTENSION

Systemic arterial hypertension (Table 4-1) is common, and its prevalence increases with age. According to the third National Health and Nutrition Examination Survey (NHANES III), 24% of the adult population of the United States has hypertension and, by age 70, the prevalence increases to more than 60%. Forty percent of patients with known hypertension either go untreated or are managed inadequately with pharmacologic therapy. Hypertension adds to the normal changes of aging by leading to a more severe form of diastolic dysfunction that may predispose the patient to congestive heart failure (CHF).

In evaluating the patient with hypertension, determining how the information will affect perioperative management is important. Patients with hypertension have a higher incidence of silent coronary artery disease (CAD) and previous myocardial infarction than the general population. A history of hypertension should be viewed in the context of the patient's general medical condition to determine the need for further evaluation of cardiac status.

A second major issue is the need for further preoperative management of the patient who presents with a markedly elevated blood pressure (diastolic greater than 110 mm Hg). Traditionally, surgery for these patients has been delayed to allow further

Table 4-1. Classification of hypertension

Category	Systolic (mm Hg)	Diastolic (mm Hg)
Normal	<130	<85
High normal	130–139	85–89
Hypertension		
Stage 1 (mild)	140–159	90–99
Stage 2 (moderate)	160–179	100–109
Stage 3 (severe)	180–209	110–119
Stage 4 (very severe)	210	120

Adapted from the Fifth Report of the Joint National Committee on Detection, Evaluation, and Treatment of High Blood Pressure (JNC V). *Arch Intern Med* 1993;153:154–183.

treatment. However, an evaluation of the original study of Goldman and Caldera, on which this recommendation is partially based, clearly shows that insufficient data exist to make such a claim. In fact, none of the patients with "uncontrolled systemic hypertension" sustained a major cardiac event. These patients may be at risk for perioperative hemodynamic lability but not for irreversible myocardial necrosis. Bedford et al. demonstrated that admission blood pressure was the best predictor of the blood pressure response to laryngoscopy. Similarly, "white-coat hypertension," in which blood pressure is normal except when taken by a health care professional, is common. These patients may have an exaggerated response to surgical stimuli and greater hemodynamic lability, but this would not lead to complications in the absence of severe CAD.

Some cases are found in which delay of surgery may be warranted based on the preoperative blood pressure. A hypertensive crisis is a medical emergency and requires treatment. A hypertensive crisis is defined as evidence of ongoing end organ damage with severely elevated blood pressure. If the patient has new symptoms of a headache or visual disturbances, the patient is at risk for a cerebral hemorrhage, and treatment before the induction of anesthesia is warranted. Similarly, elevated blood pressure of an episodic nature, particularly that associated with intermittent headaches or palpitations, should alert the anesthesiologist to the possibility of a pheochromocytoma. Because performing anesthesia and surgery on a patient with an untreated pheochromocytoma has a high rate of perioperative morbidity and mortality, further evaluation and treatment may be warranted (see Chapter 6). Although the presence of left ventricular hypertrophy is associated with a higher probability of perioperative myocardial ischemia and CAD, treatment leading to regression of left ventricular mass would require many months. Therefore, acute treatment of blood pressure is sufficient in most cases.

CONGESTIVE HEART FAILURE

CHF may be systolic (decreased ejection fraction, abnormal contraction), diastolic (elevated filling pressures, abnormal relax-

Table 4-2. New York Heart Association classification of dyspnea

Class	Description
I	Dyspnea with more than ordinary activity (e.g., prolonged exertion at work or recreation).
II	Dyspnea with ordinary activity (e.g., climbing stairs rapidly or more than one flight of stairs at normal pace, walking uphill, walking more than two blocks).
III	Marked limitation of ordinary physical activity (e.g., dyspnea walking one or two blocks, climbing one flight of stairs, "comfortable at rest").
IV	Inability to carry out any physical activity without dyspnea, short of breath at rest.

ation), or both. To date, no data exist comparing the outcomes of patients with systolic versus diastolic dysfunction, even though the therapies differ. Most of the studies performed involve patients with systolic dysfunction. In a study by Goldman et al., patients presenting for surgery with an S_3 and jugular venous distention had a 20% incidence of cardiac death and 14% incidence of serious cardiac complications.

History and physical examination are important for diagnosis and determination of the physiologic state and functional status of the patient. The New York Heart Association classification (Table 4-2) is used for determination of the functional status of the patient.

Ischemic heart disease is the most common cause of CHF. Other etiologic factors include hypertension, valvular diseases, cardiomyopathies, myocarditis, arrhythmias, pulmonary diseases (e.g., pulmonary embolism), high-output states (e.g., sepsis, severe anemia), and the nephrotic syndrome.

The most common symptom of CHF is dyspnea. Other symptoms include paroxysmal nocturnal dyspnea, orthopnea, fatigue, generalized weakness, chest pain, and nonproductive nocturnal cough. Many elderly patients complain of dyspnea. If the cause is clearly defined (e.g., documented CHF), then further testing is not warranted. In contrast, dyspnea of unknown etiology warrants a careful preoperative assessment. Physical findings of CHF include resting tachycardia, jugular venous distention, positive hepatojugular reflex, S_3 gallop, laterally displaced apical pulse, pulmonary basilar crackles, peripheral/dependent edema, unexplained weight gain, and oliguria.

Diagnostic tests that are useful include a chest radiograph (CXR) (to show cardiomegaly, pulmonary venous congestion), an electrocardiogram (ECG) (to look for ischemic changes, arrhythmia, left ventricular hypertrophy), echocardiography, and radionuclide ventriculography. Ventricular function can be assessed using echocardiography, radionuclide angiography, and contrast ventriculography. In addition to assessment of left ventricular ejection fraction (LVEF), regional wall-motion abnormalities can be discerned. During coronary angiography, contrast ventriculography can be performed. Frequently, a qualitative, rather than quantitative, assessment of LVEF is performed.

LVEF determinations have been proposed to identify patients at increased risk of postoperative myocardial complications. LVEF has been correlated with short-term and long-term prognosis in multiple studies of patients undergoing noncardiac surgery. The greatest risk of perioperative ischemic events is believed to be in patients with a resting LVEF lower than 35%, but this has not been a consistent predictor, and some studies have found that the presence of left ventricular systolic dysfunction does not predict cardiac complications after vascular surgery. Most important, a large study of patients undergoing noncardiac surgery was unable to demonstrate additive value of a preoperative echocardiogram over information based on clinical history.

Therapeutic options include medical management (therapy with angiotensin-converting enzyme or ACE inhibitors, diuretics, digoxin, nitrates, anticoagulants, β-blockers) and surgical management [revascularization for carefully selected patients with LVEF below 25% and CAD, heart transplantation, cardiomyoplasty, left ventricular reduction surgery (Batista procedure) and left ventricular assist devices]. Use of β-blockers remains controversial in CHF. In the Metoprolol in Dilated Cardiomyopathy (MDC) trial, administration of metoprolol tartrate reduced mortality from all causes combined but did not improve overall survival. Use of carvedilol has been shown to substantially improve ejection fraction and reduce mortality. The β-blockers and calcium channel blockers are therapeutic options with diastolic dysfunction, but convincing data are lacking. For patients on β-blockers chronically, this medication should be continued in the perioperative period. Use of diuretics and aggressive efforts to prevent volume overload may predispose patients to prerenal azotemia and intraoperative hypotension. Diuretics may need to be discontinued or decreased.

Patients with compensated CHF (history of CHF, but presently without jugular venous distention, crackles, and S_3) have a 5% to 7% incidence of cardiac complications, whereas those with decompensated CHF have a 20% to 30% incidence of cardiac complications. Patients with decompensated CHF should have surgery delayed if possible until their treatment is optimized with medical therapy in coordination with the primary care physician or cardiologist (or both). Detsky et al. indicated that these patients should be stabilized for more than 1 week before surgery. Patients with decompensated CHF may benefit from invasive hemodynamic monitoring to guide therapy; however, the use of pulmonary artery catheters or central venous pressure monitoring remains controversial in patients who present with well-compensated CHF.

Optimizing the medical management of CHF before an elective noncardiac surgical procedure is critical. This may require adjustments of medications on an outpatient basis or admission to a hospital. If surgery is urgent or emergent, then invasive monitoring may be of benefit. Several investigators have suggested that high-risk patients undergoing noncardiac surgery would benefit from preoperative evaluation and optimization in an intensive care unit. When such patients were evaluated solely for cardiac outcomes, however, no benefit was noted. At the present time, the optimal strategy is dependent on local factors of care. CHF is a complex and chronic disease that is notoriously difficult to manage and requires coordination among anesthesiologists and consultants for optimal perioperative outcomes.

Table 4-3. Grading of murmur intensity

Grade	Description
I	Barely audible
II	Easily audible
III	Intermediate
IV	Murmur accompanied by a thrill
V	Loudest murmur requiring stethoscope
VI	Murmur heard without a stethoscope

VALVULAR HEART DISEASE

When preoperative evaluation of a patient for noncardiac surgery reveals a murmur on chest auscultation, the first thing to determine is whether the murmur is functional or structural. Most functional murmurs, also called *systolic ejection murmurs*, are benign and occur because of turbulent blood flow across the aortic or the pulmonary outflow tracts. The murmur begins after S_1 with ejection of blood from the ventricle. As the ejection increases, the murmur augments and, as the ejection decreases, the murmur declines, which gives a crescendo-decrescendo shape to the murmur. This type of murmur is caused by high outflow states (e.g., anemia, hyperthyroidism, pregnancy, exercise), ejection into a dilated vessel beyond the valve, or increased transmission of sound through a thin chest wall. In an otherwise healthy patient, a soft systolic ejection murmur of grade I or II/VI (Table 4-3), loudest at the left sternal border, with normal S_1 and S_2, no jugular venous distention, normal arterial pulse contour, and no cardiac enlargement, is extremely unlikely to represent a hemodynamically significant cardiac lesion. If a patient gives a history of taking anorectic drugs [dexfenfluramine hydrochloride (Redux), fenfluramine hydrochloride, phentermine hydrochloride] in the past, however, and cardiac evaluation reveals a murmur, then the patient should be evaluated for valvular disease (see Chapter 15).

Murmurs from structural causes may be systolic, diastolic, or continuous, as with a patent ductus arteriosus. Description of the loudness of the murmur includes assigning a grade of I to VI (see Table 4-3). Frequently, the loudest murmurs correlate with minimal lesions, whereas severe stenosis may be associated with soft murmurs. These findings relate in part to the underlying cardiac output and degree of turbulence, with a severe stenosis and low cardiac output frequently being associated with less turbulent flow.

The location of the loudest sound along with the direction of radiation helps to identify the cardiac structure from which the murmur originates (Table 4-4). A systolic murmur from aortic stenosis is loudest in the right second intercostal space and radiates to the carotid arteries, whereas a systolic murmur from mitral regurgitation is best heard at the apex and radiates to the left axilla and base of the heart. Often, determining the origin of a murmur is difficult. In these situations, specific maneuvers that alter the cardiac hemodynamics help to identify the origin and significance of the murmur. For example:

- Deep inspiration augments venous return and accentuates murmurs in the right heart (e.g., tricuspid regurgitation).

Table 4-4. Characteristics of pathologic murmurs

Condition	Location	Timing	Description	Severity
MS	Apex	Middiastolic	Opening snap; low-pitched rumble radiates to the axilla	Intensity correlates poorly but duration correlates well
MR	Apex	Holosystolic	High pitched, blowing; loud S_3 radiates to the axilla	Significant if loud with S_3
MVP	Apex	Late systolic	Crescendo, midsystolic click	Things that decrease end-diastolic volume contractility increase the intensity and duration of the murmur
AS	Second right and left parasternal interspaces	Midsystolic	Crescendo-decrescendo diamond, radiates to the carotids; S_3 and S_4 if significant	Contour of diamond parallels the instantaneous pressure gradient; as long as cardiac output is maintained, excellent correlation seen between intensity, length, and severity
AI	Third and fourth parasternal interspace; if loudest at the right, consider aortic root	Holodiastolic	Decrescendo, blowing, high pitched, radiates to the carotids; Austin-Flint rumble at the apex	
HOCM	Apex, lower left sternal edge	Midsystolic	Reversed or single S_2 and S_4; Valsalva's maneuver increases intensity	Things that decrease diastolic volume or increase contractility increase intensity of the murmur

AI, aortic insufficiency; AS, aortic stenosis; HOCM, hypertrophic obstructive cardiomyopathy; MR, mitral regurgitation; MS, mitral stenosis; MVP, mitral valve prolapse. The patient with valvular heart disease. *Probl Anesth* 1997;9:157.
Reprinted with permission from Eisen N, Reich DL.

- Valsalva's maneuver decreases right and left ventricular filling and reduces the intensity of most murmurs except those associated with hypertrophic obstructive cardiomyopathy (HOCM) and mitral valve prolapse, in which the murmur is paradoxically accentuated with Valsalva's maneuver.
- Standing reduces left ventricular volume and accentuates murmurs of HOCM and mitral valve prolapse.
- Squatting increases venous return and systemic arterial resistance and thus afterload. This maneuver increases most murmurs except those murmurs of HOCM and mitral valve prolapse.
- Sustained hand-grip exercise increases systemic arterial blood pressure and heart rate, often accentuating murmurs of mitral regurgitation, aortic insufficiency, and mitral stenosis, but diminishing murmurs of aortic stenosis and HOCM.
- Amyl nitrate inhalation decreases systemic arterial blood pressure and afterload, thereby increasing the intensity of murmurs associated with valvular stenosis while diminishing those of aortic insufficiency and mitral regurgitation.

When a suspicion exists that the murmur is related to organic heart disease and is hemodynamically significant, a variety of noninvasive tests may be used to evaluate valvular heart disease. On many occasions, these tests have been performed previously by the patient's primary care physician, and every effort should be made to obtain the results of these tests so that duplication can be avoided.

History and Physical Examination

The history and physical examination should guide further investigation. One should attempt to determine from the patient or records whether the murmur is new. The *absence* of such a history does not establish that the murmur is indeed new. The gender of the patient is important because aortic stenosis is more common in males and mitral valve prolapse is more common in females.

A history of syncope associated with a murmur is significant because it can be due to aortic stenosis, HOCM (history of multiple syncopes), or thromboemboli from a dilated left atrium caused by mitral valve disease. Syncope can result from conduction abnormalities, often seen with structural disease of the mitral valve. Complaints of chest pain or discomfort may indicate the presence of critical aortic stenosis, HOCM, or mitral regurgitation with pulmonary congestion. Dyspnea on exertion may be secondary to aortic stenosis, HOCM, or pulmonary congestion resulting from mitral valve disease. A family history of premature sudden death, syncope, and murmur may be important clues for the diagnosis of HOCM.

The physical examination should not only focus on evaluation of valvular disease but also corroborate symptoms related to CHF, syncope, thromboembolic phenomenon, and CAD. Goldman has shown that with all forms of valvular disease the presence of CHF confirmed by preoperative physical examination is associated with a 20% risk of worsening CHF in the perioperative period. The only exception is aortic stenosis, which by itself is an independent risk factor for developing CHF postoperatively even if CHF was not present preoperatively. A thorough assessment of the severity and hemodynamic significance of the structural lesion includes evaluation of cardiac function as well as of the pulmonary, renal, and hepatic systems.

Diagnostic Testing

An ECG is important in assessing murmurs. Left ventricular hypertrophy can be from aortic insufficiency or aortic stenosis; left atrial enlargement may be from mitral valve disease; and right atrial enlargement may be from tricuspid valve disease. A CXR can provide information regarding the cardiac silhouette and pulmonary vasculature and is a useful initial test to evaluate valvular disease. An echocardiogram has proven to be one of the best noninvasive tests to evaluate a murmur. One important example of its use is with aortic stenosis, for which ECG and physical examination might fail to identify a hemodynamically significant lesion. Patients with left ventricular hypertrophy on ECG and a systolic murmur should be evaluated by echocardiography. Echocardiography can determine both the severity of the structural disease and impairment of functional status. Other noninvasive tests for evaluating valvular disease include radionuclide ventriculography and fluoroscopy.

Because each of the valvular lesions has different pathophysiologic implications for perioperative management, and the risk of surgery in a patient with aortic stenosis is extremely high, further defining the extent of valvular insufficiency, stenotic area, and flow gradient is important. Occasionally, invasive tests must be performed after thorough evaluation with a history, physical examination, and noninvasive tests. For example, if evidence of mitral regurgitation and papillary dysfunction is seen, then a cardiac catheterization should be done to evaluate for ischemic heart disease.

Mitral Stenosis

Mitral stenosis is most often secondary to rheumatic heart disease and occurs more commonly in women. Symptoms of mitral stenosis occur 10 to 20 years after the acute disease (Table 4-5). Mitral stenosis is commonly associated with mitral regurgitation. However, it is an isolated lesion in approximately 20% of patients.

Symptoms of mitral stenosis result from increased left atrial pressure and reduced cardiac output. The elevated left atrial pressure mimics symptoms of left ventricular failure, even though left ventricular contractility is normal. Pulmonary hypertension frequently develops, and right ventricular function may be compromised.

Physical findings include a diastolic rumble best heard in the apex following an opening snap. S_1 is loud, and the presence of a loud P_2 suggests pulmonary hypertension (see Table 4-4). Right ventricular overload is an ominous development and produces a right ventricular lift, jugular venous distention, ascites, hepatomegaly, and peripheral edema.

Echocardiography or cardiac catheterization may be useful to define the severity of disease. The normal adult mitral valve has

Table 4-5. Cardiac symptoms and their relationship to prognosis

Condition	Symptom onset	Symptom	Prognosis
MS	Symptoms usually occur when the valve area is <1.5 cm²	Dyspnea, PND, orthopnea, fatigue, chest pain, palpitations, hemoptysis, hoarseness, AF, embolic phenomena, RVF (ascites, peripheral edema)	20% die within 1 year of developing symptoms; NYHA class I, 85% 10-yr survival; NYHA class II, 50% 10-yr survival; NYHA class III, 20% 10-yr survival; NYHA class IV, 0% 5-yr survival
Acute MR	Immediate	Heart failure, fatigue, dyspnea, AF	Critical
Chronic MR	Usually asymptomatic for many years	Heart failure, dyspnea, AF, fatigue	Well tolerated for many years
AS	Symptoms usually occur when the valve area is <1 cm²; 15% die suddenly without previous symptoms	Angina with exertion; nitroglycerin → syncope	5 yr
		Syncope with exertion	3 yr
		Congestive heart failure	2 yr
		Sudden death: 20% of symptomatic patients, 15% of asymptomatic patients	
Acute AI	Immediate	Heart failure	Critical
Chronic AI	Usually asymptomatic for many years	Early symptoms: dyspnea, fatigue	Well tolerated for years; 50% of patients with severe AI live 10 yr; once symptoms develop, they progress rapidly; patients with palpitations have an average 5-yr survival

AF, atrial fibrillation; AI, aortic insufficiency; AS, aortic stenosis; MR, mitral regurgitation; MS, mitral stenosis; NYHA, New York Heart Association; PND, paroxysmal nocturnal dyspnea; RVF, right ventricular failure. The patient with valvular heart disease. *Probl Anesth* 1997;9:155.
Reprinted with permission from Eisen N, Reich DL.

an area of 4 to 6 cm². The stenosis is mild when the mitral valve area is 1.5 to 2.5 cm² and moderate when the area is 1.1 to 1.5 cm². Critical mitral stenosis exists when the area is 0.6 to 1.0 cm² and the resting mean transvalvular gradient is more than 10 mm Hg. With a critically stenosed mitral valve, the left atrial pressure may increase to 25 mm Hg to maintain normal cardiac output. Elevated left atrial pressure leads to increased pulmonary venous and capillary pressures, reduced pulmonary compliance, and exertional dyspnea. This may lead to pulmonary hypertension. With sustained elevated left atrial pressure, the left atrium may become dilatated, increasing the risk of clot formation. Mitral stenosis and a dilatated left atrium are associated with an increased frequency of atrial fibrillation, which also increases clot formation.

Increases in heart rate reduce left ventricular filling across a stenotic mitral valve and increase the transmitral pressure gradient. Patients can become symptomatic during activities associated with tachycardia and similarly during the perioperative period, when tachycardias are common. β-Blockers may be used to reduce heart rate to maximize hemodynamic conditions. Antiarrhythmic agents may prevent atrial fibrillation in patients in whom this arrhythmia is likely, such as those who have frequent premature atrial contractions. Those patients who develop atrial fibrillation frequently take warfarin (warfarin sodium) to prevent thrombus formation. Unrecognized mitral stenosis must be included in the differential diagnosis of pulmonary edema in the perioperative period. Antibiotic prophylaxis to prevent subacute bacterial endocarditis should be considered (see Chapter 16).

Mitral Regurgitation

Mitral regurgitation is more common than mitral stenosis and can be acute or chronic. Mitral regurgitation may be secondary to leaflet pathology (mitral valve prolapse, rheumatic heart disease, subacute bacterial endocarditis, collagen vascular diseases), subvalvular pathology (papillary muscle dysfunction, rupture of chordae tendineae), and annular dilation (left ventricular dilation secondary to CAD or cardiomyopathy). The most common cause of mitral regurgitation in the United States is mitral valve prolapse.

The clinical presentation of mitral regurgitation is more gradual than that of any other valvular lesion. Symptoms usually appear only in the late stages with onset of left ventricular dysfunction. Patients complain of fatigue, weight loss, and weakness consistent with low cardiac output. Associated symptoms of right ventricular failure from back pressure may be seen (see Table 4-5).

Chronic mitral regurgitation is compensated by eccentric cardiac hypertrophy, and cardiac enlargement is observed on physical examination. On auscultation, a holosystolic murmur is heard in the apical area with radiation to the axilla or base of the heart. An S₃ may be present and can be due to either CHF or rapid filling of the left ventricle by the large volume of blood in the left atrium (see Table 4-4).

No perfect test exists to quantify the severity of mitral regurgitation. Echocardiography provides only a semiquantitative measure, and left ventriculography provides additional but imperfect estimates of severity. Patients usually have a large left ventricular end-diastolic volume without a change in left ventricular end-diastolic pressure because of increased compliance.

When mitral regurgitation is severe, left ventricular function may be reduced, left atrial and pulmonary vascular pressures are elevated, and atrial fibrillation may be present. Mitral regurgitation is not likely to cause abrupt clinical deterioration in the perioperative period, unless associated valvular lesions (e.g., aortic stenosis) or left ventricular dysfunction is present. In the Goldman series, mitral regurgitation was a significant univariant correlate of perioperative cardiac morbidity and postoperative mortality, but the predictive value did not persist after controlling for other criteria of heart disease in a multivariate analysis. Patients with significant mitral regurgitation or mitral valve prolapse with regurgitation should receive antibiotic prophylaxis against subacute bacterial endocarditis for certain surgical procedures (see Chapter 16).

Mitral Valve Prolapse

Mitral valve prolapse, also known as *floppy valve syndrome* and *systolic click-murmur syndrome*, is a common but highly variable syndrome, most commonly seen in women 15 to 30 years of age. Patients generally remain asymptomatic but occasionally progress to severe and symptomatic mitral regurgitation. They may complain of atypical chest pain, lightheadedness, palpitations, and syncope (see Table 4-5). Men with mitral valve prolapse who are older than 55 years have the highest incidence of developing infectious and hemodynamic complications.

Preoperative evaluation should focus on identification of those patients with purely functional disease versus those with significant degeneration of the mitral valve and hemodynamically significant mitral regurgitation. The most common finding is a mid or late nonejection systolic click with or without a crescendo-decrescendo systolic murmur (see Table 4-4). Two-dimensional echocardiography is useful if it shows either thickening or a systolic displacement of the mitral valve leaflet into the left atrium; patients with these indications are at risk of developing severe mitral regurgitation or subacute bacterial endocarditis.

Management of asymptomatic patients consists of reassurance. Presence of mitral valve prolapse or an isolated click uncomplicated by other symptoms does not warrant cardiologic evaluation. Many patients with mitral valve prolapse are on β-blockers for palpitations and atypical pain, and these medications should be continued perioperatively. Antibiotic prophylaxis for subacute bacterial endocarditis should be given to high-risk patients (see Chapter 16). Appropriate treatment of other complications (symptomatic arrhythmia, symptomatic or severe mitral regurgitation, transient ischemic attacks) is warranted.

Aortic Stenosis

The natural history of aortic stenosis is usually decades long before the onset of symptoms. Aortic stenosis is most commonly an idiopathic disease resulting from degeneration and calcification of the aortic leaflets. Stenosis is more likely to develop in patients who have a congenitally bicuspid aortic valve. Rheumatic heart disease may cause aortic stenosis, which always occurs with mitral valve involvement.

The classic symptoms of aortic stenosis are angina, syncope, and CHF. The average time from onset of symptoms to death is 2 years with CHF, 3 years with syncope, and 5 years with angina. Because of the frequently fatal nature of this lesion (80% of patients who die have had symptoms for less than 4 years) and the propensity of aortic stenosis to cause sudden unexpected death (presumably from arrhythmias) in 10% of patients, surgical intervention is recommended for patients with symptomatic and hemodynamically significant aortic stenosis.

Angina may be due to CAD but is more often secondary to a supply-demand mismatch with normal coronaries. The supply is decreased by the increase in transmural pressure, and the demand is increased by the increase in afterload and myocardial hypertrophy. Patients with aortic stenosis and angina should undergo cardiac catheterization to rule out concomitant CAD. CHF can be a result of systolic dysfunction (increased afterload and decreased contractility), diastolic dysfunction (increased left ventricular wall thickness and collagen deposition), or both (see Table 4-5).

The most common physical finding in aortic stenosis is a systolic murmur, best heard over the right second intercostal space with radiation to the neck. In mild aortic stenosis, the murmur peaks early in systole and is often associated with a thrill. In severe aortic stenosis, the murmur peaks in late systole and becomes softer as cardiac output diminishes. The carotid upstroke has a diminished amplitude and slow rise (*parvus et tardus*). S_2 may be paradoxically split because of a delay in left ventricular emptying (see Table 4-4).

Critical aortic stenosis is present when the area of the aortic valve is less than 0.7 cm^2 or the mean transvalvular gradient is greater than 50 mm Hg. With critical aortic stenosis, the transvalvular gradient may not be greater than 50 mm Hg if left ventricular dysfunction is present.

Presence of moderate to severe aortic stenosis increases the risk associated with noncardiac surgery, and the American College of Cardiology/American Heart Association (ACC/AHA) guidelines for perioperative cardiac evaluation recommend that elective noncardiac surgery be postponed or canceled until aortic valve replacement or valvuloplasty is performed in patients with severe, symptomatic aortic stenosis. Studies have shown, however, that noncardiac surgery with appropriate monitoring can be performed safely in selected patients with severe aortic stenosis.

Since the Goldman study showed that aortic stenosis is an independent risk factor for postoperative morbidity, awareness of the intraoperative risk has heightened. Improvements in anesthetic techniques have resulted in a more favorable perioperative outcome in patients with severe aortic stenosis undergoing noncardiac surgery. Use of aggressive intraoperative monitoring and avoidance of adverse hemodynamic changes are important and have helped to achieve this improvement. Patients with severe aortic stenosis may benefit from intraarterial blood pressure and central venous pressure monitoring, pulmonary artery catheterization, and transesophageal echocardiography. Almost all operations requiring central neuraxial or general anesthesia in patients with severe aortic stenosis require intraarterial blood pressure monitoring. Other invasive monitoring (pulmonary artery catheterization, transesophageal echocardiography) may be indicated, depending on the severity of the surgery and the potential for significant fluid shifts or hemodynamic perturbations. Intraoperative transesophageal echocardiography can provide valuable information about valvular and myocardial anatomy and function that can facilitate anesthetic management.

Hypotension is the most detrimental hemodynamic perturbation in patients with severe aortic stenosis and should be treated promptly. If the underlying cause of hypotension is hypovolemia, then fluids should be replaced promptly to maintain an adequate preload and improve hypotension. Low tone states should be treated with phenylephrine hydrochloride. Phenylephrine does not cause tachycardia and may result in a reflex slowing of the heart rate, which is usually beneficial for patients with aortic stenosis. For the same reason, ephedrine sulfate should be avoided because it may cause undesired tachycardia, which limits the time for ejection across the stenotic aortic valve.

Controversy exists as to whether to manage asymptomatic patients with surgical or medical intervention. Limited data suggest that surgical treatment is advisable in the younger patient, whereas in elderly patients (who often have coexisting medical illnesses) the natural history of a hemodynamically significant lesion is ill defined, and a medical course of treatment may be more appropriate. Antibiotic prophylaxis for subacute bacterial endocarditis may be necessary (see Chapter 16).

Aortic Insufficiency

Aortic insufficiency results from any condition that prohibits adequate diastolic apposition of the aortic valve leaflets. Aortic insufficiency is caused by abnormalities of the aortic valve leaflets, the aortic root, or both. Valvular pathology that can result in aortic insufficiency includes rheumatic heart disease (which may lead to a fibrous, calcified aortic valve), subacute bacterial endocarditis, trauma, a bicuspid valve (which may result in aortic insufficiency or a combination of aortic stenosis and aortic insufficiency), myxomatous proliferation of the aortic valve, and collagen vascular diseases. Causes of aortic root dilation include cystic medial necrosis of the aorta (Marfan syndrome), age-related degeneration, dissection, hypertension, ankylosing spondylitis, osteogenesis imperfecta, syphilitic aortitis, and collagen vascular diseases. Aortic insufficiency may be acute (trauma, aortic dissection) or chronic. Acute aortic insufficiency is usually a surgical emergency, presenting with sudden onset of pulmonary edema and hypotension. If physical examination and echocardiography show evidence of preclosure of the mitral valve and CHF, then the patient benefits most from aortic valve replacement.

Patients with isolated chronic aortic insufficiency typically do not deteriorate abruptly in the perioperative period. Chronic aortic insufficiency produces volume overload of the left ventricle. The left ventricle dilates and undergoes eccentric hypertrophy. The enlarged left ventricle produces a large stroke volume that is ejected into the aorta. The large stroke volume causes systolic hypertension, but the regurgitant blood flow into the left ventricle during diastole produces a low diastolic pressure. The net effect is a widened pulse pressure. The murmur of aortic insufficiency is typically a high-pitched, blowing diastolic murmur after S_2, best heard over the left sternal border and accentuated when the patient leans forward. A diastolic rumble (Austin Flint murmur), best heard over the cardiac apex, is caused by the impinging of the aortic jet on the mitral valve (causing it to vibrate) and simultaneous filling of the left ventricle from the left atrium during diastole (see Table 4-4). Peripheral signs of the hyperdynamic circulation are Corrigan's or water-hammer pulse (bounding full carotid pulse with a rapid downstroke), Musset's sign (head bobbing), pistol shot sounds over the femoral artery, and Duroziez's sign (to and fro murmur after application of gentle pressure over the femoral artery).

Patients with aortic insufficiency require prophylaxis for subacute bacterial endocarditis for certain surgical procedures (see Chapter 16).

Balloon Valvuloplasty before Noncardiac Surgery

Although the long-term outcome of patients who undergo aortic balloon valvuloplasty is generally poor, due primarily to restenosis, this procedure may be used for palliation before noncardiac surgery. Balloon aortic valvuloplasty results in improvement in the severity of aortic stenosis in the majority of patients, although the procedure is not without risk. Fatal cardiac arrest complicating the procedure has been reported in 3%, but the procedural mortality may be even higher. In a report of 492 patients who underwent balloon aortic valvuloplasty, 4.9% died within the first 24 hours after the procedure and 7.5% died during the hospitalization. Acute catastrophic complications, including ventricular perforation, acute severe aortic insufficiency, cerebrovascular accident, and limb amputation have been reported in 6% of patients. The considerable procedure-related morbidity and mortality must be carefully considered before recommending this procedure to lower the risk of noncardiac surgery.

In contrast to aortic valvuloplasty, mitral balloon valvuloplasty is often a reasonable alternative to mitral valve surgery. Results have been favorable, especially in younger patients with mitral stenosis who do not have severe mitral valve leaflet thickening or significant subvalvular fibrosis and calcification.

PROSTHETIC HEART VALVES

More than 60,000 cardiac valve replacements are performed each year in the United States. Issues important in the perioperative period include managing long-term anticoagulation therapy, reducing the risk of subacute bacterial endocarditis (see Chapter 16), preventing valve thrombosis, and ruling out significant valve-related hemolysis.

The two major types of mechanical prosthetic heart valves are the caged-ball and the tilting-disk valves. The St. Jude Medical valve, a type of tilting-disk valve, is the most commonly used prosthetic valve in the world. Although mechanical prosthetic valves have greater durability than bioprosthetic valves, they are more thrombogenic. The risk of valve thrombosis is greatest in patients with caged-ball prosthetic valves (Starr-Edwards). Single tilting-disk prosthetic valves (Björk-Shiley, Medtronic-Hall, Omnicarbon) have an intermediate risk of valve thrombosis, and bileaflet tilting-disk prostheses (St. Jude Medical, CarboMedics, Edwards Duro-medics) pose the lowest risk among the mechanical valves.

Bioprosthetic valves available in the United States are porcine heterograft (Carpentier-Edwards, Hancock) and pericardial (Car-pentier-Edwards) valves. Bioprosthetic valves are usually reserved for patients older than 65 years or those for whom anticoagulation therapy is contraindicated.

The management of long-term warfarin anticoagulation therapy in the perioperative period is of major importance in patients with mechanical prosthetic valves. The risk of temporarily discontinuing anticoagulants must be weighed against the benefit of a reduced risk of perioperative bleeding. See the section "Anticoagulant and Antiplatelet Drugs" in this chapter for specific recommendations.

HYPERTROPHIC OBSTRUCTIVE CARDIOMYOPATHY

HOCM is less frequently encountered in the perioperative period. Identifying HOCM preoperatively is important, because the risk of hemodynamic compromise in the perioperative period may be increased. These patients typically have marked degrees of left ventricular hypertrophy, reduced ventricular compliance, hyperdynamic left ventricular systolic function, and systolic anterior motion of the mitral valve with or without a dynamic pressure gradient in the subaortic area.

A history of cardiac symptoms, especially chest pain, dyspnea, and syncope, should be carefully determined. The systolic murmur of HOCM is quite characteristic, and auscultation during passive leg elevation or with the patient changing from the standing to the squatting position typically demonstrates a decrease in the intensity of the murmur. Doppler and two-dimensional echocardiography are useful in evaluating these patients.

Little published information is available that defines the perioperative risk of patients with HOCM. A retrospective evaluation of patients with documented HOCM who had undergone noncardiac surgery demonstrated a high rate of perioperative CHF but no cardiac deaths. Therefore, an appropriate course is to proceed to surgery while considering additional monitoring to assess fluid status. Antibiotic prophylaxis for subacute bacterial endocarditis needs to be considered (see Chapter 16).

RHYTHM DISTURBANCES

The patient with a history of an arrhythmia or conduction delay requires careful evaluation to determine the underlying cause and planning for potential perioperative management.

Heart Block

New intraventricular conduction delays (IVCDs) frequently signify the presence of underlying CAD or may simply reflect

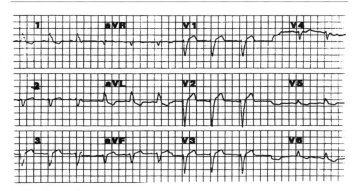

Fig. 4-1. Electrocardiogram showing left bundle branch block.

fibrosis of the conduction system. Traditionally, the view has been that a new left bundle branch block (Fig. 4-1) is pathogno-monic for CAD, whereas a right bundle branch block (Fig. 4-2) may be normal. In younger individuals, a right bundle branch block may not reflect heart disease; however, this is not the case for older patients. Therefore, further evaluation is indicated for an elderly patient with any new conduction abnormality.

In general, perioperative pacemakers are indicated for high-grade conduction abnormalities and IVCDs with associated symp-toms. In cases in which an IVCD is present without symptoms, easy access to temporary pacing equipment is advised.

In patients for whom pulmonary artery catheterization is con-sidered, a careful evaluation of the ECG for the presence of a left bundle branch block is important because of the increased proba-bility of developing complete heart block during insertion of the pulmonary artery catheter. Numerous strategies have been advo-cated for the insertion of the pulmonary artery catheter, includ-ing the use of external pacing devices in case complete heart

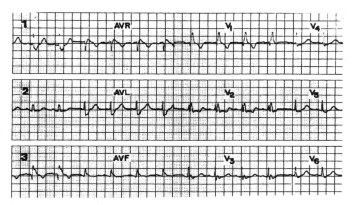

Fig. 4-2. Electrocardiogram showing right bundle branch block.

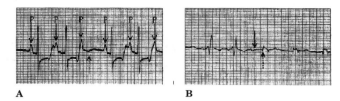

A   B

Fig. 4-3. A: An electrocardiogram (ECG) recorded from a patient with Mobitz type I block. There is progressive elongation of the PR interval until a P wave is completely blocked and a ventricular beat is dropped. B: An ECG recorded from a patient with a Mobitz type II block that occurs without progressive elongation of the PR interval. This patient has a pacemaker that is triggered by the blocked beat to sustain a regular ventricular rhythm.

block develops. Use of a pacing pulmonary artery catheter may be considered, but frequently the block develops during flotation, and adequate capture cannot be obtained in this situation. Removal of the pulmonary artery catheter frequently results in restoration of normal rhythm.

First-degree atrioventricular block exists when the PR interval is longer than 0.20 seconds at a heart rate of 60 to 100 beats per minute. The upper limits of normal for the PR interval progressively decreases as the heart rate rises. First-degree block is usually a benign abnormality and results in no significant impairment.

Two types of second-degree block have been described. The more benign, Mobitz type I block (Wenckebach block), is usually caused by atrioventricular nodal delay. As seen in Fig. 4-3, progressive prolongation of the PR interval occurs until a beat is finally blocked, after which the cycle begins again. Rarely progressing to complete heart block, Mobitz type I block can be easily abolished by the use of vagolytic agents like atropine sulfate. Mobitz type II block is the result of infranodal block and can progress to complete heart block. As seen in Fig. 4-3, a sudden interruption of atrioventricular conduction occurs, manifested as a blocked beat without progression of the PR interval. Pacemaker placement is routinely recommended for patients with Mobitz type II block.

In third-degree (complete) heart block (Fig. 4-4), all atrial beats are blocked and the ventricles are driven by a pacemaker distal to the site of the block. Complete heart block is always an indication for pacemaker placement. With high-degree heart block (second degree, Mobitz types I and II), the concern always exists that complete heart block will develop. The indications for use of a temporary pacemaker during the perioperative period are the same as those for a permanent pacemaker. The ACC/AHA guidelines advocate such an approach for temporary pacing. Although progression to complete heart block is theoretically possible, it has rarely been reported in the literature.

Supraventricular Tachycardias

The underlying mechanism of supraventricular tachycardia (SVT) is either reentry or ectopic atrial foci. In SVT owing to reen-

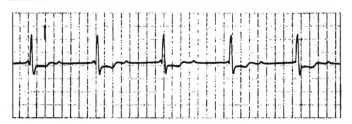

Fig. 4-4. Electrocardiogram showing infranodal third-degree heart block.

try, the mechanism involves dissociation of the conduction tissue into two pathways. One of the pathways exhibits unidirectional block and the other prolonged conduction. When a premature impulse is initiated in the atria, the impulse is conducted antegrade over the slowly conducting pathway, as the other has a unidirectional block. If the two pathways are connected, the impulse can reenter the atrial chamber in a retrograde fashion over the pathway that has a unidirectional block. Meanwhile, the pathway with the prolonged conduction has time to regain responsiveness, and the same impulse can be conducted antegrade over this pathway. Once initiated, the reentry cycle becomes self-perpetuating, resulting in SVT. This reentry mechanism has been demonstrated in the sinoatrial and atrioventricular nodes, in the His-Purkinje system, and over concealed bypass tracts in which the impulse is conducted only retrograde, in contrast to Wolff-Parkinson-White (WPW) syndrome, in which the impulse can be conducted both retrograde and antegrade (see below).

SVT of reentrant origin can occasionally be terminated by vagal maneuvers (carotid sinus massage, Valsalva's maneuver), which alter atrioventricular conduction. Pharmacologic interventions for reentry SVT include adenosine, β-blockers, calcium channel blockers, and digoxin. Nonpharmacologic interventions include atrial overdrive pacing (atrial pacer is set at a rate higher than the SVT and then abruptly terminates, which results in resumption of normal sinus rhythm). SVT due to a concealed bypass tract can be treated by ablation of the tract. Patients with hemodynamic compromise and SVT should be treated with synchronized countershock beginning at 50 J and increasing to 100 J, 200 J, and 360 J if no response is seen.

SVT may result from rapidly firing ectopic atrial foci. Here the mechanism is not reentry but rapid conduction over the atrioventricular node. Various degrees of atrioventricular block may be present that result in a slower ventricular rate. Vagal maneuvers are not effective in terminating SVT in this situation because the mechanism does not involve reentry.

WPW syndrome involves anomalous supraventricular conduction over accessory pathways that bypass the atrioventricular node. Normal sinus rhythm in WPW syndrome involves conduction and premature activation of the ventricular myocardium via the bypass tract. This results in a short PR interval (less than 0.12 seconds) and an initial slurring (delta wave) during the inscription of the QRS complex, and may be associated with a wide QRS complex (Fig. 4-5).

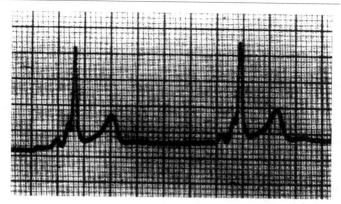

Fig. 4-5. Electrocardiogram of a patient with Wolff-Parkinson-White syndrome.

The accessory pathways in patients with WPW syndrome are capable of bidirectional conduction, which may result in a reentrant SVT. As discussed below, patients with atrial fibrillation who also have WPW syndrome may have conduction over an accessory pathway, which results in a rapid ventricular rate or ventricular fibrillation and abrupt hemodynamic compromise. Calcium channel blockers and digoxin should be used with extreme caution in patients who have WPW syndrome and SVT because they may shorten the refractory period in the accessory pathways, which can increase the ventricular rate and precipitate ventricular fibrillation. Cardioversion is indicated if hemodynamic compromise is present. β-Blockers are of little use because conduction is over accessory pathways. Procainamide hydrochloride or lidocaine can aid in this situation by increasing the refractory period of the accessory pathway and slowing conduction. Radiofrequency catheter or surgical ablation of the accessory pathway offers a permanent cure in patients with WPW syndrome and SVT/atrial fibrillation.

Atrial Fibrillation

Patients with atrial fibrillation (Fig. 4-6) may have one of the following patterns, with the presentation often progressing over time. Atrial fibrillation may be intermittent (paroxysmal), persistent (able to be cardioverted), and permanent (resistant to cardioversion). A few patients with atrial fibrillation who have undergone successful conversion to sinus rhythm with electrical or pharmacologic cardioversion are maintained on antiarrhythmic drugs. These drugs should be continued in the perioperative period if the atrial fibrillation is adequately controlled.

The other strategy in management of atrial fibrillation is rate control. This can be achieved either pharmacologically or by nonpharmacologic methods (catheter ablation, placement of a permanent pacemaker). Pharmacologic agents that are used to control the ventricular rate in atrial fibrillation by slowing down conduction at the atrioventricular node are digoxin, β-blockers, and cal-

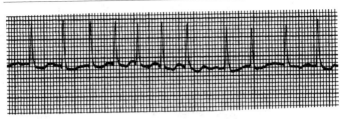

Fig. 4-6. Electrocardiogram showing atrial fibrillation.

cium channel blockers. These drugs should be continued in the perioperative period.

Two groups of patients with atrial fibrillation need further evaluation. The first group are patients with atrial fibrillation who have an inappropriately fast ventricular response (more than 150 beats per minute). This may be due to atrioventricular conduction across accessory pathways, including WPW syndrome (Fig. 4-7).

The other group of patients with atrial fibrillation who deserve special mention are those with inappropriately slow ventricular rates (less than 90 beats per minute) in the absence of treatment with pharmacologic agents to slow atrioventricular conduction. These patients should be suspected of having underlying atrioventricular nodal disease, and this may be a manifestation of sick sinus syndrome (SSS) (see below).

The patient with atrial fibrillation represents a unique challenge because of the risk of thromboembolism. Patients may be on varying degrees of anticoagulation therapy depending on their thrombotic risk. Stroke may be a devastating complication of an embolic phenomenon, and the goal must be to balance the risk of stroke against the risk of bleeding if anticoagulation is continued. See the section "Anticoagulant and Antiplatelet Drugs" below for specific recommendations.

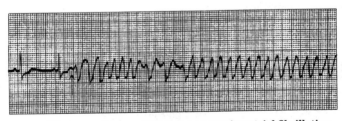

Fig. 4-7. Electrocardiogram (ECG) demonstrating atrial fibrillation with conduction over an aberrant pathway in a patient with Wolff-Parkinson-White syndrome. The ventricular response exceeds 300 beats per minute in some portions of the ECG, and the rhythm is irregularly irregular, which is characteristic of atrial fibrillation.

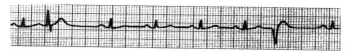

Fig. 4-8. Electrocardiogram showing multifocal premature ventricular complexes.

Ventricular Arrhythmias

Many patients are found to have ventricular premature beats (VPBs) (Fig. 4-8) during preoperative testing, and a dilemma often exists as to whether further evaluation is necessary. VPBs are differentiated from premature atrial contractions by their origin. A VPB originates in the ventricle, resulting in a wide QRS complex (longer than 0.12 seconds) because of abnormal ventricular depolarization and repolarization. A premature atrial contraction originates in the atrium, resulting in a P wave and an unchanged QRS complex. VPBs can be classified and graded according to the morphology, frequency, and other characteristics proposed by Lown (Table 4-6).

The Lown classification has limitations in stratifying the risk of sudden cardiac death. For example, both couplets and ventricular tachycardia are better indicators of risk of sudden death than R-on-T VPBs. A clinically useful classification has been developed that is based on the nature of the arrhythmia, any underlying heart disease, and the potential for sudden cardiac death. Contributing factors (hypokalemia, hypomagnesemia, acidosis, alkalosis, endocrine abnormalities, drug toxicities) should be ruled out. Myocardial ischemia and CHF should be considered. Based on these factors, patients with VPBs may be classified as follows:

Benign: Patients with benign ventricular arrhythmias (e.g., single VPBs) but without structural heart disease or hemodynamic compromise are at no risk for sudden cardiac death or future major arrhythmic events.

Potentially lethal: Patients with more than 30 VPBs per hour and nonsustained ventricular tachycardia usually have underlying structural heart disease, although no hemodynamic compromise is present. They are at moderate to high risk for sudden cardiac death or a major arrhythmic event.

Lethal: Patients with lethal ventricular arrhythmias (sustained ventricular tachycardia, ventricular fibrillation, syncope, and reduced LVEF) usually have underlying structural heart disease and are hemodynamically compromised. They are at very high risk for sudden cardiac death.

Patients with benign VPBs do not warrant further cardiac evaluation, and treatment is primarily to relieve symptoms. Patients with potentially lethal or lethal arrhythmias, however, are at high risk for sudden death. These patients should have further cardiac evaluation (electrophysiologic testing, signal-averaged ECG, cardiac catheterization) and pharmacologic treatment (antiarrhyth-

Table 4-6. Lown's grading of ventricular premature beats (VPBs)

Grade	Description
1	Uniform VPB (<30/h)
2	Uniform VPB (>30/h)
3	Multiform VPB
4a	Couplets (two consecutive VPBs)
4b	Ventricular tachycardia (three or more consecutive VPBs)
5	R-on-T VPB (potential to progress to ventricular tachycardia)

mic agents) or nonpharmacologic intervention (ablative operation, implantation of a cardioverter defibrillator). Many patients with a history of arrhythmia and sudden death are implanted with a cardioverter defibrillator, a topic that is addressed later in this chapter. When patients are on antiarrhythmic agents, one must understand the class of medication and potential intraoperative medications that can be used (see the section "Antiarrhythmic Drugs" below). Patients with VPBs and heart disease should have electrolyte levels and an ECG evaluated preoperatively.

Sick Sinus Syndrome

Patients with SSS may be asymptomatic but commonly present with syncope or palpitations. In SSS, the automaticity of the sinus node is diminished and inappropriate sinus bradycardia occurs, often associated with varying degrees of sinoatrial block or even sinus arrest. Frequently, the bradycardia is punctuated with SVT (bradycardia-tachycardia syndrome). Figure 4-9 presents ECGs recorded over several days in a patient with SSS. The ECG in the first panel shows sinus arrest with a junctional rhythm of 50 beats per minute. The ECG in the middle panel (recorded 5 days later) shows atrial fibrillation. The ECG in the bottom panel (recorded 12 days later) shows SVT at a rate of 130 beats per minute.

Patients with SSS can be difficult to manage intraoperatively because of their inability to respond with appropriate ventricular rates to the stress of surgery and anesthesia, or their propensity to develop tachyarrhythmias. Moreover, the already diminished automaticity of the sinus node may be depressed further by anesthetic and vagotonic agents. These patients should be monitored carefully and may require transvenous pacing. Although pacing is the treatment of choice for symptomatic bradycardia, it is less predictable in suppressing SVTs. Patients with SVT may benefit from the use of pharmacologic agents that slow atrioventricular conduction (digoxin, β-blockers, calcium channel blockers), in addition to pacemaker placement.

PACEMAKERS

Pacemakers are designated with a five-letter code (clinically, only the first three may be used). The first three letters describe

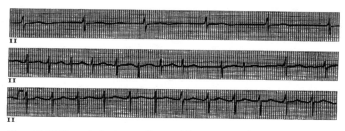

Fig. 4-9. Different electrocardiographic patterns observed over a 2- to 3-week period in a patient with bradycardia-tachycardia syndrome.

the basic antibradycardia functions and the last two describe the programmability and the antitachycardia functions. See Table 4-7 for pacemaker classification.

The indication for the initial pacemaker placement should be determined. The status of and treatment for CHF, CAD, valvular heart disease, arrhythmias, and concomitant diseases like hypertension and diabetes mellitus should be known and optimized. On physical examination, the location, shape, and size of the pulse generator should be determined. Occasionally, the pulse generator may become mobile and loose as a result of external manipulation by the patient. Pacemaker function should be evaluated preoperatively, and the last time the device was checked by the pacemaker clinic should be determined. Preoperative tests should include an ECG, CXR, and electrolyte studies. The ECG should be reviewed for appropriate sensing, pacing, and capture by the pacemaker. Capture may be confirmed by feeling the patient's pulse simultaneously with ECG monitoring. Specific evaluation should include the type, model, and mode of function of the device in place. Usually this can be obtained from the history or from the identification card provided to the patient by the pacemaker clinic. If the patient does not have a card or cannot provide information, an overpenetrated radiograph of the device will usually reveal the pacemaker identification code or the initials or name of the manufacturer.

More than 460,000 individuals in the United States have permanent cardiac pacemakers. Knowing the type of pacemaker is important for guiding perioperative management if issues arise. A conservative recommendation is that a pacemaker be interrogated within 2 months of an elective procedure. Indications for use of perioperative pacemakers and management of preexisting devices are generally based on expert opinion, because no established evidence-based guidelines are currently available.

Rate modulation, which is an important component of many pacemakers, is used when the intrinsic heart rate is unable to accelerate to meet demand (e.g., during exercise). Atrial chronotropic incompetence is defined as inability to exceed 70% of maximum predicted heart rate for a given level of metabolic demand or inability to reach a heart rate of 100 beats per minute during exercise. Rate-adaptive pacemakers respond to activity, minute ventilation, and temperature. Activity-sensing pacemakers respond by increasing heart rate at the onset of exercise and decreasing heart rate with rest. These pacemakers detect mechanical forces or vibrations from body movements, which are transformed to elec-

Table 4-7. Classification of pacemakers

I: chamber paced	V = Ventricle
	A = Atrium
	D = Dual
II: chamber sensed	V = Ventricle
	A = Atrium
	D = Dual
	O = None
III: response to sensing	I = Inhibited
	T = Triggered
	D = Dual
	O = None
IV: programmability and rate modulation	P = Programmable and/or output
	M = Multiprogrammable
	C = Communicating
	O = None
	R = Rate modulated
V: tachyarrhythmia function	P = Pacing
	S = Shock
	D = Dual (pacing and shock)
	O = None

trical energy that controls the heart rate. Respiratory-dependent pacemakers respond by calculating the minute ventilation. Temperature-sensing pacemakers have a special lead that detects a change in blood temperature secondary to changes in metabolic activity.

Whether the pacemaker has rate modulation capabilities should be determined preoperatively, and this function should be turned off before induction. What will be the mode of a pacemaker when a magnet is applied and removed must also be determined. The anesthesiologist should arrange for the cardiologist or pacemaker service to interrogate the pacemaker postoperatively.

A magnet should not routinely be used during surgery because the pulse generator may become unpredictably reprogrammed. However, with nonprogrammable pacemakers, it may be safe to use a magnet to provide transient asynchronous pacing should the pacemaker malfunction. Typically, a ring magnet is used for this function. The location and orientation of the pacemaker generator should be ascertained by palpation. A baseline ECG should be obtained. The patient should always be placed on a cardiac monitor and intravenous access should be maintained during this procedure. The magnet is applied directly over the pacemaker generator, and a repeat ECG is compared to the baseline. After a few seconds' delay, the pacemaker converts to an asynchronous mode. If the alignment of the magnet is incorrect, it may cause intermittent pacing in the asynchronous mode. If placement of a magnet corrects an underlying problem (e.g., bradycardia associated with failure to pace, pacemaker-mediated tachycardia, or runaway pacemaker), then the magnet should be left in place, and a cardiology consult should be sought for reprogramming of the pacemaker. A plan should always be in place for alternative emergency pacing and defibrillation. Emergency pacing can be achieved by esophageal, transthoracic, or transvenous techniques.

Electrocautery with unipolar and, rarely, bipolar systems may interfere with pacemakers by causing oversensing. In this case, the recommendation is that the electrocautery electrode be at least 4 to 6 in. away from the pacemaker to minimize electrical interference. A pacemaker can be programmed to a fixed-rate mode to avoid interference problems. However, one should be aware that a fixed-rate mode can cause R-on-T phenomena and precipitate an undesirable tachyarrhythmia (e.g., ventricular tachycardia). In cases of emergent surgery or situations in which the pacemaker is not able to be interrogated, a magnet can be placed over the pacemaker and an ECG recorded to evaluate the backup mode and function of the pacemaker. Prophylaxis for subacute bacterial endocarditis is not recommended for patients with permanent pacemakers before noncardiac surgery.

IMPLANTABLE CARDIOVERTER DEFIBRILLATORS

The preoperative evaluation of the patient with an implantable cardioverter defibrillator (ICD) should focus on the cause of the arrhythmogenic potential. This may be related to underlying CAD or other structural problems. The evaluation should focus on the need for further evaluation of the CAD and decisions regarding perioperative monitoring.

In addition to defining the underlying cause, determining the type of ICD in place is important. Many different devices currently exist, and they are constantly changing. The first-generation devices had only defibrillation capability without any programmability. Second-generation devices had limited programmability, whereas third-generation devices provided antibradycardia pacing, antitachycardia pacing, low-energy cardioversion, and standard defibrillation capabilities. The fourth-generation devices have a different electrode configuration with similar capabilities. Because multiple causes of inhibition or triggering can occur intraoperatively, the standard anesthetic management is to turn the devices off. Therefore, knowing the type of device is important, because a magnet may have variable effects and the device may have to be selectively deprogrammed. If the type of ICD is unknown, a radiograph may allow visualization of the manufacturer's name. At the completion of surgery, the device should be reactivated. Therefore, surgery on a patient with an ICD may not be appropriate in all locations if facilities to program and reprogram the device are not available.

An ICD should be deactivated preoperatively if electrocautery will be used during surgery. This is done because the ICD can misinterpret electrocautery as an arrhythmia and discharge inappropriately or suspend arrhythmia detection. A cardiologist should be consulted for deactivation of the ICD preoperatively and reactivation of the device postoperatively.

PATIENT WITH A TRANSPLANTED HEART

In patients with a transplanted heart, in addition to assessment of the overall status of the patient and any associated disease processes, preoperative evaluation should focus on the functional status of the transplanted heart. The transplanted heart is denervated; therefore, autonomic reflexes as well as pain

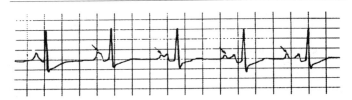

Fig. 4-10. Electrocardiogram demonstrating two sets of P waves in a patient with a heart transplant. The P waves indicated by the arrows are from the recipient sinus node. The P waves preceding the QRS complex are from the donor heart.

from ischemia are absent. Patients with transplanted hearts undergo periodic angiography to evaluate CAD and echocardiography to determine deterioration of myocardial function. The most recent results should be documented.

Patients with a transplanted heart are preload dependent and have a decreased adaptation to exercise and decreased ventricular compliance. They have 50% to 70% of the exercise capacity of normal individuals of the same gender and age. In a patient with a heart transplant, the ECG occasionally shows two sets of P waves, as seen in Fig. 4-10. The sinoatrial node of the recipient remains intact and still has autonomic regulation, but the impulses are not conducted to the donor heart. The donor sinoatrial node is denervated and does not have direct autonomic regulation, and these impulses are conducted to the ventricles.

The patient with a heart transplant should be evaluated for evidence of rejection, especially in the first 3 months when the incidence is highest. Low cardiac output and dysrhythmias may be due to rejection and should be evaluated by echocardiography and ECG. Endomyocardial biopsy may be needed to confirm rejection, which may require high-dose immunosuppressive therapy.

Immunosuppressive therapy should be continued in the perioperative period. Although immunosuppressants are given in combination to minimize dose-related toxicity of individual agents, significant side effects are still associated with their use. Glucocorticoids can cause adrenal suppression and glucose intolerance, and preoperative evaluation should include measurement of serum glucose level and a plan for administration of stress doses of steroids perioperatively (see Chapter 15). Patients on azathioprine (Imuran) and antilymphocyte globulin should have a complete blood count to detect myelosuppression and leukopenia. Cyclosporine is a nephrotoxic agent and can cause elevated blood urea nitrogen (BUN) and creatinine levels, electrolyte abnormalities, and hypertension. Immunosuppressed patients are at a greater risk of opportunistic infections and should have minimal exposure to sources of nosocomial infection (e.g., central and intravascular catheters, mechanical ventilators).

CAROTID BRUIT

The presence of a carotid bruit does not predict severity or location of carotid artery disease. It is an indicator of systemic atherosclerosis and CAD. The patient with a carotid bruit is at risk for a perioperative stroke. The absolute risk is difficult to quantify because few objective data related to loudness of the bruit and perioperative events are available. In fact, louder bruits may reflect less critical stenosis but more turbulent flow, whereas soft bruits may reflect tight stenosis but more laminar flow.

The presence of a carotid bruit signals an increased risk of stroke but does not correlate with location or mechanism of the stroke. The Asymptomatic Carotid Atherosclerosis Study was halted by the National Institute of Neurological Disorders and Stroke because a clear benefit was seen in favor of surgery (for asymptomatic, good-risk patients operated on by a surgeon whose record of surgical mortality and morbidity is less than 3%) for patients with carotid stenosis of 60% or greater as measured by diameter reduction.

Patients who have a carotid bruit with a history of transient ischemic attacks (TIAs), lacunar strokes, nondisabling cortical stroke in the territories supplied by the internal carotid artery, or ophthalmic TIAs should be evaluated for carotid artery disease. The North American Symptomatic Carotid Endarterectomy study revealed a clear benefit of carotid endarterectomy (for stroke prevention) for patients with high-grade stenosis of 70% or more who had had a nondisabling stroke or TIA in the past 6 months. Carotid endarterectomy is acceptable but not proven treatment for patients with a TIA or a nondisabling stroke in the past 6 months and a stenosis of 50% to 69%. Carotid endarterectomy is of uncertain benefit in patients who have experienced a TIA or mild nondisabling stroke and have stenosis of less than 50%.

Carotid ultrasonography is highly sensitive (greater than 95%) for hemodynamically significant stenosis. Cerebral angiogram is the gold standard test, but carries a risk of stroke or death of 0.5% to 1.2%. Magnetic resonance angiography complements carotid ultrasonography because of high specificity and sensitivity but has a substantial cost. Transcranial Doppler ultrasonography does not directly evaluate the degree of carotid stenosis but is often used in conjunction with carotid ultrasonography to assess the intracranial circulation. All patients with symptomatic carotid stenosis should undergo noncontrast computed tomography or magnetic resonance imaging to rule out the possibility that the symptoms are due to infarction from stenosis in another territory. Other diagnostic tests include single photon emission computed tomography, positron emission tomography, and computed tomographic angiography.

Routine evaluation of an asymptomatic bruit is indicated before noncardiac surgery only if the patient is scheduled for major surgery with anticipation of significant blood loss or fluid shifts. An asymptomatic carotid bruit also should be evaluated if the patient has symptoms of angina or a history of significant CAD, severe peripheral vascular disease, history of prior carotid endarterectomy, or contralateral carotid artery occlusion. Patients should be questioned carefully about TIAs (amaurosis fugax, tingling or numbness of the face or extremities). Often these transient symptoms are not recognized by patients to be of any significance.

PREOPERATIVE MANAGEMENT OF DRUG THERAPY

To provide an optimal anesthetic and optimal control of adverse hemodynamic perturbations, one must understand a patient's preexisting drug therapy. Review of limited data suggests that it is safe to continue the vast majority of drugs until the time of surgery, especially in cases in which withdrawal could lead to adverse hemodynamic changes.

β
β-Blockers

β-Blockers are most commonly used to treat cardiac diseases, especially CAD, hypertension, SVT, and HOCM. Patients taking β-blockers should have these drugs continued throughout the perioperative period. Withdrawal of β-blockers can lead to hypertension, tachycardia, and relapse of tachyarrhythmias, and can worsen or precipitate ischemia by altering oxygen supply-demand balance. Use of these drugs is not without a note of caution, however. Giving β-blockers in combination with calcium channel blockers or class I antiarrhythmic drugs (quinidine, procainamide hydrochloride, disopyramide phosphate) carries a risk of prolonging atrioventricular conduction, resulting in complete heart block. β-Blockers decrease hepatic blood flow and can prolong the effects of drugs metabolized by the liver.

Alpha₂-Adrenergic Agonist Drugs

The alpha₂-adrenergic agonists control blood pressure by a centrally mediated stimulation of alpha₂ receptors, which causes a decrease in sympathetic outflow. This class of drugs includes clonidine, methyldopa, guanabenz acetate, and guanfacine hydrochloride. Withdrawal from these drugs may result in rebound hypertension. If the patient is taking an oral medication, methyldopa administered parenterally or clonidine administered via a transdermal patch can be substituted. Studies have shown that alpha₂ agonists decrease anesthetic requirements and decrease the hemodynamic lability frequently seen in hypertensive patients. Clonidine decreases analgesic requirements and provides sedation and anxiety reduction. Other possible benefits include attenuation of opiate withdrawal and decreased postoperative shivering, both of which may have adverse hemodynamic effects and precipitate or worsen ischemic heart disease.

Alpha-Adrenergic Antagonist Drugs

The alpha-adrenergic antagonist drugs include prazosin hydrochloride given for hypertension and terazosin hydrochloride given for benign prostatic hyperplasia. No significant studies have been conducted of the perioperative use of these drugs. Theoretically, these drugs can cause tachycardia through unopposed beta-adrenergic activity. However, especially in the case of prazosin hydrochloride, which is an alpha₁-adrenergic antagonist, the prejunctional alpha₂ receptors are still intact and through negative feedback stimulation will blunt the tachycardia.

Angiotensin-Converting Enzyme Inhibitors and Angiotensin II Receptor Antagonists

Angiotensin-converting enzyme (ACE) inhibitors include captopril, lisinopril, enalapril maleate (oral), enalaprilat (intravenous), and benazepril hydrochloride. Angiotensin II receptor antagonists are losartan potassium and valsartan. These drugs are indicated for hypertension, CHF (afterload reduction, cardiac remodeling), post–myocardial infarction (improved survival), and diabetic nephropathy. No contraindications exist to continuing ACE inhibitors perioperatively when patients are taking them long term. Patients taking ACE inhibitors are more sensitive to hypovolemia, and some patients, especially those with renal insufficiency, may develop hyperkalemia. Preoperative evaluation should include evaluation of electrolyte, BUN, and creatinine levels in these patients.

Calcium Channel Blockers

Calcium channel blockers are used to treat hypertension (nifedipine), SVT (verapamil hydrochloride, diltiazem hydrochloride) and ischemic heart disease, especially vasospastic angina. Controversial studies have been done regarding continuation of calcium channel blockers in the perioperative period. Controversies also exist regarding the safety of using calcium channel blockers in patients with CAD (some well-designed prospective studies are underway). These drugs do not have the same rebound effects from withdrawal as do the β-blockers. Pending further investigations, one can continue these drugs perioperatively if patients take these drugs long term. Calcium channel blockers potentiate nondepolarizing neuromuscular blocking agents. Verapamil hydrochloride and diltiazem hydrochloride potentiate the depression of cardiac contractility and atrioventricular conduction block by the volatile anesthetics. Some of the newer agents (e.g., amlodipine besylate) have less negative inotropic effect. Nifedipine can potentiate the vasodilatory effect of volatile agents. Calcium channel blockers combined with β-blockers can lead to complete heart block.

Antiarrhythmic Drugs

Most antiarrhythmic drugs should be continued through the perioperative period. Some of the antiarrhythmic drugs (class I, quinidine, procainamide hydrochloride) can potentiate the inhalational agents and cause myocardial depression. Class I antiarrhythmics can potentially promote arrhythmias (torsades de pointes), and preoperative evaluation should include an ECG to measure the QT interval. The QT interval represents the duration of ventricular systole and is measured from the beginning of the QRS complex to the end of the T wave. The normal QT interval, corrected for heart rate (QTc), is usually less than 0.425 second. QTc is calculated by dividing the QT interval by the square root of the R-R interval.

Some inhalational agents decrease liver biotransformation of drugs. Because most of the antiarrhythmic drugs are metabolized in the liver, consideration should be given to reducing the dosages of these drugs. Long-term use of amiodarone hydrochloride can cause serious side effects. Patients should undergo periodic evaluation (every 4 to 6 months) to detect pulmonary toxicity (by pulmonary function tests, CXR) and thyroid dysfunction (by measurement of thyroid profile; see Chapter 6). Concomitant use of amiodarone hydrochloride with warfarin can potentiate the anticoagulant effect. Amiodarone hydrochloride can increase the serum concentration of digoxin, quinidine and procainamide. Amiodarone hydrochloride is a myocardial depressant with a half-life of 30 days. It can cause bradycardia (atropine resistant), atrioventricular block, and severe hypotension. Planning for surgery should include preparation for pacing and cardiac support.

Digoxin

Digoxin is used for both CHF and atrial fibrillation. Patients taking digoxin long term can be continued on this drug perioperatively. Normal therapeutic levels are 1.5 to 2.0 ng per mL. Digoxin has a high toxic to therapeutic dose ratio. Patients at risk for toxicity include those with hypovolemia, electrolyte abnormalities, renal failure, or hypothyroidism; elderly patients; and those who are on other drugs (diuretics, antiarrhythmics). Serum potassium levels may fluctuate in patients who are on diuretics or are critically ill, predisposing to digoxin toxicity. Any dysrhythmia in the presence of digoxin should be considered a manifestation of digoxin toxicity. Paroxysmal atrial tachycardia with 2:1 atrioventricular block is pathognomonic of digoxin toxicity (Fig. 4-11).

Other side effects of digoxin toxicity include VPBs, bigeminy, junctional tachycardia, second-degree atrioventricular block, ventricular tachycardia, nausea, anorexia, vomiting, diarrhea, altered mental status, agitation, lethargy, scotoma, and altered perception of color vision. Preoperative prophylactic digitalization of patients with diminished cardiac reserve who are at risk for development of atrial fibrillation remains controversial. All patients on digoxin should have potassium levels checked and hypokalemia corrected preoperatively.

Diuretics

The major categories of diuretics include loop diuretics (furosemide), thiazides (hydrochlorothiazide), osmotic diuretics (mannitol), related sulfonamide compounds (indapamide), and potassium-sparing diuretics (spironolactone). Volume depletion and hypokalemia may predispose patients to dysrhythmias. Other problems that can be seen with diuretics are hyponatremia, hypomagnesemia, hypocalcemia, and hyperglycemia. Diuretics are generally discontinued or the doses reduced preoperatively to avoid hypovolemia, prerenal azotemia, and intraoperative hypotension. For patients taking diuretics, electrolytes should be evaluated preoperatively.

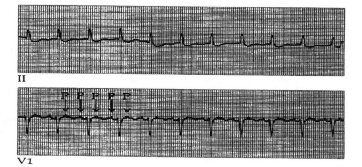

Fig. 4-11. Electrocardiogram demonstrating paroxysmal atrial tachycardia with 2:1 block in a patient with digoxin toxicity. Atrial rate is 200 beats per minute, and ventricular rate is 100 beats per minute.

Anticoagulant and Antiplatelet Drugs

Evaluation of a patient on anticoagulant and antiplatelet drugs must be individualized. Each situation is unique and should be considered in its totality. When a patient is taking warfarin (Coumadin), 4 days are required for the international normalized ratio (INR; see Chapter 7) to reach 1.5 in most cases. An INR of 1.5 or less is adequate for surgical hemostasis. If the INR is 2.0 to 3.0, four scheduled doses of warfarin should be withheld to allow the INR to fall to 1.5 or less before surgery. If the INR is higher than 3.0 or if the desired INR for surgery is less than 1.3, then warfarin should be withheld for a longer period. The INR should be measured the day before surgery, and if the INR is 1.8 or higher, vitamin K in a dose of 1 mg intravenously or subcutaneously can be given. Prothrombin time and partial thromboplastin time should be determined preoperatively.

Elective surgery should be avoided for 1 month after an arterial embolism. If surgery is necessary during the first month, then the patient should be admitted to the hospital and intravenous heparin should be given until 6 hours before surgery. In patients with mechanical heart valves and nonvalvular atrial fibrillation who have *not* had a recent embolism, the risk of embolism is not high enough to warrant preoperative intravenous administration of heparin. Low-dose subcutaneous heparin or low-molecular-weight heparin in high-risk venous thromboembolism prophylactic doses is recommended for hospitalized patients with mechanical heart valves or atrial fibrillation. However, hospitalization for the sole purpose of administering subcutaneous heparin or administration of subcutaneous heparin to outpatients is not necessary. In cases of emergency surgery for fully anticoagulated patients with mechanical heart valves or atrial fibrillation, consultation with a cardiologist is recommended.

Patients treated with fibrinolytic agents such as tissue plasminogen activator may benefit from administration of antifibrinolytic drugs (e.g., aprotinin, ε-aminocaproic acid) to control bleeding. Patients on aspirin (acetylsalicylic acid) should usually discontinue this drug 7 days preoperatively because aspirin irreversibly affects platelet function for 1 week. If the risk of stopping this drug is high, however, or urgent surgery is required, the patient can be continued on low-dose aspirin (less than 650 mg per day) until 48 hours before surgery. Approximately 70,000 platelets per cubic millimeter are produced daily and only 30,000 to 50,000 functioning platelets per cubic millimeter are required for normal clotting. Platelet transfusions can be given (with associated risks of transfusion). Aspirin therapy is not a significant risk factor for developing a spinal or epidural hematoma. Preoperative anticoagulation therapy (with warfarin, heparin), however, presents a significant risk of bleeding with regional anesthesia, and potentially devastating neurologic injury can result from a hematoma. Heparin is started postoperatively for patients at high risk for thromboembolism.

CASE STUDY

A 55-year-old man is scheduled to have a right inguinal herniorrhaphy. Preoperative evaluation reveals a history of syncope while walking on a treadmill 2 months previously, for which he did not seek medical care. Previous to this, he had good exercise capacity and walked on a treadmill at a brisk pace for 30 minutes daily. He relates that over the last 6 months he has been feeling progressively fatigued and short-winded with a feeling of chest heaviness at the end of his workout. Currently, he is limited to only 5 minutes of exercise. He blames his symptoms on job-related stress and feelings of depression. He has a history of hypertension and hyperlipidemia, and a 45 pack-year smoking history. His medications include atenolol, pravastatin sodium, and aspirin.

Physical examination reveals a blood pressure of 152/90 mm Hg and heart rate of 62 beats per minute. He has a slow-rising, low-amplitude pulse with a delayed sustained peak palpated at the brachial and carotid arteries. The cardiac apical beat on palpation is displaced laterally, is forceful, and is sustained during systole. A systolic thrill is present at the base of the heart and along the carotid arteries. Auscultation reveals a soft S_1, an S_4, and an ejection systolic crescendo-decrescendo murmur, loudest at the second right intercostal space, graded III/VI with radiation to the carotids. ECG shows a sinus rhythm with left ventricular hypertrophy. Hematocrit is 41%, total cholesterol is 241 with a low-density lipoprotein level of 162, and CXR is normal.

A history of syncope always raises the possibility of cardiac disease. Cardiac syncope is due to impaired cerebral perfusion, which can be caused by an arrhythmia or diminished cardiac output. Syncope after exertion may be due to aortic stenosis because of limitation of the cardiac output by the stenotic valve or by an associated arrhythmia. HOCM is usually associated with a history of multiple episodes of exertional syncope. Exertional syncope may be due to myocardial ischemia that causes a low cardiac output or a dysrhythmia. Less commonly, exertional syncope can be caused by pulmonary hypertension, a left atrial myxoma, or obstruction of the cardiac output by a large intracardiac mass. Syncope due to arrhythmias (atrial fibrillation, ventricular tachycardia, ventricular fibrillation, high-degree atrioventricular block) without structural heart disease is usually sudden and nonexertional.

An echocardiogram was done to further evaluate this patient's systolic murmur. The echocardiogram revealed an ejection fraction of 46%, mild inferior wall hypokinesis, and severe aortic stenosis with an aortic valve area of 0.7 cm^2 and a peak gradient of 68 mm Hg. The average survival time of patients with untreated aortic stenosis with syncope is 3 years. Because of this prognosis and the high incidence of sudden death in patients with aortic stenosis (possibly due to arrhythmias), this patient needs repair or replacement of his aortic valve. Surgical intervention (valvuloplasty or aortic valve replacement) is usually recommended for symptomatic patients with hemodynamically significant aortic stenosis. Because of his history of possible angina, a cardiac catheterization is indicated to evaluate his coronary arteries before surgery.

Moderate to severe aortic stenosis increases the risk of noncardiac surgery, and the recommendation is generally that the aortic stenosis be corrected first. However, this might not be an option in certain situations in which the need to undergo noncardiac surgery is urgent. Studies have shown that, although a certain risk is involved, proceeding with noncardiac surgery is possible in selected patients with significant aortic stenosis.

General anesthesia is usually recommended over epidural or spinal anesthesia for patients with critical aortic stenosis because central neuraxial anesthesia can precipitate hypotension by sympathetic blockade and a reduction of preload and afterload. Several cases have been reported, however, in which epidural and continuous spinal catheter anesthesia have been used successfully in these patients. Epidural anesthesia usually is preferred over spinal anesthesia in this situation because the onset of hypotension is more gradual. Regional anesthesia may provide some significant benefits over general anesthesia. Direct laryngoscopy and intubation induce significant hemodynamic perturbations, which can be avoided by a regional technique. Patients can stay awake during regional anesthesia and communicate symptoms (chest pain, shortness of breath). Regional anesthesia avoids the need for positive-pressure ventilation; such ventilation can decrease preload, afterload, and cardiac output, which can be deleterious in a patient with significant aortic stenosis.

Regardless of the type of anesthesia, patients with critical aortic stenosis require careful intraoperative management. If large fluid shifts are anticipated or a high-risk surgical procedure is planned (e.g., thoracotomy), a pulmonary artery catheter or transesophageal echocardiography should be used to guide fluid and volume management, so that decreases in preload, afterload, and cardiac output can be avoided. Intraarterial blood pressure monitoring is recommended, and hypotension should be treated promptly, either with fluid boluses (for decreased central filling pressures) or with vasoactive drugs (phenylephrine). Ephedrine should be used with caution because it may cause undesirable tachycardia that limits time for ejection across a stenotic aortic valve and may precipitate myocardial ischemia.

In summary, because this patient is scheduled for an *elective* hernia repair, he should have an aortic valve replacement to correct his critical aortic stenosis before his herniorrhaphy. He needs a cardiac catheterization to evaluate his coronary anatomy because he will be undergoing cardiac surgery and cardiopulmonary bypass. If the hernia repair were urgent (e.g., if strangulation or small bowel obstruction were present), however, then one should proceed with surgery using invasive monitoring. Intraarterial blood pressure monitoring (necessary for almost any procedure requiring central neuraxial or general anesthesia in a patient with critical aortic stenosis) and either a pulmonary artery catheter or transesophageal echocardiography (if significant fluid shifts or blood loss are anticipated) are indicated. Subacute bacterial endocarditis prophylaxis guidelines should be followed (see Chapter 16).

BIBLIOGRAPHY

Bedford R, Feinstein B. Hospital admission blood pressure: a predictor for hypertension following endotracheal intubation. *Anesth Analg* 1980;59:367–370.

Bourke ME. The patient with pacemaker or related device. *Can J Anaesth* 1996;43:24–41.

Braunwald E. Heart failure. In: Isselbacher KJ, Braunwald E, Wilson JD, et al., eds. *Harrison's principles of internal medicine*, 13th ed. New York: McGraw-Hill, 1994:998–1008.

Braunwald E. Valvular heart disease. In: Isselbacher KJ, Braunwald E, Wilson JD, et al., eds. *Harrison's principles of internal medicine*, 13th ed. New York: McGraw-Hill, 1994:1052–1065.

Carabello BA, Crawford FA. Valvular heart disease. *N Engl J Med* 1997;337:32–41.

Etchells E, Bell C, Robb K. Does this patient have an abnormal systolic murmur? *JAMA* 1997;277:564–569.

Gohlke-Barwolf C, Acar J, Burckhardt D, et al. Guidelines for prevention of thromboembolic events in valvular heart disease. Ad Hoc Committee of the Working Group on Valvular Heart Disease, European Society of Cardiology. *J Heart Valve Dis* 1993;2:398–410.

Goldman L, Caldera DL. Risks of general anesthesia and elective operation in the hypertensive patient. *Anesthesiology* 1979;50:285–292.

Guidelines for evaluation and management of heart failure. Report of the American College of Cardiology/American Heart Association Task Force on Practice. *Circulation* 1995;92:2764–2784.

Hanson E, Neerhut R, Lynch C. Mitral valve prolapse. *Anesthesiology* 1996;85:178–195.

Hayes SN, Holmes DRJ, Nishimura RA, Reeder GS. Palliative percutaneous aortic balloon valvuloplasty before noncardiac operations and invasive diagnostic procedures. *Mayo Clin Proc* 1989;64:753–757.

Horlocker TT, Wedel DJ, Schroeder DR. Preoperative antiplatelet therapy does not increase risk of spinal hematoma. *Anesth Analg* 1995;80:303–309.

Kearon C, Hirsh J. Management of anticoagulation before and after elective surgery. *N Engl J Med* 1997;336:1506–1511.

Mangano DT. *Preoperative cardiac assessment*. Philadelphia: JB Lippincott Co, 1990:141–163.

Notarius CF, Levy RD, Tully A, et al. Cardiac vs. noncardiac limits to exercise after heart transplantation. *Am Heart J* 1998;135:339–348.

O'Keefe JH, Shub C, Rettke SR. Risk of noncardiac surgical procedures in patients with aortic stenosis. *Mayo Clin Proc* 1989;64:400–405.

Potyk D, Raudaskoski P. Preoperative cardiac evaluation for elective noncardiac surgery. *Arch Fam Med* 1998;7:164–173.

Rauck RL. The anticoagulated patient. *Reg Anesth* 1996;21:51–56.

Schneck MJ. Stroke prevention and screening for surgical interventions in carotid artery disease. *Hosp Med* 1998;34:22–36.

Torsher LC, Rettke SR, Brown DL. Risk of patients with severe aortic stenosis undergoing noncardiac surgery. *Am J Cardiol* 1998;81:448–452.

Pulmonary Disease

Kenneth E. Shepherd and William E. Hurford

This chapter outlines the pertinent history, physical findings, diagnostic testing algorithms, and management of patients with lung diseases, including **asthma, cystic fibrosis (CF), sleep apnea syndrome (SAS),** and **chronic obstructive pulmonary disease (COPD).** A brief discussion of **lung volume reduction surgery** and **lung transplantation** is included. The chapter also discusses the approach to patients who present with a **history of tobacco use** or **shortness of breath (dyspnea)** and patients with **restrictive lung disease** and **pulmonary vascular disease.** Diseases of the upper airway (above the larynx), diseases of the larynx and large airway (extrinsic compression or tracheomalacia), and management of the airway are important issues covered in other chapters and therefore are only mentioned here. This chapter outlines how to optimize medical management (when to use corticosteroids, intensify bronchodilator regimens, etc.) and how to identify patients who may present a high risk for surgery. The chapter concludes with a case study of a complex patient.

The chapter not only provides a framework that allows the anesthesiologist to perform an appropriate examination but also enables the anesthesiologist to know when, in the rarest of circumstances, to request a consult without having done too little or having ordered too many expensive, irrelevant tests. The information in this chapter enables evaluation of patients with pulmonary diseases so as to all but eliminate the need for input from pulmonologists.

DEFINITIONS, ETIOLOGY, AND PATHOPHYSIOLOGY

Asthma is a chronic inflammatory airway disease process in which cellular and chemical mediators augment airway inflammation, bronchial smooth muscle tone, mucus production, edema of airways, and airway bronchoconstrictor responsiveness. The typical hallmark of asthma is the episodic occurrence of bronchospasm characterized by wheezing and shortness of breath (with improvement after the use of bronchodilators). The underlying defect that causes asthma remains largely unknown, and the disease probably has several different pathogenic mechanisms that vary in importance from person to person. Bronchoconstriction is precipitated by unknown triggers or obvious events such as allergen exposure; viral infection; administration of medications; and instrumentation of the larynx, trachea, and airways.[1-3]

COPD is a disorder characterized by abnormal tests of expiratory flow that do not change appreciably over several months of observation. The obstruction to airflow may be either structural or functional but usually is due to localized disease of the larger airways. Bronchiectasis and CF are excluded, as is asthma. Tobacco use is by far the most important risk factor for COPD. Alpha$_1$-antitrypsin deficiency, other familial or genetic processes, and dusty occupational environments are other well-established risk factors. Childhood respiratory illness may render some people susceptible to COPD in later life. All of these latter-mentioned influences, however, although well-established risks for COPD, are minor compared to that of cigarette smoking.

Three disorders are currently incorporated in COPD. These are emphysema, chronic bronchitis, and peripheral airway disease. Although any individual patient is likely to have some combination of these conditions, the dominant clinical and pathophysiologic feature of COPD is always limitation of expiratory airflow rate. COPD characteristically affects middle-aged and elderly persons. These patients may present with dyspnea, cough, wheezing, sputum production, and recurrent respiratory infections.[4] Emphysema, chronic bronchitis, and peripheral airway disease are discussed in this chapter as if they were separate entities.

Emphysema is defined pathologically by the American Thoracic Society[5] as "a condition of the lung characterized by abnormal permanent enlargement of the airspaces distal to terminal bronchioles, accompanied by destruction of their walls, and without obvious fibrosis." It is recognized *in vivo* by a decreased diffusing capacity (for carbon monoxide) on pulmonary function tests (PFTs) and reduced lung parenchymal density on chest radiography (CXR) or computed tomography (CT).[6] The pathogenesis of emphysema in smokers is incompletely known but stresses inherited or acquired proteolytic activity against extracellular matrix proteins. Damage to elastic fibers leading to alveolar wall enlargement and septal destruction appears to be the critical event.[7]

Chronic bronchitis is defined clinically[5] and refers to the condition experienced by patients who have chronic (occurring on most days for at least 3 months of the year for at least 2 successive years) or recurrent excess bronchial mucus secretion (not due to other diseases such as bronchiectasis) leading to severe impairment in expiratory flow rates. The lung pathology of chronic bronchitis primarily includes large airway mucus gland hyperplasia and airway inflammation.[6] It is generally due to cigarette smoking.

A variety of morphologic abnormalities have been identified in the peripheral airways[5] of patients with COPD. These include inflammation of the terminal and respiratory bronchioles, fibrosis and narrowing of airway walls, and goblet cell changes (metaplasia) of the epithelium of bronchioles.[5] Structure-function correlations suggest that these changes in the peripheral airways contribute to airflow obstruction in COPD.[5]

CF is a genetic disease diagnosed when a patient has an elevated sweat chloride concentration (greater than 60 mEq per L) and chronic pulmonary disease of appropriate character. The disease also is diagnosed if the patient has pancreatic insufficiency and has a history of CF diagnosed in a parent, sibling, or first cousin. The fundamental physiologic defect is a failure of cyclic adenosine monophosphate (cAMP) regulation of airway chloride transport. The pulmonary disease in CF is characterized by chronic and suppurative inflammation leading to progressive airway obstruction.[8]

Dyspnea is a symptom (not a specific disease state) defined as an uncomfortable sensation of breathing. It is associated with conditions in which the respiratory drive is increased or the respiratory system is subject to a mechanical load. The cause(s) of dyspnea are complex and our understanding of dyspnea has not reached the point at which a specific disease (pulmonary or nonpulmonary) can be linked conclusively with a specific pathophysiologic mechanism of dyspnea.[9,10] One must remember that dyspnea can be due to cardiac disease without intrinsic lung disease.

Lung transplantation is a treatment, not a cure, for a variety of end-stage lung diseases, including COPD. As the number of transplants continues to increase and survival improves, patients with complications related to the transplanted lung(s) as well as lung transplant patients with unrelated disorders undergo procedures more frequently.[11] Transplantation is impractical in the vast majority of patients with COPD, largely due to advanced age and coexisting nonpulmonary disease.

The other surgical procedure recommended for selected patients with COPD is lung volume reduction surgery. Lung volume reduction surgery may improve ventilatory function beyond that achieved by intense medical management in some patients with COPD. It may be useful as a primary therapy for patients with COPD or as a bridge to lung transplantation. Selection of patients and surgical techniques have not been standardized, however. Results of this surgical procedure are not predictable at present, and a determination of its role in the treatment of COPD awaits data from current ongoing multicenter studies.[7]

The pathophysiologic entities capable of inducing **pulmonary vascular disease** range from COPD to interstitial fibrosis (see individual discussions of COPD and restrictive lung diseases). This is a broad topic and includes: (a) pulmonary embolism; (b) pulmonary hypertension; (c) pulmonary heart disease (cor pulmonale, defined here as right ventricular dysfunction or hypertrophy secondary to disease of the lung or its blood vessels), often due to COPD or interstitial fibrosis; (d) congenital and acquired pulmonary arteriovenous aneurysms; and (e) neoplasia of the pulmonary vascular bed.[2] If extensive, any of these disorders may lead to pulmonary hypertension.[2] Rather than detail all these categories, this chapter mentions pulmonary thromboembolism but focuses on the features of pulmonary vascular changes in COPD and restrictive diseases and refers the reader to specific sections in this chapter and other texts[2] for additional information.

Restrictive lung diseases are discussed in a general way in this chapter. In restrictive diseases, the complicated differential diagnosis can be simplified by recognizing five basic pathophysiologic categories: disorders involving the thoracic cage (e.g., kyphoscoliosis); disorders involving the respiratory muscles; and interstitial, alveolar, and pleural abnormalities.[12] The interstitial diseases comprise a large part of this disease category. Interstitial diseases comprise more than 150 disorders of known etiologies (e.g., environmental and occupationally related disorders as well as those of infectious cause due to mycobacteria) and unknown etiologies.[13] Idiopathic pulmonary fibrosis is a group of progressive interstitial diseases of unknown etiology[14] that make up a large proportion of the interstitial lung diseases seen clinically. The underlying similarities in the interstitial diseases are damage to the alveolar walls and interstitium with a subsequent inflammatory alveolitis and eventual fibrosis of the architecture of the lung.[13]

Simple smoking is used in this chapter to denote tobacco use by patients who are smokers but are asymptomatic. Generally, no specific quantity of cigarette smoking is included in the definition, but in this chapter up to one pack per day is considered significant. Although no formal consensus has been reached regarding the appropriate American Society of Anesthesiologists Physical Status (ASA-PS) classification for asymptomatic smokers, these patients—especially those with 10 pack-years or more of tobacco exposure (where pack-years equals the number of packs per day times the number of years of smoking)—may be at risk for both pulmonary and nonpulmonary perioperative complications.[15,16] Smoking causes hypersecretion of mucus, dysfunction of ciliary activity, small airway inflammation, increased lung closing volume, and increased bronchial reactivity.[15]

Distinguishing between smoking exposure in active smokers and in prior smokers is important. The acute effects on hemodynamics due to nicotine and carbon monoxide appear to be largely reversible after a period of 12 hours.[15] In contradistinction to these acute cardiopulmonary effects, many of the disturbances of lung function take longer to resolve.[15] Lung function may return toward normal in smokers after a long period of abstinence (longer than 8 weeks).[15] This may lead to decreased perioperative complications in former smokers.

SAS is defined as the occurrence of 30 or more periods of apnea (complete cessation of airflow for 10 seconds or longer) over a 7-hour period of nocturnal sleep due to central apnea (loss of medullary respiratory drive with no respiratory muscle movement), peripheral apnea (obstruction of the upper airway in the presence of continuous respiratory muscle effort), or both (a central respiratory pause followed by an obstructed airway with respiratory muscle efforts). Patients with SAS typically have a history of snoring and complain of excessive daytime sleepiness. Although the disorder is more common and more severe in men, SAS that occurs during rapid eye movement sleep is more common in women.[17] The depressant effects of general anesthetics and epidural opioid analgesics on respiration assume a greater importance in patients with SAS.[18–20] (See Chapter 15 for more information on SAS.)

The subject matter is treated here as though each entity existed alone and without coexisting pulmonary abnormalities. This is clearly overly simplistic. Obviously, many patients have aspects of obstructive, reactive, restrictive, and vascular disease combined. In these patients, the management is generally a sum of the approaches to each separate disease, except for dynamic hyperinflation and patients receiving supplemental oxygen. One must be particularly concerned with dynamic hyperinflation, or breath stacking, in patients with severe lung disease. This occurs when end-expiratory volume encroaches on total lung capacity (discussed in the section on PFTs) due to an increase in ventilatory drive and expiratory flow limitation, restricting the tidal volume.[21] The only mechanism to increase ventilation is to increase frequency of breathing. This establishes a cycle that further increases intrathoracic pressure, increases end-expiratory lung volume, decreases tidal volume, increases respiratory frequency, and decreases alveolar ventilation.[21] This cycle leads to cardiovascular and respiratory failure, and often the cause is not readily recognized. Another exception to the rule of "simply the sum of approaches to each separate disease" is patients receiving supplemental oxygen, who may need to receive additional evaluation.

HISTORY

History taking[22] should elicit background features and specific symptoms referable to the pulmonary system. Critical information includes exposure to cigarettes, infectious organisms, and occupational and environmental agents, as well as current medication use and allergies. Pertinent symptoms and signs are cough, sputum character and amount, hemoptysis, wheezing, dyspnea, exercise tolerance, and chest tightness or pain. Evaluation of nutritional status is important because weight loss is a reversible factor influencing the prognosis of patients with COPD[23] and may have important implications in CF. Ascertaining whether recent changes have occurred in these symptoms is imperative. If positive responses are obtained to questions about the symptoms listed, then more detailed questions should be asked. For example, if the patient has a productive cough, the clinician should determine how much sputum is expectorated. Because patients may swallow sputum instead of spitting it out in large quantities, such patients' risks may be underestimated if the correct questions are not asked.

Exercise tolerance and dyspnea are often difficult to quantitate during history taking because they are, to a large degree, subjective.[2] A classification of dyspnea (Table 5-1) as well as the following examples are included to assist with functional status assessment. Strenuous exercise normally produces shortness of breath and a sensation of dyspnea.[2] For example, if the patient is able to climb two flights of stairs carrying a 22-pound load (e.g., two bags of groceries) at a rapid pace (54 ft per minute), no respiratory impairment is likely to be present.[2] On the other hand, if the patient

Table 5-1. Modified Medical Research Council dyspnea scale

Grade	Description
1	Not troubled by breathlessness except with strenuous exercise.
2	Troubled by shortness of breath when hurrying on the level or walking up a slight hill.
3	Walks slower than people of the same age on the level because of breathlessness or has to stop for breath when walking at own pace on the level.
4	Stops for breath after walking approximately 100 yd or after a few minutes on the level.
5	Too breathless to leave the house or breathless when dressing or undressing.

Reprinted with permission from Mahler DA, Weinberg DH, Wells CK, Feinstein AR. The measurement of dyspnea: contents, interobserver agreement, and physiologic correlates of two new clinical indexes. *Chest* 1984;85:751–758.

exhibits shortness of breath at rest or with minimal activity (e.g., eating or dressing) or a rapid decline in exercise tolerance, significant pulmonary impairment is suggested. With mild respiratory disease between impairment and normal function, assessing the significance of subjective complaints is more difficult. Of note, when the patient reports subjective exercise tolerance at some level less than "normal," CF, COPD, restrictive disease, pulmonary vascular disease, or dysfunction of a transplanted lung is likely. When exercise tolerance is more variable, bouts of asthma are possible.[2] Formalized cardiorespiratory testing[2] may be needed to quantitate the degree of impairment and determine whether it is cardiac or pulmonary in origin, or whether poor exercise performance is due to poor motivation, obesity, deconditioning, or some combination of these factors. A history of severe dyspnea or peripheral edema would lead one to suspect hypoxemia (especially if the hematocrit is elevated) or cor pulmonale. Learning of any previous pulmonary diagnoses and the results of any specialized testing is important.[24]

Asthma

For asthma, the most important historical questions relate to wheezing, coughing, and sputum production. If asthma is suspected, the presence of episodic or nocturnal dyspnea; chest tightness on awakening; coughing; breathlessness; or wheezing in response to exercise, cold air, viral infection, or irritants (e.g., cigarette smoke or fumes) should be ascertained.[3,24,25] A history of difficult-to-control asthma requiring corticosteroid therapy, hospitalization requiring intensive care unit (ICU) admission or mechanical ventilation, and severe bronchospasm with a previous anesthetic suggest an increased risk for perioperative complications.

Chronic Obstructive Pulmonary Disease

Exposure to cigarette smoke and pollutants (environmental or occupational) is important to elicit from patients with known or suspected airflow limitation. Important symptoms to evaluate are wheezing, coughing, and the quantity of sputum production.[24] Although no absolute quantities of sputum production add specific prognostic information, patients with COPD that produce sputum daily and especially those with a recent increase in the quantity of purulent sputum have an increased risk of postoperative pulmonary complications. Patients with a history of respiratory failure unrelated to surgery that has required intubation of the trachea and mechanical ventilatory support have an elevated risk of complications postoperatively.

Cystic Fibrosis

The course of patients with CF is determined by the chronic, suppurative, obstructive nature of their pulmonary disease, which may lead to weight loss, hemoptysis, pneumothorax, hypoxemia, and cor pulmonale. Questioning should elicit the extent of these features of CF.

Unexplained Dyspnea

The common complaint of dyspnea can be attributable to a wide spectrum of pulmonary (and nonpulmonary) causes. The most common nonpulmonary causes are cardiac, neuromuscular, or psychogenic disorders. In general, pulmonary processes that cause dyspnea are classified into restrictive disorders, pulmonary vascular disease, or obstructive airway diseases. Determining an accurate pulmonary diagnosis begins with the focused history outlined above, with an attempt to elicit the historical features of asthma or COPD. Given the nonspecificity of the symptoms, however, specialized tests of respiratory and cardiac function are often necessary.[9]

Lung Transplantation

In evaluating patients who may be potential lung (or heart-lung) transplant candidates, the history taking is as discussed in each of the individual disease categories. However, the anesthesiologist should focus on the severity of the chronic disease. One should ensure that the patient is experiencing functional decline while receiving maximum optimal medical therapy for the disease, that no further medical or surgical therapy is available, and that survival is limited.[26]

Potential transplant candidates may have other medical conditions or therapies that constitute relative contraindications (e.g., age older than 65 years, severe kyphoscoliosis, use of 20 mg or more of prednisone per day, current requirement for invasive mechanical ventilation) or absolute contraindications (e.g., infection with human immunodeficiency virus, renal dysfunction with a creatinine clearance of 50 mg per mL per minute or less) to isolated lung or heart-lung transplantation.[26] The history must include a general medical review to elicit important coexisting medical conditions in addition to the pulmonary disease–specific inquiry as detailed in the guidelines of the American Thoracic Society.[26]

Although the pulmonary history of patients who have undergone single or double lung (or heart-lung) transplants may differ somewhat in focus, one should inquire about airway complications, infection, rejection, and the development of neoplasms.[11] One should ascertain if nonpulmonary side effects of immunosuppression such as renal insufficiency, hematologic impairment, Cushing's disease, or osteoporosis are present. Although the summary given here is brief, a full discussion is beyond the scope of this chapter, and the reader is referred to the article by Trulock.[11]

Vascular Disease

Pulmonary vascular diseases occur in a variety of clinical circumstances. In patients with prolonged bed rest, underlying malignancy, or congestive heart failure, dyspnea is the most reliable symptom of pulmonary thromboembolism.[2] Additional symptoms of pulmonary embolism include pleuritic chest pain, hemoptysis, and syncope.[2]

Restrictive Disease

Restrictive lung diseases have variable clinical features. In most patients with idiopathic pulmonary fibrosis, the presentation is insidious, with a progressive course spanning several years. The presenting symptoms[13] generally include a dry cough and a history of episodic dyspnea not associated with exacerbations of asthma, COPD, or congestive heart failure. As the disease progresses, the episodes of nonproductive cough and dyspnea become longer and more frequent, with associated constitutional symptoms such as fatigue, weight loss, and arthralgias.[13] Patients with idiopathic pulmonary fibrosis have a median survival of 5 years after diagnosis.[27]

Simple Smoking

Simple smokers are, by definition, asymptomatic, but they should be questioned carefully as outlined above for symptoms of COPD, asthma, and dyspnea and for pack-years of tobacco use.

Sleep Apnea Syndrome

Patients with sleep apnea syndrome often present with a history of snoring, gasping, and choking while asleep; morning headache; hypersomnolence; impaired daytime performance; intellectual deterioration; or changes in personality. A history from a family member can be helpful. None of these features, however, is invariably present.[18]

PHYSICAL FINDINGS

General Focused Examination

The focused examination should include inspection of the nose, throat, upper airway, neck, chest, spine, and extremities; determination of vital signs; and palpation, percussion, and auscultation of the lungs.[2,24,28] See Chapter 14 for a description of evaluation of the airway.

Inspection

The nose and throat should be inspected carefully because lower respiratory tract diseases often are associated with upper respiratory tract abnormalities. Rhinorrhea and nasal polyps should not be present. The upper airway should be free of tumors, strictures, and inflammation. The trachea should be midline and mobile. An examination of the neck veins (internal jugular) should be performed to estimate the central venous pressure (CVP). When the patient is positioned at 45 degrees above the horizontal, a jugular venous pulse should be 4 cm or less above the sternal angle (corresponding to a CVP of 9 cm of water, the upper limits of normal).[29] Use of accessory muscles of respiration should be noted. The configuration of the chest (e.g., anteroposterior diameter) should be assessed. Chest expansion and whether it is equal bilaterally should also be noted. The ability to blow out a match is a bedside test to reliably estimate forced expiratory flows. Pursed-lipped breathing is abnormal. Kyphoscoliosis should not be present. The extremities should be assessed for the presence of clubbing, cyanosis, and edema.

Vital Signs

Pulsus paradoxus, which is the normal difference in the systolic blood pressure between expiration and inspiration (normally less than 15 mm Hg), should be determined. The respiratory rate should be 12 to 20 breaths per minute.

Palpation

The cardiac apical impulse should be located; it is normally in the left midclavicular line.

Percussion

The chest should be resonant, and the diaphragm should move 2 to 4 cm between maximal inspiration and expiration.

Auscultation

Breath sounds should be equal bilaterally with normal intensity and a lack of adventitious (abnormal) sounds. Wheezing may indicate bronchospasm. Causes of bronchospasm include, but are not limited to, asthma, anaphylaxis (characterized by skin urticaria, upper airway obstruction, cardiovascular collapse), foreign body in the airway (look for altered consciousness as a risk for aspiration), congestive heart failure ("cardiac asthma" with an elevated CVP, a left-sided S_3, peripheral edema), pneumonia (characterized by cyanosis, use of accessory muscles, crackles on examination), and pneumothorax (characterized by decreased breath sounds on one side). The patient should be able to expire the entire vital capacity (forced expiration) in less than 4 seconds and easily blow out a match. Usually a forced expiratory time of longer than 4 seconds denotes airway obstruction. Young, motivated subjects, however, may be able to expire a greater residual volume (exceeding the 4-second limit), and this would reflect normal respiratory function. The heart sounds should be normal with no murmurs or gallops.

Asthma

The upper respiratory tract should be assessed for nasal polyps, inflammation, postnasal drainage, and chronic or acute infection. The overall thoracic configuration should be evaluated for a barrel shape as a sign of hyperinflation. Assessment should be made of inappropriate respiratory muscle use, the neck accessories, intercostal spaces (for bulging) during expiration, and the abdominal muscles during quiet expiration. The CVP should be estimated. An increased CVP, an enlarged liver, and peripheral edema may reflect right heart failure. The value of the CVP assessment in patients with severe expiratory limitation is diminished, however. A pulsus paradoxus of more than 15 mm Hg suggests airflow limitation. When the chest volume is increased due to hyperinflation, the cardiac apical impulse often is displaced toward the xiphoid, is less intense, and is diffused over a wider area. If the percussed sound is more hollow than normal, this hyperresonance may reflect hyperinflation. Hyperinflation leads to flaring of the intercostal and the supraclavicular spaces. Crackles that begin early in inspiration are likely to be associated with airway obstruction. Rhonchi denote large airway secretions. Expiratory wheezing generally occurs in the presence of bronchospasm and is an important finding in asthma. Although wheezing can occur with asthma in both the inspiratory and expiratory phases, inspiratory wheezing may indicate upper airway obstruction. Distant heart sounds may be due to hyperinflation. A loud closure of the pulmonic valve (P_2), a right heart gallop (S_3 or S_4), and murmurs of tricuspid and pulmonary insufficiency suggest pulmonary hypertension and right heart dysfunction (cor pulmonale).

Chronic Obstructive Pulmonary Disease

The principal findings in COPD involve expiratory airflow limitation and are outlined in the section on asthma. One should inspect for pursed-lip breathing, although its significance in perioperative medicine has not been validated. The value of CVP assessment in patients with severe expiratory obstruction is diminished. If distention of neck veins is apparent, however, an additional cause may be superior vena cava obstruction from a coexisting lung cancer, especially if the upper extremity veins are dilatated.

Cystic Fibrosis

The physical findings in cystic fibrosis relate to airflow limitation as outlined in the asthma discussion. One should look for kyphosis and malnutrition by an overall assessment of body habitus (see Chapter 16).

Unexplained Dyspnea

No pathognomonic physical findings are apparent in cases of unexplained dyspnea. The physical findings of severe airflow limitation and right heart failure (cor pulmonale) should be sought as described in the asthma section.

Lung Transplantation

Patients who have undergone lung transplantation should have signs of the previous thoracotomy. If the patient is a unilateral recipient, the chest may be asymmetric. Expect the smaller side to expand more. Breath sounds are shifted from midline by a hyperexpanded native lung crowding the transplanted one. Neck vein distention may reflect right heart failure or pulmonary venous obstruction.[11] The respiratory rate and degree of pulsus paradoxus may indicate airway obstruction or bronchospasm as outlined in the asthma section above. The presence of adventitious (abnormal) breath sounds should be determined. Crackles may suggest infection or rejection, and an isolated wheeze may indicate a bronchial anastomotic stenosis.[11] One must remember that unilateral diseased lung may influence physical findings after single lung transplantation.

Pulmonary Vascular Disease

Pulmonary embolism has few characteristic physical findings.[2] However, tachycardia and tachypnea are almost invariably present. Other physical findings include crackles, arrhythmias, diaphoresis, and wheezing.[2] Cor pulmonale may be present with massive pulmonary embolism (see section on COPD). Findings may include a right ventricular gallop (S_3), a gallop that increases with inspiration, and an accentuated pulmonary valve closure sound (P_2).[2]

Restrictive Lung Disease

Restrictive lung diseases may have various physical findings depending on the cause (e.g., curvature of the spinal column in kyphoscoliosis) and the stage of the process. Early in the course of interstitial lung disease, the physical examination is often unremarkable[13] or only crackles can be heard on auscultation. As interstitial fibrosis progresses, physical findings include tachypnea, finger clubbing, inspiratory crackles, and evidence of cor pulmonale (discussed in the COPD section).[13]

Simple Smoking

The physical examination may be normal for simple smokers, but patients should be evaluated for evidence of COPD, asthma, and dyspnea.

Sleep Apnea

No specific physical findings are diagnostic of patients with sleep apnea. However, obesity, advanced age, and airway shape and size[30] may be suggestive. Assessment of coexisting airflow limitation and signs of right heart failure should be sought, as described in the asthma section.

DIAGNOSTIC TESTING

Chest Radiograph

Although various publications[31–33] can assist the clinician in deciding on preoperative CXR examinations, the patient population is important in determining preoperative policy. See Chapter

2 for recommendations on ordering CXRs. In patients unable to stand, an anteroposterior CXR can be obtained.

Important findings on the CXR include: (a) hyperinflation with flattened diaphragms, decreased vascular markings, and blebs (consistent with COPD), (b) airspace consolidation (an important predictor of ventilation/perfusion, or $\dot{V}/\dot{Q}$, mismatch and hypoxemia), and (c) specific lesions such as tracheal deviation or narrowing (possibly causing dyspnea or difficulty with intubation).[4]

Electrocardiogram

An electrocardiogram (ECG) is not routinely indicated as a screening test before noncardiac surgery in young patients without symptoms, signs, or other disease states associated with cardiopulmonary disease (see Chapters 3 and 4). Patients in whom an ECG would be helpful include (a) asymptomatic, healthy men 40 years or older and women 50 years or older, (b) patients with lung carcinoma, (c) patients having intrathoracic surgery,[21] and (d) patients with severe COPD as defined in Table 5-2.

Electrocardiographic signs of significant pulmonary dysfunction include low voltage and poor R wave progression (due to hyperinflation),[2] right-axis deviation (an axis between 90 and 180 degrees), P pulmonale (characterized by high, peaked P waves 2.5 mm or larger in leads II, III, or a V lead[2]), right ventricular hypertrophy (R/S ratio greater than 1 in lead V_1[2]), and right bundle branch block (sign of pulmonary hypertension).[4]

Arterial Blood Gas Measurement

The indications for preoperative arterial blood gas (ABG) sampling and analysis are imprecisely defined.[31] Room-air ABGs may be indicated in patients being considered for a lung resection and in patients with a history of smoking and associated dyspnea before coronary artery bypass grafting and upper and lower abdominal surgery.[34]

Normal resting values of oxygenation decline with age by 3 to 4 mm Hg per decade after age 20 years. An arterial partial pressure of oxygen (PaO_2) less than 80 mm Hg (at sea level) is abnormal at any age. Hypoxemia suggests significant pulmonary dysfunction and an increased risk for postoperative pulmonary complications. Although classification of hypoxemia based on PaO_2 is arbitrary, a value of 60 to 80 mm Hg usually is indicative of mild hypoxemia; 45 to 59 mm Hg indicates moderate hypoxemia, and less than 45 mm Hg, severe hypoxemia.[35] Likewise, ABG sampling that shows carbon dioxide retention (arterial partial pressure of carbon dioxide, or $PaCO_2$, greater than 45 mm Hg) is a marker of end-stage lung disease and increased dead space ventilation, and suggests that the patient has little or no pulmonary reserve. The patient with an elevated $PaCO_2$ is at increased risk for postoperative pulmonary complications.

Pulmonary Function Tests

PFTs[12] can provide important information about the character and severity of the lung disease. PFTs encountered clinically usually

Table 5-2. Grading the severity of chronic obstructive pulmonary disease (COPD)

	TLC (% predicted)	FEV$_1$/FVC (% predicted)	DLCO (% predicted)	PaO$_2$ (mm Hg)	PaCO$_2$ (mm Hg)	ECG	CXR
Mild COPD	80–99	65–79	65–79	60–79	Normal	Normal	Mild hyperinflation
Moderate COPD	100–119	50–64	50–64	45–59	40–44	Normal (may be signs of pulmonary HTN)	Moderate hyperinflation (may be signs of pulmonary HTN)
Severe COPD	>120	<50	<50	<45	>45	Pulmonary HTN (may be normal)	Severe hyperinflation; signs of pulmonary HTN often present

CXR, chest radiograph; DLCO, diffusing capacity for carbon monoxide; ECG, electrocardiogram; FEV$_1$, forced expiratory volume in 1 second; FVC, forced vital capacity; HTN, hypertension; PaCO$_2$, partial pressure of carbon dioxide; PaO$_2$, partial pressure of oxygen; TLC, total lung capacity. See text for definitions of pulmonary function tests and for description of signs of pulmonary HTN on ECG and CXR.

are obtained from spirometry. Spirometry measures volumes and flow rates of gas expired from total lung capacity (TLC; measured separately, when indicated, by body plethysmography and helium dilution) versus time.

In the forced vital capacity (FVC) maneuver, the patient exhales forcefully and maximally from TLC (the amount of air in the chest after a full inspiratory effort). The FVC is the maximal amount of gas that can be exhaled after a maximal inhalation. The amount of gas exhaled in the first second of the FVC is known as the FEV_1. Although the FVC and the FEV_1 are valuable indicators of lung function (or dysfunction), their ratio is a more sensitive index of airway obstruction. Diffusing capacity for carbon monoxide (DLCO) gives information about the surface area of the lung available for gas exchange (i.e., the amount of functioning capillary bed in contact with functioning alveoli); decreases in the DLCO correlate well with loss of lung tissue secondary to emphysema (see Table 5-2).

In restrictive diseases, spirometry usually demonstrates a decrease in vital capacity and normal or increased expiratory flow rates.[12] TLC and DLCO are less than 80% predicted.

Although PFTs, particularly spirometry, are easy to perform, are informative, and are obtained before many types of surgical operations for the purpose of anticipating perioperative pulmonary complications, they have been shown clearly to assist in decision making in a limited number of situations. One review[36] of many papers indicated that performance of preoperative spirometry before abdominal operations had no relation to postoperative complications because the studies had significant flaws. However, when a history and physical examination uncover a history of cigarette smoking, dyspnea, or evidence of uncharacterized lung disease, preoperative PFTs may assist in making a specific diagnosis and assessing the degree of impairment. PFTs are obtained routinely for patients being evaluated for major lung resection. As no absolute cutoff values have been established for safe surgery at other anatomic sites, routine PFTs cannot be recommended in patients being prepared for other procedures (unless they have independent indications for PFTs such as uncharacterized lung disease).[34] A possible exception to this rule is that spirometry may be indicated in patients with asthma or COPD to assess their baseline function and determine if preoperative therapies have optimized lung function (e.g., maximized FVC). PFTs also are recommended preoperatively to confirm the response to bronchodilator therapy for asthmatic patients and optimization of lung function in patients with COPD.

A general consensus from the literature is that expiratory flow parameters are the most reliable predictors of postoperative pulmonary complications.[37] For example, limited expiratory flow rates (e.g., a peak expiratory flow rate of less than 60 L per minute) indicates severe flow limitation and obstruction due to COPD or asthma[2] and a greater risk for perioperative pulmonary complications. If this level of severity is found, ABG measurements should be obtained, even for patients undergoing nonpulmonary resection surgery, despite the known imperfect relationship between abnormal PFTs and abnormal ABGs.

In some circumstances, patients with suboptimal preparation present for semiurgent surgery. These patients are at a higher risk for postoperative pulmonary complications, a topic addressed in an excellent text on perioperative management.[38]

Specialized Investigations

The preoperative use of chest CT, magnetic resonance imaging, exercise testing to assess maximal oxygen consumption, V/Q scans to select nonperfused regions for resection, and differential bronchospirometry[2,34] are inadequately studied in most types of surgeries except thoracic surgery. Therefore, their use must be highly selective.

PATIENTS AT RISK: IDENTIFICATION AND TREATMENT

Postoperative pulmonary complications are defined rather broadly and inconsistently in different publications. Postoperative pulmonary complications are of various severity and importance but most commonly include atelectasis, tracheobronchial secretion retention, pneumonia, hypoxemia, and acute respiratory failure. Other postoperative complications are bronchospasm and pulmonary embolism. Pulmonary complications have been reported to occur in 5% to 10% of the general surgical population and in up to 22% of preoperatively identified high-risk patients.[39]

Providing an accurate assessment of perioperative pulmonary risk for the patient and surgeon is difficult in many circumstances with no absolutes or systematic reviews for guidance. A rational assessment, however, can usually be made based on the following evidence.

Risk Assessment

History

Both pulmonary and nonpulmonary[40] factors are important in assessing the risks of anesthesia and surgery. Age, obesity, smoking history, type and anatomic location of the anticipated surgical procedure, type and duration of the anesthetic, and coexisting disease (pulmonary and nonpulmonary) can influence perioperative risks.[4,16,39,41]

The risk of perioperative pulmonary complications increases with age for patients older than 60 years. This increased risk is due to the higher prevalence of coexisting nonpulmonary diseases[40] and the effects of aging on the respiratory system (e.g., loss of elastic lung recoil, increased prevalence of functional airway closure, gradual decrease of the maximal expiratory flow, and impairment of the protective airway reflexes).[16]

Obesity increases the risk of pulmonary complications, with the degree of risk proportional to the degree of obesity.[16] A decreased expiratory reserve volume, an increased closing volume, and an increased risk of sleep apnea promote atelectasis and intrapulmonary shunting (resulting in hypoxemia). Decreased postoperative mobility may lead to an increased risk of deep venous thrombosis and pulmonary embolism.

The incidence of perioperative pulmonary complications increases in direct proportion to cigarette consumption above a threshold of 10 pack-years.[16,41] The risks of postoperative atelectasis, pneumonia, hypoxemia, and bronchospasm are increased by cigarette smoking—even in the absence of preoperative symptoms or physical findings.[16,41]

The incidence of pulmonary complications is influenced by the surgical site and type of surgical procedure. The risk of pulmonary complications is increased approximately threefold after a thoracotomy (and increases further after resection of lung tissue) or after nonlaparoscopic upper abdominal surgery.[41] The complication rate after a lung resection is influenced by the severity of COPD, the degree to which the thoracic bellows function is impaired by the surgical procedure, and the amount of functional lung tissue that is resected.[16] Nonabdominal, nonthoracic surgical procedures usually have a low risk of pulmonary complications.[16,41]

The incidence of pulmonary complications is influenced by the type and duration of anesthesia.[16,38,41] Inhaled anesthetic agents, especially if administered in cool, dry gases, decrease mucociliary transport and promote the retention of airway secretions.[16] When possible, administration of general anesthesia without intubation may decrease the risk of postoperative bronchospasm.[39] Shortening the duration of general anesthesia may decrease the risk of a prolonged recovery room or ICU admission.[39] Regional anesthesia may be the best choice for patients with pulmonary disease when the site of operation is peripheral. This seems to be the case almost without exception in those having peripheral nerve blocks. It is known that spinal and epidural anesthesia can be associated with important pulmonary complications.[42,43] The literature had been inconsistent regarding pulmonary complications in patients having spinal or epidural anesthesia due to insufficient numbers of patients in single-institution studies.[42] A metaanalysis, however, has shown that postoperative analgesia with either epidural opioids or local anesthetics improves pulmonary function and decreases the incidence of pulmonary complications compared with the use of systemic opioids after a variety of procedures.[42]

Other factors that may influence the incidence of pulmonary complications include the severity (see Table 5-2) and stability of pulmonary disorders (e.g., a recent increase in productive cough or poorly controlled asthma with wheezing) as well as nonpulmonary factors (e.g., spontaneous or provokable myocardial ischemia or poor exercise tolerance).[39–41]

Physical Examination

Important physical findings suggesting an increased incidence of perioperative pulmonary complications include obesity, cyanosis, tachypnea, pulsus paradoxus when vital signs are measured, displacement of the maximal cardiac impulse toward the xiphoid process, hyperresonance to percussion, prolonged expiration, and wheezing on auscultation.[4]

Diagnostic Testing

Testing must be individualized depending on the complexity of the clinical situation, using guidelines discussed in the diagnostic testing section. In general, indicators of perioperative pulmonary complications in lung resection surgery are related to abnormalities found in PFTs and ABGs. Although no spirometric values exist that absolutely contraindicate abdominal surgery,[41] in general, an FEV_1 of less than 2 L suggests that the patient is at increased risk for pulmonary complications.[16] A paradoxical response[44] or a significantly positive response to bronchodilators may indicate suboptimal control of reactive airway disease (asthma or asthmatic bronchitis) and a greater likelihood of perioperative bronchospasm. For pulmonary resection surgery undertaken without additional testing, an FEV_1 of 2 L or more or greater than 60% of the predicted normal value[45] is preferred for a pneumonectomy and an FEV_1 of 1.5 L for a lobectomy.[16] Other experts suggest different FEV_1 values for pneumonectomy and lobectomy and modify these further depending on whether surgery is performed on the right or left lung. One should keep in mind that predicted postoperative lung function (FEV_1) applies to long-term pulmonary function. The correlation between predicted pulmonary function and actual short-term and long-term pulmonary function after pneumonectomy is good.[46] After lobectomy, however, an early disproportionate loss of pulmonary function occurs, followed by significant improvement with time.[46]

ABGs are often analyzed before surgery in patients with moderate to severe abnormalities on PFTs and in those being evaluated for lung resection.[16] The $PaCO_2$ appears to be the best measure of effective ventilation; $PaCO_2$ values above 45 mm Hg are associated with a high risk of postoperative pulmonary complications, including acute respiratory failure.[4,16]

For patients being evaluated for lung resection who have PFT or ABG abnormalities suggesting an inability to tolerate the proposed removal of the lung, additional specialized tests are often performed. The preferred method to predict residual lung function after lung resection surgery involves the use of quantitative $\dot{V}/\dot{Q}$ lung scanning to clarify the function of the proposed resectable lung in relation to the residual lung.[16] The imaging technique used is the same as in the evaluation of pulmonary embolism and involves the use of inhaled and intravenously injected radionuclides. Instead of focusing on areas with normal ventilation and abnormal perfusion (as in the diagnosis of pulmonary embolism), the total amount of radioactivity is quantitated and the percentages of ventilation and perfusion to each individual lung (or lung region) is determined to predict residual lung function. The FEV_1 from PFTs is obtained and is the only other value needed in this calculation. Residual FEV_1 is predicted by multiplying the FEV_1 by the percentage of radioactive counts from the nonoperative lung (or lung region) and can be calculated[2] as follows:

$$\text{Predicted postoperative } FEV_1 = FEV_1 \times [(\text{radioactive counts in nonoperative lung})/(\text{total counts from both lungs})]$$

Thus, for a patient being assessed for a pneumonectomy who has a preoperative FEV_1 of 1.8 L and a quantitativee $\dot{V}/\dot{Q}$ scan with 60% to the nonoperative lung, one would predict that after pneumonectomy the patient would have an FEV_1 of 1.8 L × 0.6 (60%) or 1.1 L.

A calculated predicted postoperative FEV_1 of at least 0.8 L[16] or more than 40% of the predicted normal value[45] suggests that the patient has sufficient lung tissue to tolerate the procedure.[41] Debate exists, however, as to whether an FEV_1 of less than 0.8 L contraindicates a lung resection.[41] A cutoff value of 0.6 L may be more appropriate given improvements in perioperative support techniques.[41] Of note, selection criteria for patients being evaluated for lung volume reduction surgery may differ from those for patients being considered for resection of more functional lung tissue; at present, however, determination of specific criteria awaits the results of ongoing multicenter trials.[7] A low predicted postoperative FEV_1 remains a marker for a high risk of perioperative pulmonary complications.[41] Determination of diffusion capacity and measurement of exercise-related oxygen uptake hold promise for better risk stratification in this patient population,[45] but at the present time insufficient data exist to generally recommend these tests.[45]

Summary

Pulmonary factors alone cannot precisely predict the likelihood of perioperative pulmonary complications. A comprehensive medical assessment[40] should be performed to assist in predicting a patient's risk of perioperative complications. Composite scoring systems, such as the modified Shapiro classification of perioperative risk (Table 5-3) and the ASA-PS, seem to be better predictors of postoperative pulmonary complications than PFTs alone, probably because they include both pulmonary and nonpulmonary factors,[39] especially cardiac disease[47] with ASA-PS scores of 3, 4, and 5 associated with increased perioperative complications.

Risk Modification

The risk of perioperative pulmonary complications can be decreased through a program of preoperative therapy (Table 5-4). Assessment of the success of such therapy and reassessment of risk may be indicated after several days or weeks of a therapeutic program if the patient's clinical condition (e.g., a pneumonia under treatment) warrants this and the surgical condition allows a delay.

Although therapeutic programs need to be individualized, they often consist of preoperatively teaching respiratory maneuvers such as deep breathing, coughing, and selective use of intermittent positive-pressure breathing[48] that will be used postoperatively. Cessation of smoking for at least 8 weeks,[15] bronchodilator therapy to reduce wheezing, and measures to control tracheobronchial secretions and infection can reduce the incidence and severity of perioperative pulmonary complications.[16,41] Intraoperative and postoperative measures can also reduce pulmonary complications and are discussed in the following sections.

Preoperative Plans

Figure 5-1 shows an algorithm for an approach, discussed in detail above, to preoperatively identify patients at risk for perioperative pulmonary complications and suggests prophylactic measures to decrease these risks. In this section, premedication is discussed.

The goals of premedication are to optimize pulmonary function, allay anxiety, and facilitate a smooth induction of anesthesia.[4] Oxygen therapy, if required preoperatively, should be

Table 5-3. Shapiro's classification of perioperative risk based on preoperative factors

Test results or system reviewed	Points
Expiratory spirogram	
Normal (%FVC + %FEV$_1$/FVC) >150	0
%FVC + %FEV$_1$/FVC = 100–150	1
%FVC + %FEV$_1$/FVC <100	2
Postbronchodilator FEV$_1$/FVC <50%	3
Preoperative FVC <20 mL/kg	3
Cardiovascular system	
Normal	0
Controlled hypertension; MI >2 yr ago	0
Dyspnea on exertion, orthopnea, PND, CHF, angina	1
Nervous system	
Normal	0
Confused, obtunded, agitated, spastic, uncoordinated, bulbar dysfunction	1
Significant muscle weakness	1
Arterial blood gases	
Acceptable	0
PaCO$_2$ >50 mm Hg or PaO$_2$ <60 mm Hg on room air	1
Metabolic pH abnormality, pH >7.50 or <7.30	1
Postoperative ambulation	
Expected within 36 hr	0
Expected to be confined to bed for at least 36 hr	1
Maximum total points	**7**

CHF, congestive heart failure; FEV, forced expiratory volume; FVC, forced vital capacity; MI, myocardial infarction; PaCO$_2$, partial pressure of carbon dioxide; PaO$_2$, partial pressure of oxygen; PND, paroxysmal nocturnal dyspnea.
Adapted with permission from Shapiro BA, Kacmarek RM, Cane RD, et al. *Clinical application of respiratory care,* 4th ed. St. Louis: Mosby–Year Book, 1991:429–432.

Table 5-4. Measures to decrease the risk of postoperative pulmonary complications

Preoperative
   Instruction in respiratory maneuvers
   Smoking cessation
   Bronchodilator administration
   Antibiotic treatment for infections
   Chest physiotherapy
Postoperative
   Lung expansion maneuvers
   Chest physiotherapy
   Epidural analgesia for thoracic incisions, thoracoscopy, and abdominal aortic aneurysm surgery

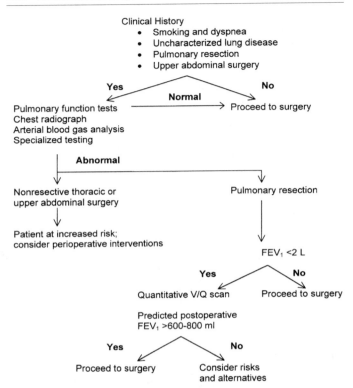

Clinical History
- Smoking and dyspnea
- Uncharacterized lung disease
- Pulmonary resection
- Upper abdominal surgery

Yes / **Normal** / **No**

Pulmonary function tests
Chest radiograph
Arterial blood gas analysis
Specialized testing → Proceed to surgery

Abnormal

Nonresective thoracic or upper abdominal surgery

Patient at increased risk; consider perioperative interventions

Pulmonary resection

FEV_1 <2 L

Yes / **No**

Quantitative V/Q scan / Proceed to surgery

Predicted postoperative FEV_1 >600–800 ml

Yes / **No**

Proceed to surgery / Consider risks and alternatives

Fig. 5-1. Algorithm for risk assessment of perioperative pulmonary complications. (FEV_1, forced expiratory volume in 1 second; V/Q, ventilation/perfusion.) (Modified with permission from Mohr DN, Lavender RC. Preoperative pulmonary evaluation. *Postgrad Med* 1996;100:241–256.)

continued during transport to the operating room. If the patient is receiving bronchodilators or if wheezing is present in an asthmatic patient who is not receiving bronchodilator therapy, then bronchodilators and, on occasion, corticosteroids should be administered preoperatively. In patients with asthma, the risk of intraoperative hypoxemia and other pulmonary complications is reduced if wheezing is eliminated preoperatively.[41] Other pulmonary medications such as inhaled or systemic corticosteroids (see Appendix) may need to be started or continued. If the patient is at risk for aspiration, appropriate medications to alkalinize gastric contents, decrease gastric volume, and increase gastric emptying are recommended. Benzodiazepines and narcotics should be used judiciously (if at all) and are best avoided in patients with sleep apnea or severe pulmonary dysfunction.[4] Corticosteroids may be needed for acute pulmonary exacerbations (bronchospasm)[49,50] or, in "stress doses," (defined in Corticosteroids, below) for those whose hypopituitary-adrenal axis is suppressed from recent corticosteroid therapy (see Chapter 15). The duration of prior corticosteroid therapy, the highest dose given, and the total cumulative dose often are assessed but are imperfect predictors of the severity of bronchospasm or hypopituitary-adrenal suppression. Predicting which patients will experience perioperative adrenal insufficiency is difficult, except that adults receiving only inhaled corticosteroids rarely need systemic corticosteroids in the perioperative period to prevent adrenal insufficiency (see Corticosteroids, below, for specific corticosteroid dosage recommendations to prevent adrenal insufficiency).

Special Anesthetic Considerations

Anesthetic measures that may decrease pulmonary complications include intraoperative control of airway secretions with airway humidification and warming, prevention of aspiration, maintenance of bronchodilation, intermittent hyperinflation of the lungs, shortening of the duration of anesthesia, and avoidance of general anesthesia and tracheal intubation when clinically appropriate (especially in patients with asthma).[16,39]

Less invasive surgical procedures may be selected if the risk of pulmonary complications is high,[41] but evidence to support such an approach is generally lacking. Regional anesthesia, including peripheral nerve blocks or local anesthesia, may be an appropriate choice for patients with significant pulmonary dysfunction if the surgical site is peripheral. Spinal or epidural anesthesia is a reasonable choice for lower extremity surgery of short duration. This approach may not be possible if the patient is unable to lie flat. Regional techniques using high spinal or epidural blockade or neuraxial opioid administration may not always be appropriate because these techniques can be associated with motor blockade of the intercostal muscles and retention of secretions, inability to cough, atelectasis, hypoxemia, dyspnea, and respiratory arrest.[4,18,43] This is especially the case for patients with COPD and an active cough who, in addition to being unable to lie flat, lose intercostal and abdominal muscle use. In addition, if the patient has an increased respiratory rate due to anxiety or dyspnea, this can lead to air trapping with cardiovascular effects (hypotension) as well as worsening gas exchange and respiratory status.

Combined epidural and general anesthesia may be useful in certain surgical procedures (see Case Study that follows). This technique of general anesthesia supplemented with epidural anesthesia and postoperative epidural analgesia ensures airway control, permits intraoperative mechanical ventilation of the lungs and postoperative pain control, and may significantly reduce pulmonary complications.[51,52] This technique, however, has not uniformly been shown to decrease respiratory morbidity[52–54] and does not eliminate the possibility of acute postoperative respiratory failure related to the effects of residual anesthetics on the control of respiration,[19] especially in patients with certain coexisting diseases (e.g., hypothyroidism or sleep apnea).

Patients at high risk for perioperative pulmonary complications should be admitted to a monitored postoperative unit and have pulmonary therapies (see Table 5-4) and pain management therapies instituted expeditiously to decrease the incidence and severity of complications.[4]

Case Study

A 50-year-old man presents for a Nissen repair (esophagogastric fundoplasty) of a hiatal hernia. He has a 40 pack-year smoking history (quitting 4 weeks previously when a theophylline preparation was prescribed for wheezing), a clinical diagnosis of COPD, wheezing, and a hiatal hernia. The patient is unaware of any reflux of gastric contents into the oropharynx or lungs. The rest of the review of systems is negative. He has no drug allergies. His medications include a long-acting theophylline preparation, a histamine$_2$ (H$_2$) blocker, and antacids as needed. His H$_2$ blocker therapy was begun when an endoscopy showed distal esophageal mucosal erosions. He has noted a slight increase in both wheezing and heartburn since taking the theophylline preparation.

On physical examination, he is noted to be of normal weight and breathing comfortably. He has normal vital signs with no pulsus paradoxus. His airway is Mallampati class I (see Chapter 14). His CVP is normal. The maximal cardiac impulse is palpated in the left midclavicular line. The chest is slightly hyperresonant to percussion. Air entry is equal bilaterally, but breath sounds are slightly diminished. Wheezing is noted diffusely, and forced expiratory time is 5 seconds.

A complete blood cell count is normal (hematocrit 46%); a CXR, obtained because of his 40 pack-year tobacco use[55] and because the surgical procedure involves the chest,[31] shows mild hyperinflation; an ECG (obtained because the patient is a man over the age of 40)[31] is normal. Spirometry shows an FEV$_1$ of 3.3 L (66% of normal), an FEV$_1$/FVC ratio of 66%, and a postbronchodilator increase in FEV$_1$ of 15%.

Impression

The patient has mild COPD (FEV$_1$/FVC ratio that is 66% of the predicted value) with a component of airway tone reversibility as shown by a response to bronchodilators. He has a hiatal hernia with reflux by history and by endoscopy, which was noted to involve only the lower portion of the esophagus. The bronchospasm appears due to stimulation of esophageal mucosal receptors ("reflex" bronchoconstriction in response to acid reflux),[56] which is worsened by theophylline[56] and H$_2$ blocker therapy[4] and possibly is secondary to an inflammatory process of the airways.[57] Because this is elective surgery and the patient's care is not optimized, the surgery is postponed for 4 weeks after a thorough discussion with the surgeon and the patient.[58] The patient is told to refrain from smoking (a minimum of 8 weeks of smoking cessation is needed to minimize perioperative pulmonary complications)[15] and discontinue his H$_2$ blocker. H$_2$ blockers may exacerbate bronchospasm in patients with reactive airways because blockade of H$_2$ receptors may result in unopposed H$_1$-mediated bronchoconstriction.[4] He is to stop taking theophylline because it may decrease lower esophageal sphincter tone and promote reflux.[56] He is to begin inhaled steroids on a routine schedule,[57] use a beta$_2$-adrenergic agonist inhaler as needed for wheezing,[1] and begin an H$^+$,K$^+$-adenosinetriphosphatase inhibitor[56] to treat gastric acid reflux. He is scheduled to return in 4 weeks for reevaluation.

Four Weeks Later

The patient returns with much improved symptoms of reflux and no further episodes of wheezing. He has been compliant with his medication regimen and has not smoked for 4 weeks. On physical examination, the only significant change is the absence of wheezing. The patient is instructed to refrain from oral intake after midnight except to take his H^+,K^+-adenosinetriphosphatase inhibitor with a sip of water. He is to continue his corticosteroid inhaler and beta$_2$-adrenergic bronchodilator. He will be given 30 mL of sodium citrate to drink before induction of anesthesia and several inhalations of an anticholinergic medication such as ipratropium bromide[4] or a beta$_2$-adrenergic agonist. General risks related to anesthesia and specific risks related to his gastric reflux (e.g., the possibility of aspiration, pneumonia, and subsequent acute respiratory distress syndrome), his COPD, and reactive airway disease (bronchospasm, need for supplemental oxygen, respiratory failure) should be discussed. Preoperatively he should be taught the respiratory maneuvers (see Table 5-4) he will need to perform postoperatively to decrease pulmonary complications. Epidural placement for postoperative analgesia should be offered. Because he is at risk for pulmonary aspiration, the trachea will need to be intubated with fiberoptic guidance while the patient is awake[59] or after a rapid sequence induction with cricoid pressure. If an awake intubation procedure is selected, it should be discussed with the patient.

Postoperative Management

The patient should be monitored in an ICU or other monitored postoperative unit for complications[4,59] such as atelectasis, aspiration, mediastinal hemorrhage, pneumothorax, hemothorax, hypoxemia, bronchospasm, hypoventilation, recurrent laryngeal nerve injury, esophageal anastomotic leak, and pain.[59]

COMMONLY USED RESPIRATORY MEDICATIONS

Beta-Adrenergic Agonist Drugs

Beta-adrenergic agonist drugs include nonselective drugs with effects on both beta$_1$-adrenergic and beta$_2$-adrenergic receptors (e.g., isoetharine, isoproterenol hydrochloride, epinephrine) and selective beta$_2$-adrenergic agonists (e.g., short-acting albuterol, long-acting salmeterol xinafoate) that avoid cardiac chronotropic and inotropic effects. This class of drugs causes bronchodilatation by augmenting cAMP-mediated relaxation of bronchial smooth muscle. In addition to reversing the bronchospastic component in reactive airway diseases, these drugs may have beneficial effects on mucociliary function. Although inhaled beta-adrenergic agonists have been a common component of management of asthma and COPD (e.g., asthmatic bronchitis) for many years, concern has arisen that their regular use may be detrimental to disease control by increasing airway responsiveness. In addition, they can have adverse cardiovascular and metabolic effects (e.g., hypokalemia) and occasionally precipitate acute bronchospasm. These drugs should be used only when necessary. They remain useful in preventing bronchoconstriction that can be induced by instrumentation of the trachea or inhalation of anesthetic gases.[60,61] The usual dose of albuterol is two inhalations from a metered-dose inhaler (90 mg per activation of the inhaler).[62]

Anticholinergic Drugs

Anticholinergic drugs include glycopyrrolate and ipratropium bromide. These drugs bronchodilate by blocking formation of cyclic guanosine monophosphate (cGMP) and are useful in both asthma and COPD. With the usual bronchodilator doses, no drying of secretions or interference with mucociliary clearance occurs. Although their onset of action is slower than that of beta agonists, the effects last longer. They are particularly effective in preventing reflex bronchoconstriction due to intubation of the trachea.[63,64] Usual doses of nebulized glycopyrrolate are 0.4 to 0.8 mg by nebulizer.[4] For ipratropium bromide, the usual dose is two puffs from a metered-dose inhaler.[4]

Methylxanthines

The methylxanthines aminophylline and theophylline are commonly used drugs in the management of chronic airway diseases. Although several mechanisms explain their antiinflammatory, immunomodulatory, and bronchodilator actions, nonspecific inhibition of phosphodiesterase isoenzymes (which increases cAMP) and nonselective antagonism of adenosine receptors are likely to be the most important. Because of frequent undesirable side effects (nausea, tachycardia, arrhythmias), a low toxic to therapeutic dose ratio, and a lack of objective efficacy data, their perioperative use should be individualized. Adding a volatile anesthetic and administering beta agonists or anticholinergics are more efficacious therapies for intraoperative and perioperative bronchospasm than use of methylxanthines.[65] Doses of theophylline are in the range of 300 to 1,500 mg per day.[4]

Cromolyn Sodium and Nedocromil Sodium

The mechanisms of action of **cromolyn sodium** and **nedocromil sodium** are not fully defined. They are known to stabilize mast cell membranes and blunt the acute release of preformed bronchospastic mediators. They are of no utility in the acute management of bronchospasm and have limited perioperative use[4,60]; no "usual" dose is recommended.

Leukotriene Receptor Antagonists

Leukotriene receptor antagonists and inhibitors of leukotriene synthesis are medications with antiinflammatory effects that have been approved for prophylaxis and maintenance treatment of chronic asthma.[66–70] Evidence suggests that blocking leukotriene effects on specific receptors and blocking the formation of leukotrienes are effective clinical strategies in the treatment of some patients with asthma. Specific recommendations for the perioperative use of these drugs cannot be made[67] because a specific benefit has not been determined.[66]

Corticosteroids

Steroids are often used in the short term and over the long term by patients with respiratory diseases. Inflammation is present even in patients with mild asthma, and inhaled corticosteroids are used on a long-term basis for patients with all degrees of disease severity. Virtually all asthma outcome parameters, including hospitalization rates, are improved with the use of inhaled corticosteroids.[71] Occasionally, patients with asthma or asthmatic bronchitis are treated with short bursts or long-term oral (systemic) corticosteroids due to treatment failure of other drugs, including inhaled corticosteroids. Chronic systemic corticosteroid use may cause adverse metabolic, endocrine, and infection-related effects. Even short courses of oral and inhaled corticosteroids are associated with rare systemic problems (glucose intolerance, psychosis).[1]

Although the mechanisms of action of corticosteroids in the lung are complex and incompletely defined, these drugs reduce airway inflammation and hyperresponsiveness, mucus secretion, smooth muscle constriction, and edema, at least in part by decreasing the numbers of eosinophils, T cells, and mast cells, and modulate β receptor responsiveness and cytokine gene expression within the bronchial mucosa.[72] Corticosteroids inhibit the formation of inflammatory leukotrienes. Although augmentation of bronchodilator sensitivity may occur rapidly (within an hour) after intravenous administration of corticosteroids,[73] full clinical effects may not be seen for several hours.

Perioperatively, corticosteroids are given to treat bronchospasm and for adrenal replacement in many patients who have recently taken these medications. Glucocorticoid administration should be based on the severity of asthma, previous corticosteroid use, magnitude of the surgical stress, and the known glucocorticoid production rate associated with that anticipated degree of stress and should be augmented if postoperative complications occur. In patients with poorly controlled asthma, administration of corticosteroids is often indicated to control and reduce bronchospasm before surgery. Corticosteroids used selectively in the perioperative period have been shown to be efficacious and have low complication rates.[74] Usual doses in the perioperative period are 40 to 50 mg of intravenous methylprednisolone every 4 to 6 hours.[4]

A consensus paper[75] makes concise recommendations for the dose and duration of parenteral corticosteroid supplementation for "stress dose replacement." For a minor stress, a total dose of 25 mg, given preoperatively, is recommended; for moderate stress, 50 to 75 mg is recommended, and for major stress, up to 150 mg of hydrocortisone should be given for 1 to 3 days.[75,76] These doses and durations are substantially less than the usual dose of 100 mg of hydrocortisone every 8 hours, which was based on empirically derived recommendations[4] (see Chapter 15).

Hypopituitary-adrenal suppression is very rarely reported in patients who receive inhaled corticosteroids via pressurized metered-dose inhalers[76] with usual doses of 168 to 840 μg of beclomethasone dipropionate or 400 μg of budesonide daily.[77] Withholding additional perioperative corticosteroids during minor or moderate surgical procedures appears to be safe in these patients, as long as their clinical course is uncomplicated.[76]

Mucolytics

Medications ranging from nebulized saline to acetylcysteine and deoxyribonuclease are used to decrease mucus viscosity and facilitate mobilization and expectoration of retained airway secretions. These medications are commonly used in CF patients.[4,8]

Miscellaneous and Experimental Drugs

Numerous medications approved for other indications, such as magnesium, methotrexate sodium, colchicine, and cyclosporine, are occasionally used in patients with various lung disorders, including idiopathic pulmonary fibrosis,[26] and in patients whose bronchospasm is inadequately controlled by or intolerant of the usual pulmonary medications listed above. These medications and other novel therapies undergoing investigation, such as inhaled nitric oxide for patients with asthma[60] and pulmonary hypertension, have considerable potential as therapy for respiratory diseases and in the future may be proven clinically useful.[78]

REFERENCES

1. Rees J, Price J, eds. *ABC of asthma*, 3rd ed. Nailsea, England: British Medical Journal Publishing Group, 1995:1–46.
2. George RB, Light RW, Matthay MA, Matthay RA. *Chest medicine*, 2nd ed. Baltimore: Williams & Wilkins, 1990:1–494.
3. Folkerts G, Busse WW, Nijkamp FP, et al. Virus-induced airway responsiveness and asthma. *Am J Respir Crit Care Med* 1998; 157:1708–1720.
4. Shepherd KE. Specific considerations with pulmonary disease. In: Hurford WE, Bailin MT, Davison JK, et al., eds. *Clinical anesthesia procedures of the Massachusetts General Hospital*, 5th ed. New York: Lippincott–Raven Publishers, 1997:35–46.
5. American Thoracic Society Medical Section of the American Lung Association. Standards for the diagnosis and care of patients with chronic obstructive pulmonary disease (COPD) and asthma. *Am Rev Respir Dis* 1987;136:225–244.
6. Repine JE, Bast A, Lankhorst I. The Oxidative Stress Study Group. Oxidative stress in chronic obstructive pulmonary disease. *Am J Respir Crit Care Med* 1997;156:341–357.
7. Senior RM, Anthonisen NR. Chronic obstructive pulmonary disease (COPD). *Am J Respir Crit Care Med* 1998;157:S139–S147.
8. Davis PB, Drumm M, Konstan MW. Cystic fibrosis. *Am J Respir Crit Care Med* 1996;154:1229–1256.
9. Gillespie DJ, Staats BA. Unexplained dyspnea. *Mayo Clin Proc* 1994;69:657–663.
10. Manning HL, Schwartzstein RM. Pathophysiology of dyspnea. *N Engl J Med* 1995;333:1547–1553.

11. Trulock EP. Lung transplantation. *Am J Respir Crit Care Med* 1997;155:789–818.
12. Clausen JL. Pulmonary function testing. In: Bordow RA, Moser KA, eds. *Manual of clinical problems in pulmonary medicine*, 2nd ed. Boston: Little, Brown and Company, 1985:9–17.
13. Edwards P. Obstructive and restrictive diseases. In: Murray MJ, Coursin DB, Pearl RG, Prough DS, eds. *Critical care medicine: perioperative medicine*. New York: Lippincott–Raven Publishers, 1997:427–439.
14. Katzenstein ALA, Myers JL. Idiopathic pulmonary fibrosis: clinical relevance of pathologic classification. *Am J Respir Crit Care Med* 1998;157:1301–1315.
15. Egan TD, Wong KC. Perioperative smoking cessation and anesthesia: a review. *J Clin Anesth* 1992;4:63–72.
16. Okeson, GC. Pulmonary dysfunction and surgical risk. *Postgrad Med* 1983;74:75–83.
17. Research identifies gender differences in COPD and sleep apnea. *Pulm Rev* 1998;3:22.
18. Ostermeier AM, Roisen MF, Hautkappe M, et al. Three sudden postoperative respiratory arrests associated with epidural opioids in patients with sleep apnea. *Anesth Analg* 1997;85:452–460.
19. Dahan A. General anesthesia and control of respiration. *Semin Anesth* 1996;15:328–334.
20. Strohl KP, Redline S. Recognition of obstructive sleep apnea. *Am J Respir Crit Care Med* 1996;154:279–289.
21. Macklem PT. The mechanics of breathing. *Am J Respir Crit Care Med* 1998;157:S88–S94.
22. Sackett DL, Rennie D. The science of the art of clinical examination. *JAMA* 1992;267:2650–2652.
23. Annemie M, Schols WJ, Slangen J, et al. Weight loss is a reversible factor in the prognosis of chronic obstructive pulmonary disease. *Am J Respir Crit Care Med* 1998;157:1791–1797.
24. Holleman DR, Simel DL. Does the clinical examination predict airflow limitation? *JAMA* 1995;273:313–319.
25. Gal TJ. Bronchial hyperresponsiveness and anesthesia: physiologic and therapeutic perspectives. *Anesth Analg* 1994;78:559–573.
26. American Thoracic Society. International guidelines for the selection of lung transplant candidates. *Am J Respir Crit Care Med* 1998;158:335–339.
27. Douglas WW, Ryu JH, Swensen SJ, et al. Colchicine versus prednisolone in the treatment of idiopathic pulmonary fibrosis. *Am J Respir Crit Care Med* 1998;158:220–225.
28. Pasterkamp H, Krahan SS, Wodica GR. Respiratory sounds. *Am J Respir Crit Care Med* 1997;156:974–987.
29. Cook DJ, Simel DL. Does this patient have abnormal central venous pressure? *JAMA* 1996;275:630–634.
30. Leiter JC. Upper airway shape. Is it important in the pathogenesis of obstructive sleep apnea? *Am J Respir Crit Care Med* 1996;153:894–898.
31. Sox HC. *Common diagnostic tests: use and interpretation*, 2nd ed. Philadelphia: American College of Physicians, 1990:1–441.
32. Archer C, Levy AR, McGregor M. Value of routine perioperative chest x-rays: a meta-analysis. *Can J Anaesth* 1993;40:1022–1027.
33. Sagel SS, Evens RG, Forrest JV, Bramson RT. Efficacy of routine screening and lateral chest radiographs in a hospital-based population. *N Engl J Med* 1974;291:1001–1004.
34. Zibrac JD, O'Donnell CR, Marton K. Indications for pulmonary function testing. *Ann Intern Med* 1990;112:763–771.
35. Tisi GM, Menn SJ. Evaluation of arterial blood gases and acid-base homeostasis. In: Bordow RA, Moser KM, eds. *Manual of clinical problems in pulmonary medicine*, 2nd ed. Boston: Little, Brown and Company, 1985:24–28.
36. Lawrence VA, Page CP, Harris GD. Preoperative spirometry before abdominal surgery. *Arch Intern Med* 1989;149:280–285.

37. Tisi GM. Preoperative identification and evaluation of the patient with lung disease. *Med Clin North Am* 1987;71:399–412.
38. Murray MJ, Coursin DB, Pearl RG, Prough DS. *Critical care medicine: perioperative management*. New York: Lippincott–Raven Publishers, 1997:1–794.
39. Wong DH, Weber EC, Schell MJ, et al. Factors associated with postoperative pulmonary complications in patients with severe chronic pulmonary disease. *Anesth Analg* 1995;80:276–284.
40. Merli GJ, Weitz HH. Approaching the surgical patient: role of the medical consultant. *Clin Chest Med* 1993;14:205–210.
41. Mohr DN, Lavender RC. Preoperative pulmonary evaluation. *Postgrad Med* 1996;100:241–256.
42. Ballantyne JC, Carr DB, deFerranti S, et al. The comparative effects of postoperative analgesic therapies on pulmonary outcome: cumulative meta-analyses of randomized, controlled trials. *Anesth Analg* 1998;86:598–612.
43. Wang CY, Ong GSY. Severe bronchospasm during epidural anaesthesia. *Anaesthesia* 1993;48:514–515.
44. Shepherd KE, Johnson DC. Bronchodilator testing: an analysis of paradoxical responses. *Respir Care* 1988;33:667–671.
45. American Thoracic Society/European Respiratory Society. Pretreatment evaluation of non-small-cell lung cancer. *Am J Respir Crit Care Med* 1997;156:320–332.
46. Ali MK, Mountain CF, Ewer MS, et al. Predicting loss of pulmonary function after pulmonary resection for bronchogenic carcinoma. *Chest* 1980;77:337–342.
47. Hurford WE, Lynch KE, Strauss HW, et al. Myocardial perfusion as assessed by thallium-201 scintigraphy during the discontinuation of mechanical ventilation in ventilator-dependent patients. *Anesthesiology* 1991;74:1007–1016.
48. The Intermittent Positive Pressure Breathing Trial Group. Intermittent positive pressure breathing therapy of chronic obstructive pulmonary disease. *Ann Intern Med* 1983;99:612–620.
49. McFadden ER Jr. Dosages of corticosteroids in asthma. *Am Rev Respir Dis* 1993;147:1306–1310.
50. Corbridge TC, Hall JB. The assessment and management of adults with status asthmaticus. *Am J Respir Crit Care Med* 1995;151:1296–1316.
51. Yeager MP, Glass DD, Neff RK, et al. Epidural anesthesia and analgesia in high-risk surgical patients. *Anesthesiology* 1987;66:729–736.
52. Christopherson R, Norris EJ. Regional versus general anesthesia. *Anesthesiol Clin North Am* 1997;15:37–47.
53. Baron JF, Bertrand M, Barre E, et al. Combined epidural and general anesthesia versus general anesthesia for abdominal aortic surgery. *Anesthesiology* 1991;75:611–618.
54. Christopherson R, Beattie C, Frank SM, et al. Perioperative morbidity in patients randomized to epidural or general anesthesia for lower extremity vascular surgery: perioperative ischemia randomized anesthesia trial group. *Anesthesiology* 1993;79:422–434.
55. Sweitzer BJ, Palmer-Toy DE, Einaudi EM, Bitzer AM. Guidelines for preoperative laboratory testing: report of an MGH Task Force. *Turnaround Times* 1996;5:13–19.
56. Pope CE II. Acid-reflux disorders. *N Engl J Med* 1994;331:656–660.
57. Paggiaro PL, Dahle R, Bakran I, et al. Multicentre randomised placebo-controlled trial of inhaled fluticasone propionate in patients with chronic obstructive pulmonary disease. *Lancet* 1998;351:773–780.
58. Quill TE, Brody H. Physician recommendations and patient autonomy: finding a balance between physician power and patient choice. *Ann Intern Med* 1996;125:763–769.
59. Oberhelman HA. Esophageal surgery. In: Jaffe RA, Samuels SI, eds. *Anesthesiologist's manual of surgical procedures*. New York: Lippincott–Raven Publishers, 1996:291–304.

60. Peterfreund RA. Pathophysiology and treatment of asthma. *Curr Opin Anaesth* 1994;7:284–292.
61. Weinberger M, Hendeles L. Theophylline in asthma. *N Engl J Med* 1996;334:1380–1388.
62. Nelson HS. Beta-adrenergic bronchodilators. *N Engl J Med* 1995;333:499–506.
63. Wu SC, Hildebrandt J, Isner PD, et al. Efficacy of anticholinergic and β-adrenergic agonist treatment of maximal cholinergic bronchospasm in tracheally intubated rabbits. *Anesth Analg* 1992;75:777–783.
64. Walker FB, Kaiser DL, Kowal MB, Suratt PM. Prolonged effect of glycopyrrolate in asthma. *Chest* 1987;91:49–51.
65. Siafakas NM, Stoubou A, Haviaras V. Effect of aminophylline on respiratory muscle strength after upper abdominal surgery: a double blind study. *Thorax* 1993;48:693–697.
66. O'Byrne PM, Israel E, Drazen JM. Antileukotrienes in the treatment of asthma. *Ann Intern Med* 1997;127:472–480.
67. Horowitz RJ, Mcgill KA, Busse WW. The role of leukotriene modifiers in the treatment of asthma. *Am J Respir Crit Care Med* 1998;157:1363–1371.
68. Calhoun WJ. Summary of trials with zafirlukast. *Am J Respir Crit Care Med* 1998;157:S238–S246.
69. Drazen J. Clinical pharmacology of leukotriene receptor antagonists and lipoxygenase inhibitors. *Am J Respir Crit Care Med* 1998;157:S233–S237.
70. Montelukast for persistent asthma. *Med Lett* 1998;40:71–73.
71. Blais L, Ernest P, Boivin JF, Suissa S. Inhaled corticosteroids and the prevention of readmission to hospital for asthma. *Am J Respir Crit Care Med* 1998;158:126–132.
72. Bentley AM, Hamid Q, Robinson DS, et al. Prednisolone treatment in asthma. *Am J Respir Crit Care Med* 1996;153:551–556.
73. Tan KS, Grove A, McLean A, et al. Systemic corticosteroid rapidly reverses bronchodilator subsensitivity induced by formoterol in asthmatic patients. *Am J Respir Crit Care Med* 1997;156:28–35.
74. Kabalin CS, Yarnold PR, Grammer LC. Low complication rate of corticosteroid-treated asthmatics undergoing surgical procedures. *Arch Intern Med* 1995;155:1379–1384.
75. Salem M, Tainsh RE, Bromberg J, et al. Perioperative glucocorticoid coverage: a reassessment 42 years after emergence of a problem. *Ann Surg* 1994;219:416–425.
76. Lamberts SWJ, Bruning HA, de Jong FH. Corticosteroid therapy in severe illness. *N Engl J Med* 1997;337:1285–1292.
77. van der Molen T, Meyboom-de Jong B, Mulder HH, Postma DS. Starting with a higher dose of inhaled corticosteroids in primary asthma treatment. *Am J Respir Crit Care Med* 1998;158:121–125.
78. Scientific Advisory Council of the American Lung Association/American Thoracic Society. Update: future directions for research on diseases of the lung. *Am J Respir Crit Care Med* 1998;158:320–334.

Endocrine Disorders

Stephanie L. Lee and Robert A. Peterfreund

Patients frequently present for preoperative evaluation with endocrine conditions (e.g., thyroid disorders) as the primary reason for surgery. More commonly, concomitant endocrine disease (e.g., diabetes mellitus) complicates anesthetic and surgical management of a patient. Although fulminant, life-threatening manifestations of endocrine disease are unusual, physiologic perturbations in the perioperative period may precipitate endocrine crises. These can contribute to intraoperative and postoperative morbidity and mortality. To anticipate and prevent perioperative complications from an endocrine disorder, underlying conditions should be thoroughly evaluated before surgery.

DIABETES MELLITUS

Diabetes mellitus (DM) is the condition of a relative or absolute lack of insulin, which leads to hyperglycemia and other metabolic abnormalities. Although all tissues are potentially affected by DM, atherosclerotic vascular, renal, and nervous system effects are of greatest relevance to the anesthesiologist.

Two types of DM have been generally recognized. *DM type 1*, also known as *insulin-dependent, juvenile-onset,* or *ketosis prone DM*, is characterized by immune-mediated destruction of the pancreatic β cells that produce insulin. Patients depend on exogenous insulin to regulate metabolism. These patients tend to present at younger ages, are not obese, and have normal sensitivity to insulin. Lack of insulin may precipitate diabetic ketoacidosis, a complex and potentially life-threatening metabolic derangement. In *DM type 2*, also known as *adult-onset* or *non–insulin dependent DM*, target cells are resistant to insulin. The pancreas is relatively deficient in insulin secretion. Patients take medications that enhance the release of endogenous insulin, increase sensitivity to the effect of insulin on target cells, reduce hepatic production of glucose, or decrease absorption of carbohydrates by the intestine. They may require insulin (in large doses) because of tissue resistance to the glucose-lowering effects of insulin. These patients tend to be obese and of older age. They are prone not to diabetic ketoacidosis but rather to hyperglycemic hyperosmolarity. A third class of diabetic patients comprise a group intermediate to those with the traditional type 1 and type 2 DM. These patients have partial autoimmune destruction or surgical removal of insulin-producing cells but generate enough insulin to prevent diabetic ketoacidosis under normal conditions.

Hyperglycemia may result from other conditions affecting the pancreas, such as hemochromatosis and chronic pancreatitis. Other endocrine derangements, including pheochromocytoma, glucagonoma, acromegaly, hyperthyroidism, and adrenal gluco-corticoid excess promote hyperglycemia. Stressful situations such as surgery elevate the levels of counterregulatory hormones (catecholamines, growth hormone, cortisol), resulting in a signifi-cant increase in resistance to insulin-mediated glucose disposal that may last for several days.

Interview and History

The cause of a patient's hyperglycemia (DM types 1 and 2, other endocrinopathy) should be specifically identified by the his-tory. The preoperative evaluation must elicit details about the hyperglycemic condition, including the extent of involvement of other organ systems and the medical regimen followed by the patient. The patient should be questioned about symptoms attributable to cerebrovascular, cardiovascular, and peripheral vascular disease. Patients with DM may not experience classic cardiac chest pain but rather may be prone to "silent" myocardial ischemia. The interviewer should have a high index of suspicion for an ischemic cardiac condition in a diabetic patient with long-standing disease or other risk factors for cardiovascular disease (peripheral vascular disease, smoking, hypertension, elevated cholesterol, family history). Symptoms attributable to diabetic autonomic neuropathy (orthostatic hypotension, spastic bladder, gastroparesis) should be elicited. Any history of diabetic ketoaci-dosis (type 1 DM) or hyperglycemic, hyperosmolar coma (type 2 DM) should be ascertained. Patients should be questioned about the frequency, severity, and symptoms of hypoglycemic episodes. Some patients with long-standing type 1 DM in tight control have repeated episodes of asymptomatic hypoglycemia and failure of counterregulatory mechanisms that results in *hypoglycemic unawareness*, even when blood glucose levels are dangerously low. Particularly in patients with type 2 DM, complicating inter-current conditions such as hypertension, hyperlipidemia, or obe-sity should be ascertained.

Physical Examination

The physical examination begins with an assessment of body habitus (height, weight) and vital signs. Orthostatic changes in blood pressure and heart rate, and loss of beat-to-beat heart rate variation with respiration may indicate autonomic nervous sys-tem dysfunction. Patients with peripheral vascular disease often exhibit discrepancies in blood pressure at different sites of mea-surement. Blood pressures in both arms should be compared. Examination of peripheral pulses (presence or absence, quality, bruits) provides information about vascular pathology and infor-mation for planning invasive monitoring cannulation sites. In the obese patient, peripheral venous cannulation sites and anatomic landmarks for nerve blocks may be difficult to identify, and these should be noted. DM patients are prone to skin lesions from infection or ischemia. Because of positioning considerations dur-ing surgery, the location of skin lesions should be documented.

Cutaneous lesions overlying sites for nerve blocks may eliminate some options for regional anesthesia. Preexisting sensory deficits may complicate attempts to assess the adequacy of a regional anesthetic.

Diagnostic Testing

Minimum testing includes electrocardiography (ECG), measurement of glucose and electrolyte levels, and a complete blood cell count. The preoperative ECG provides information about ischemic cardiac disease and serves as a baseline for comparison should cardiovascular or hemodynamic complications develop. An electrolyte panel provides information about volume, osmolarity and acid-base status, glycemic control, and renal function. Additional testing may include measurement of hemoglobin A_{1C} or total glycosylated hemoglobin levels to evaluate glucose control over the preceding 3 months. The desired level is 1% or less above normal and indicates good long-term control. Higher levels suggest possible poor patient compliance or the need for adjustment of the medical regimen. With conventional therapies, hemoglobin A_{1C} levels are within the normal range only when diabetics under tight control experience frequent episodes of hypoglycemia.

The history, physical examination, and minimum laboratory data may indicate that more extensive testing is needed. Diabetic patients with peripheral vascular disease as a surgical or comorbid condition commonly have coronary or neurovascular disease, and vice versa. Detailed cardiac evaluations (stress testing, angiography, etc.) or vascular evaluations (pressure or flow studies, angiography) may be indicated before surgery.

Preoperative Medication and Instructions

Diabetics often have complex medical regimens. Compliance with preoperative instructions may be problematic, particularly when drug dosing (e.g., the insulin regimen) is altered. Providing written instructions for the patient coming to the hospital on the day of surgery is useful. Patients with severe diabetic retinopathy or cataracts, however, may not be able to read instructions handwritten in typical physician fashion.

Patients treated for other conditions such as hypertension or angina should be instructed to take their regular medications before coming to the hospital on the day of surgery. Diabetics with gastroparesis may benefit from preoperative administration of metoclopramide, perhaps with a histamine$_2$ (H_2) antagonist. Patients unable to take oral medications can be treated with parenteral substitutes (topical nitrates, intravenous beta-adrenergic blockers, calcium channel blockers, H_2 antagonists).

Management of the hypoglycemic regimen is far more complicated. Hypoglycemia, with symptoms possibly masked by concurrent use of beta-adrenergic blockers, is a potential complication in patients taking nothing by mouth for extended periods. Classically, patients treated with oral hypoglycemic agents have been instructed to discontinue their use before surgery, with the last dose taken on the preceding day. Use of sulfonylurea agents with very long half-lives (e.g., chlorpropamide) is associated with hypoglycemia in the fasting patient. These drugs should be stopped several days in advance of elective surgery, and shorter acting agents (e.g., glipizide or repaglinide) should be used. Newer oral agents (acarbose, metformin hydrochloride, troglitazone) used as single-agent therapy do not carry a risk of hypoglycemia in the fasting patient and do not need to be shaped before surgery (Table 6-1).

Management of patients on insulin is complex. For patients hospitalized before surgery, the typical recommendation is first to establish an intravenous line containing dextrose (D_5) and then to administer subcutaneously one-third to one-half of the usual morning dose of long-acting insulin preparations such as insulin zinc suspension (Lente insulin) or isophane insulin suspension (NPH insulin) to the fasting patient. The usual dose of short-acting insulins (regular, lispro) should be held. Further control can be achieved using finger-stick blood glucose determinations combined with a sliding scale regimen of regular insulin (administered subcutaneously every 4 to 6 hours).

An alternative recommendation is simultaneous intravenous infusion of glucose and regular insulin. Unlike intermittent subcutaneous injections of long-acting insulins, which may have varied absorption depending on the perfusion state, continuous intravenous infusion allows rapid adjustment of doses. Most adult type 2 diabetic patients can be maintained at a blood glucose level of 120 to 180 mg per dL with an infusion of regular insulin at 1 to 2 units per hour with an intravenous drip of D_5-containing fluid at 100 mL per hour. The dose of insulin may vary threefold to fivefold depending on other factors that raise insulin requirements (e.g., steroid therapy, obesity, infection). Renal insufficiency reduces insulin requirements.

Patients prone to diabetic ketoacidosis (those with type 1 DM) or patients known to be particularly susceptible to hypoglycemia probably should be admitted to the hospital before the day of surgery. The medical regimen should be designed in consultation with the patient's primary care physician or endocrinologist. Simultaneous intravenous infusion of glucose and insulin is the best way to maintain glucose in the desired range of 120 to 180 mg per dL. Patients presenting to the hospital on the day of surgery should take one-half of the usual morning dose of long-acting insulin. The short-acting insulins should not be administered. No additional insulin is necessary for 6 to 8 hours unless the patient becomes hyperglycemic. To avoid diabetic ketoacidosis, patients must receive additional insulin after 6 to 8 hours, even if they are still fasting and have normal blood sugar levels.

Implications for Perioperative and Anesthetic Management

In general, patients with DM should be the first cases of the day. This minimizes the time patients must take nothing by mouth and hastens their return to a routine diet and medical regimen. Glucose determinations are indicated for any fasting diabetic patient, but especially for patients who take their hypoglycemic medications. Concurrent use of beta-adrenergic antagonists, heavy sedation, or general anesthesia may mask signs or symptoms of hypoglycemia. Determinations of serum glucose level intraoperatively and in the recovery area should be considered.

Table 6-1. Agents used to treat diabetes mellitus

Agent	Time to onset (h)	Peak (h)	Duration of action (h)
Insulin (subcutaneous administration)			
Lispro (Humalog)	≤ 0.25	1	3.5–4.5
Regular	0.5–1.0	1–5	5–8
Prompt insulin zinc suspension (Semilente)	0.5–3.0	2–10	12–16
Isophane insulin suspension (NPH)	1–4	4–12	24–28
Insulin zinc suspension (Lente)	1–3	6–15	22–28
Protamine zinc	1–6	14–24	≥ 36
Extended insulin zinc suspension (Ultralente)	2–8	10–30	≥ 36
Sulfonylurea[a]			
Tolbutamide (Orinase, Oramide)	1		6–12
Glipizide (Glucotrol)	1		6–12
Glipizide XL	1–4		10–24
Acetohexamide (Dymelor)	1		8–12
Tolazamide (Tolinase)	4–6		10–15
Glyburide (Micronase, DiaBeta)	1–4		10–24
Glimepiride (Amaryl)	1		18–24
Chlorpropamide (Diabinese)	1		24–72
α-Glucosidase inhibitor[b,c]			
Acarbose (Precose)	Immediate		<0.3
Biguanide[c,d]			
Metformin hydrochloride (Glucophage)	1		8–12
Thiazolidinedione[c,d]			
Troglitazone (Rezulin)	1		24
Rosaglitazone (Avandia)	1		24
Pioglitazone (Actos)	1		24
Meglitinide[a,e]			
Repaglinide (Prandin)	≤ 0.25	1	3–4

[a]Increases insulin secretion.
[b]Nonsystemic. Delays digestion and absorption of complex carbohydrates from the intestine.
[c]When used as the *sole agent* for treatment, hypoglycemia (insulin reaction) is unlikely; may be taken on the morning of surgery.
[d]Inhibits hepatic glucose production and/or increases peripheral tissue sensitivity to insulin. No increase in insulin secretion.
[e]Closes adenosine triphosphate–dependent potassium channels, depolarizing pancreatic β cells and leading to calcium channel opening and enhanced insulin release. Nonsulfonylurea.

The anesthetic plan should consider the risks posed by cardiac, vascular, renal, and neurologic consequences of DM. Perioperative management may include the placement of additional intravenous cannulae for monitoring, fluid administration, or drug delivery. Some anesthesiologists feel that diabetic patients are relatively sensitive to spinal anesthetic agents, so that doses of local anesthetics should be reduced. However, no firm data exist to support this view. Epinephrine-containing solutions of local anesthetics should be avoided in peripheral blocks (e.g., ankle blocks) because of the risk of poor perfusion from diabetic microvascular disease. Meticulous attention to aseptic technique is essential because of the susceptibility to infection. Careful positioning of the diabetic patient is important because of the propensity for poor perfusion in extremities. This increases the risk of skin lesions and subsequent infection at pressure points.

THYROID DISORDERS

Hormones secreted from the thyroid gland are essential for fetal development, normal growth, sexual maturation, cardiac and central nervous system (CNS) function, and the regulation of temperature and metabolic rate. Directly relevant to the anesthesia preoperative evaluation are (a) the location and function of ectopic thyroid tissue, (b) anatomic complications from abnormal glands, (c) benign versus malignant character of thyroid tumors, and (d) alterations of thyroid function that influence responses to the stress of surgery and to anesthetics.

The thyroid gland is part of the hypothalamic-pituitary-thyroid axis. Thyrotropin-releasing hormone (TRH) from the hypothalamus is the most important positive regulator of thyroid-stimulating hormone (TSH), which is secreted by the pituitary gland. TSH has multiple effects on the thyroid gland, resulting in increased production and secretion of the thyroid hormones thyroxine (T_4) and triiodothyronine (T_3). Elevated thyroid hormone levels normally exert negative feedback control over the release of TRH and TSH. In states of thyroid hormone excess, TSH levels should be suppressed. Conversely, TSH levels should be elevated in hypothyroidism unless coexisting CNS disease is present. T_4 is the major secreted form of thyroid hormone. It is converted by peripheral tissues into the metabolically active hormone T_3. The majority of T_4 and T_3 molecules are bound to a group of thyroid hormone–binding proteins in the blood, the most important of which is thyroxine-binding globulin. The small amount of free (unbound) thyroid hormone (less than 0.1% of total T_4), however, is the biologically active molecule.

The physiologic effects of thyroid hormone include a general increase in most of the body's metabolic processes. Thyroid hormone increases carbohydrate, lipid, and drug metabolism. Protein anabolism and catabolism increase with an enhanced production of heat. Synergistic actions of thyroid hormone and catecholamines stimulate the cardiovascular system with elevated heart rate, blood pressure, and cardiac output, which removes metabolic waste and excess heat. As a result of alterations in the cardiovascular system and in metabolic activities of the liver, the kinetics and dynamics of drugs may vary depending on thyroid status.

Table 6-2. Clinical features of hypothyroidism

Symptoms
  Fatigue
  Sleepiness
  Depression
  Cold intolerance
  Hoarseness
  Dry skin
  Weight gain
  Constipation
  Irregular menses, menorrhagia
  Paresthesias
  Carpal tunnel syndrome
Signs
  Slow movement
  Slow speech
  Hoarseness
  Bradycardia
  Dry, sallow skin
  Periorbital edema
  Nonpitting edema (myxedema)
  Delayed relaxation of deep tendon reflexes
  Enlarged tongue
  Hypertension (especially diastolic)
  Low-voltage electrocardiogram
  Enlarged cardiac silhouette on chest radiograph

The incidence of thyroid disorders increases with age. Thyroid enlargement with goiter becomes more prevalent and, at age 60, 50% of the population has at least one thyroid nodule by ultrasound examination. Primary hypothyroidism, the relative lack of production of thyroid hormone, is far more common in women (incidence of approximately 12% by age 60) than in men. Primary hyperthyroidism, defined as a state of increased synthesis of thyroid hormone, is also more common in women but occurs at a lower frequency. Thyrotoxicosis is the condition in which levels of thyroid hormone are elevated regardless of etiology and includes states of increased hormone synthesis or excessive ingestion of exogenous hormone.

The elderly often have blunted responses to thyroid dysfunction. This is termed *"apathetic" hypothyroidism* or *"apathetic" hyperthyroidism*. Evidence of any change in mental status with memory loss or confusion should prompt an evaluation with a TSH measurement (see Diagnostic Testing, below) to check for hypothyroidism. Also, a TSH level should be obtained if an elderly patient exhibits unexplained weight loss or new-onset atrial tachydysrhythmia to rule out hyperthyroidism.

Interview and History

The first recognition of thyroid disease may be made during the anesthesia evaluation, based on the patient's presenting symptoms and signs (Tables 6-2 and 6-3) and the clinician's index of suspi-

Table 6-3. Clinical features of thyrotoxicosis

Symptoms
  Nervousness
  Fatigue
  Weakness
  Increased perspiration
  Tremor
  Palpitations
  Increased appetite
  Weight loss despite increased appetite
  Frequent bowel movements, diarrhea
  Irregular menses
Signs
  Hyperkinesis
  Tachycardia, atrial fibrillation
  Systolic hypertension
  Warm, moist skin
  Tremor
  Proximal muscle weakness
  Eyelid retraction
  Lid lag
  Stare
Signs with specific causes
  Diffuse goiter (Graves' disease)
  Thyroid eye disease—proptosis, chemosis, injection (Graves' disease)
  Localized myxedema (Graves' disease)

cion. More commonly, patients present for preoperative evaluation with a history of an adequately treated or inadequately treated (overtreated or undertreated) thyroid disorder.

The hypothyroid patient should be questioned to determine the cause of the condition, which may be inflammatory, postsurgical, postablative, or due to pituitary insufficiency. The hormone replacement regimen should be documented. Recent changes in therapy, symptoms, and the results of thyroid tests should be ascertained. Typical thyroid hormone replacement is 1.6 μg per kg per day. Doses in adults are typically 75 to 125 μg per day. Deviations from this range should suggest the possibility of overtreatment or undertreatment, malabsorption, or patient noncompliance. Persistence of symptoms attributable to hypothyroidism (see Table 6-2) suggests undertreatment. Patients with mild hypothyroidism may have only minor or nonspecific symptoms. Questioning may elicit evidence of excessive thyroid hormone replacement (see Table 6-3).

Patients with a neck mass or goiter should be specifically questioned about symptoms suggesting anatomic airway compromise, including changes in voice, dyspnea, orthopnea, chronic cough, and dysphagia.

Physical Examination

The examination of patients with thyroid disorders should include measurement of vital signs with particular attention to heart rate and rhythm, body weight and habitus, and a careful search for evidence of heart failure. Physical signs of hypothyroidism (see Table 6-2) or hyperthyroidism (see Table 6-3) should be specifically sought, depending on the presenting history. A thorough evaluation of the head and neck is essential to identify airway compromise (e.g., a deviated or narrowed trachea, enlarged tongue, vocal cord paresis) or the presence of intraoral thyroid tissue (the "lingual thyroid"), which may complicate laryngoscopy and intubation. Critical mediastinal obstruction by a goiter is indicated by a positive Pemberton's sign, which consists of facial plethora sometimes accompanied by syncope when the arms are elevated above the head for 1 to 2 minutes. Patients with Graves' ophthalmopathy may exhibit proptosis with or without conjunctival edema (chemosis). This should be noted because of the enhanced risk for ocular injury under general anesthesia.

Diagnostic Testing

A constellation of tests exists to evaluate thyroid status. In the absence of known hypothalamic or pituitary dysfunction, TSH level is the most reliable measure of thyroid function in the non–chronically ill patient without significant weight loss. Patients with weight loss, chronic inflammatory diseases (e.g., rheumatoid arthritis), or chronic infections (e.g., bronchitis) can have a suppressed TSH level. However, these patients do not have hypothyroidism. This condition is known as *euthyroid sick syndrome*. Assays for total T_4 or T_3 measure both free (bioactive) and protein-bound (biologically inactive) hormones. To correct for alterations in thyroid hormone–binding proteins, the total thyroid hormone level is multiplied by a correction factor, often termed *THBR*, T_3U, or T_3RU, to yield the free T_4 index. The free T_4 index is an *estimate*, not a direct measure, of the free T_4 level. Normal ranges for basic thyroid function tests vary from one institution to another, so that local standards should be used to interpret results.

Additional evaluation of the patient with known or suspected thyroid disease may include imaging studies of the neck or chest (ultrasonography, radiography, computed tomography, magnetic resonance imaging) to evaluate anatomic abnormalities. Cardiac studies (ECG, echocardiogram) may be indicated to evaluate rhythm disturbances or ventricular function, or confirm the presence of a pericardial effusion. Electrolyte levels should be evaluated as hypothyroidism decreases free water excretion, which results in hyponatremia. Excess perspiration or insensible losses in thyrotoxic states contribute to volume depletion with possible electrolyte abnormalities.

Evaluation of thyroid hormone levels must consider the possible effects of intercurrent conditions on the determinations. Levels of thyroxine-binding globulin, albumin, and other thyroid-binding proteins vary with physiologic changes such as pregnancy, or disease states such as hepatitis, and influence the level of total (free plus protein-bound) thyroid hormone. Diphenylhydantoin, high-dose furosemide, and salicylates can displace T_4 from binding proteins, which results in low levels of total thyroid hormone. In general, the active or free thyroid hormone is present in normal concentrations, as reflected by a normal TSH level.

Preoperative Medication and Instructions

T_4 has a long half-life (7 to 10 days), and most patients receiving this drug can miss several days of therapy without adverse consequences. Therefore, patients need not take their usual T_4 dose on the day of surgery. Patients receiving antithyroid drugs such as propylthiouracil or methimazole (Tapazole) should be instructed to take their usual doses on the day of surgery and resume therapy as soon as possible because these agents have short half-lives (6 to 8 hours). No intravenous formulations of these medications are available. Propylthiouracil may be crushed and administered as a slurry via a gastric tube. Methimazole can be administered as a suppository formulated by the hospital pharmacy. Patients should take their usual doses of medications such as digoxin or β-blockers used to treat cardiac rate and rhythm disturbances associated with hyperthyroidism. The purpose of continuing therapy with these drugs is to blunt exaggerated hemodynamic responses.

Propylthiouracil and methimazole have an average onset of effect of 7 to 10 days, and a stable euthyroid condition may not be achieved for several weeks. Newly diagnosed, moderately or severely hyperthyroid patients with Graves' disease requiring urgent surgery may be treated with high-dose antithyroid drugs, iodine, and β-blockers. Patients who are hyperthyroid from a toxic multinodular goiter or toxic adenoma, or patients intolerant of propylthiouracil or methimazole because of unacceptable side effects such as agranulocytosis, may be treated with combinations of high-dose adrenergic blockers and glucocorticoids. Administration of these preparations should be carried out in consultation with an endocrinologist. Anesthetized patients with severe untreated or partially treated thyrotoxicosis are at risk for the physiologic decompensation of "thyroid storm" (see next section). This condition is fatal in 25% to 40% of cases.

Implications for Perioperative and Anesthetic Management

Elective surgery should be postponed until patients are euthyroid and on a stable medical regimen. In cases in which surgery is urgent, preparation should be initiated to manage cardiac disturbances, airway issues, and metabolic abnormalities.

In the untreated hyperthyroid patient, glucocorticoid therapy should be considered because of the rapid metabolism of cortisol and the risk of relative adrenal insufficiency with surgical stress or thyroid storm. Hyperthyroidism results in chronic volume depletion as a result of diaphoresis or diarrhea, and unusually large volume replacement may be indicated. Preoperative sedation may alleviate anxiety and blunt an already activated sympathetic nervous system. Anesthetic agents with sympathomimetic properties (pancuronium bromide, ketamine hydrochloride) should be avoided or used with care. Because of muscle weakness associated with hyperthyroidism, cautious administration of neuromuscular blocking agents is indicated to prevent prolonged responses. A propensity for thyroid storm precipitated by anesthesia and surgery should be considered.

The newly diagnosed hypothyroid patient does not need to be treated before surgery. Generally these patients do well with no significantly increased perioperative morbidity. However, hypothyroid patients may exhibit an exaggerated sensitivity to sedative or hypnotic agents and narcotics. These drugs should be carefully titrated to effect with incremental small doses to avoid excessive sedation or respiratory depression. In the severely hypothyroid patient, depressed myocardial function, coagulation disturbances, hypothermia, hypoglycemia, and respiratory insufficiency should be recognized and appropriate management strategies devised.

Patients unable to resume their oral thyroid replacement within a week after surgery may require intravenous therapy. The typical intravenous dose of T_4 is approximately 50% of the customary oral dose. Intravenous T_3 is not recommended for replacement therapy. Planning for intravenous thyroid replacement must take into account the clinical situation, however, particularly the presence of cardiac disease. Thyroid hormone increases cardiac work and oxygen consumption. Thyroid hormone replacement may precipitate cardiac ischemia in the presence of coronary artery disease.

Thyroid storm is a state of cardiovascular or nervous system decompensation in a patient with severe hyperthyroidism after a destabilizing event such as surgery, myocardial infarction, stroke, infection, or trauma. Thyroid storm is associated with the signs and symptoms of extreme thyrotoxicosis (see Table 6-3). These include fever out of proportion to any evidence of infection, tachydysrhythmia often resistant to pharmacologic therapy, cardiovascular collapse with hypotension, dehydration (from fever, perspiration, or diarrhea), and alterations in mental status, which range from confusion and agitation to psychosis and ultimately stupor and coma. The first line of treatment is cardiovascular resuscitation with volume replenishment. β-Blockers for tachycardia should be given only after rehydration. Antithyroid medication is used in large doses. Propylthiouracil (300 to 400 mg, by mouth or by gastric tube every 4 hours) is preferred over methimazole because propylthiouracil prevents conversion of T_4 to T_3 (T_3 is 100 times more bioactive than T_4). Patients with Graves' disease (but not patients with toxic multinodular goiter) are also treated with iodine (saturation of potassium iodide, 5 drops, every 6 hours) with the dose given at least 1 hour *after* the administration of propylthiouracil. Fever is treated with acetaminophen and external cooling. The heat-generating effects of shivering may be prevented by administration of meperidine hydrochloride. Administration of high-dose glucocorticoids (dexamethasone, 2 mg, every 6 hours) partially inhibits release of thyroid hormone and prevents relative adrenal insufficiency resulting from the physiologic stress and increases in glucocorticoid metabolism seen with thyrotoxicosis. Management of thyroid storm should be carried out in consultation with an endocrinologist.

DISORDERS OF CALCIUM METABOLISM

Calcium is a critical ion for coagulation, neurotransmitter and hormone secretion, neuromuscular excitability, muscle contraction, hormone action, and enzyme function. Bone is the primary reservoir of calcium stores (99% of total). Quantitatively minute amounts of calcium playing critical roles in normal physiology are found in the extracellular fluid and within cells. In the bone, 99% of calcium is complexed in the solid crystal phase and 1% is in a rapidly exchangeable pool. This pool is in equilibrium with extracellular calcium. The extracellular pool is the source of biologically active calcium for crucial cellular processes. Approximately 50% of the extracellular calcium is complexed with proteins (primarily albumin and globulin). The remainder exists as calcium ion. The level of ionized calcium is tightly regulated in the plasma at approximately 1.2 mmol per L (5 mg per dL) by a complex integration of parathyroid hormone (PTH), bioactive 1,25-dihydroxyvitamin D, and daily calcium intake. Total plasma calcium concentration depends on the level of the binding proteins.

Calcium sensors in the parathyroid gland control the release of PTH, an 84-amino-acid peptide whose secretion depends on magnesium ions. PTH secretion is activated by hypocalcemia and elevated phosphorous levels. Hypercalcemia and 1,25-dihydroxyvitamin D (calcitriol) normally suppress PTH secretion. PTH increases the mobilization of calcium from bone, increases calcium reabsorption and phosphorus excretion in the renal tubules, and increases the 1-hydroxylation of 25-hydroxyvitamin D to 1,25 dihydroxyvitamin D (active form) in the kidney. The net effect of PTH is to increase extracellular calcium. In hyperparathyroidism, PTH is elevated. Three types of hyperparathyroidism are recognized: primary, secondary, and tertiary hyperparathyroidism. Hypercalcemia is associated with primary and tertiary hyperparathyroidism. In secondary hyperparathyroidism, PTH levels are elevated but serum calcium remains normal or slightly low.

One must recognize that an excess or deficiency of the serum calcium disrupts normal physiology of nerves, muscles, and coagulation. This disruption can profoundly affect perioperative hemodynamics, surgical hemostasis, and responses to anesthetic agents. The severity of the clinical effects of hypocalcemia or hypercalcemia depends on the absolute level of ionized calcium and the rapidity with which the abnormality occurs. Chronic hypocalcemia may have few clinical signs or symptoms, whereas rapidly developing hypocalcemia may have impressive clinical effects.

Hypocalcemia

Patients with moderately severe hypocalcemia present with neuromuscular irritability. Symptoms include perioral or acral paresthesias and spontaneous tetany. Acute, severe hypocalcemia is a medical emergency associated with death from laryngeal spasm or grand mal seizures. The treatment is immediate intravenous administration of calcium chloride or calcium gluconate. Common causes of hypocalcemia are listed in Table 6-4. Preoperative patients with rhabdomyolysis, pancreatitis, sepsis, burns, fat embolism syndrome, recent massive transfusion, or renal insufficiency are at risk for hypocalcemia.

Interview and History

Hypocalcemia is asymptomatic until calcium falls to nearly critical levels. Patients first note acral paresthesias. The most

Table 6-4. Hypocalcemia: causes, signs, and symptoms

Causes
Hypoparathyroidism
  Primary
  Surgical
  Idiopathic
  Autoimmune
  Hypomagnesemia
  Peripheral resistance (pseudohypoparathyroidism)
  Hemosiderosis
  Amyloidosis
Hyperphosphatemia
  Renal failure
  Rhabdomyolysis
  Chemotherapy/tumor lysis
  Phosphate therapy
Vitamin D deficiency
  Liver failure
  Renal failure
  Lack of sun exposure
  Dietary deficiency
Intestinal malabsorption
Anticonvulsant therapy
Hypoalbuminemia
Osteoblastic metastases
Contrast media containing EDTA
Loop diuretics
Critical illness
  Alkalosis
  Burns
  Toxic shock
  Pancreatitis
  Fat embolism
Massive transfusion (citrate intoxication)
Signs and symptoms
Muscle spasms
  Stridor
  Laryngospasm
  Carpal/pedal spasm
  Chvostek's sign
  Trousseau's sign
  Tetany
Weakness
Hypotension
Congestive heart failure
Dysrhythmia
Altered mental status
Paresthesias (acral, perioral)
Apnea
Catechol resistance
Seizures

EDTA, ethylenediamine-tetraacetic acid.
Particularly when symptomatic, hypocalcemia should be treated if total calcium is less than 8.0 g/dL. Of note, alkalosis decreases *ionized* calcium 0.1 mg/dL (0.25 mEq/L) for every increase of 0.1 pH unit. Total calcium is not affected by pH changes.

common setting for symptomatic hypocalcemia is postsurgery, particularly after total or subtotal thyroidectomy or four-gland parathyroid exploration or removal. Patients usually present 12 to 24 hours postoperatively. Any patient with a history of neck surgery, however, should be evaluated for signs and symptoms of hypocalcemia (see Table 6-4). In renal failure (because of elevated levels of phosphorus sequestering calcium) or vitamin D deficiency, a secondary PTH elevation occurs to elevate calcium levels back to normal. Patients with endocrine dysfunction from autoimmune destruction (hypothyroidism, early menopause, DM type I associated with vitiligo or pernicious anemia) should be screened for hypocalcemia. Hypocalcemia from vitamin D deficiency is often asymptomatic because calcium levels decline slowly and a compensatory increase in PTH mobilizes bone calcium to maintain nearly normal serum calcium levels.

Physical Examination

Neuronal irritability can be detected by tapping the facial nerve below the zygoma. In hypocalcemic patients, this results in ipsilateral contractions of the facial muscle with twitching of the corner of the mouth (Chvostek's sign). Carpal spasm of the hand (Trousseau's sign) can be elicited by 3-minute occlusive pressure with a blood pressure cuff. Long-standing hypocalcemia with hyperphosphatemia and PTH deficiency is associated with calcification of the basal ganglia with extrapyramidal signs. Cataracts and deposition of calcium in the lens may be seen.

Diagnostic Testing

Evaluation of calcium status is typically determined by measuring total serum calcium and albumin levels. A rough correction for protein-binding abnormalities can be made by assuming a change in total calcium of 0.8 mg per dL (0.2 mmol per L) for every 1 mg per dL change in albumin from 4.0 mg per dL. Ionized calcium levels are a more accurate indicator of calcium homeostasis. The measurement is greatly affected by specimen handling, so that ionized calcium is not usually measured in the routine setting. In the operating room or intensive care unit, with immediate processing and analysis, ionized calcium levels may be reliable. Acidosis increases the level of ionized calcium and alkalosis decreases ionized calcium levels. Ionized calcium changes 0.1 mg per dL (0.25 mEq per L) for every 0.1 pH unit. Total calcium is not affected by pH changes. Concomitant assessment of acid-base status may be important in analyzing a clinical situation.

An elevated serum phosphorus level with normal renal function supports the diagnosis of hypoparathyroidism. Renal function and phosphorous and magnesium levels should be evaluated in hypocalcemic patients. Hypocalcemia can cause cardiac conduction disturbances. ECG abnormalities include prolonged QT intervals and marked QRS and ST changes. These can mimic changes associated with an acute myocardial infarction or conduction abnormalities. Ventricular dysrhythmia is a rare complication of hypocalcemia.

Preoperative Medication and Instructions

Patients with chronic hypocalcemia should continue their usual medications before surgery. Calcium levels plummet within 4 to 6 hours after missed doses of calcium and vitamin D supplements (calcitriol, in particular). If hypocalcemia is associated with hypomagnesemia, magnesium should be replaced orally as magnesium oxide. Vitamin D deficiency is treated with a variety of vitamin D metabolites. Commonly used supplements include calcitriol (25-hydroxyvitamin D) and ergocalciferol (1,25-hydroxyvitamin D). This therapy should probably be undertaken in consultation with an endocrinologist. Oral calcium supplementation for severe hypocalcemia is 1,500 to 3,000 mg daily. The most common agent for calcium therapy, calcium carbonate (40% elemental calcium by weight), requires stomach acid for absorption. Calcium carbonate should be taken with meals, especially by elderly patients who often have impaired gastric acid secretion. Occasionally, achlorhydric patients do not absorb calcium carbonate, and calcium citrate should be used instead (21% elemental calcium by weight). After serum calcium reaches the low normal range, urinary calcium should be assessed to avoid nephrolithiasis.

Implications for Perioperative and Anesthetic Management

Hypocalcemia disrupts the coagulation cascade and may contribute to problems with hemostasis. Cardiac rhythm or conduction disturbances, decreased contractility, and peripheral vasodilation are associated with hypocalcemia. Hypocalcemia can contribute to perioperative hemodynamic disturbances. Compromised neuromuscular function should be anticipated, and sensitivity to muscle relaxants may increase. Patients may require postoperative intubation and ventilation if hypocalcemia impairs neuromuscular function. Acute hypocalcemia (serum calcium less than 7.5 mg per dL, normal albumin), especially associated with symptoms, neurologic or cardiovascular instability, or coagulopathy, is a medical emergency requiring immediate therapy. Treatment is with elemental calcium (~100 mg calcium, intravenously, administered as 10 mL of a 10% solution of calcium gluconate, 4 mL of a 10% solution of calcium chloride, or 5 mL of a 22% solution of calcium gluceptate over 15 to 20 minutes). The initial dose is followed by a continuous infusion of elemental calcium at 15 mg per kg over 8 to 12 hours (ten ampules of 10% calcium gluconate in 500 mL D_5-half normal saline) with close monitoring of serum calcium levels every 2 hours. After stabilizing the patient, treatment is directed to the cause of the hypocalcemia.

Hypercalcemia

Hypercalcemia can be categorized as either parathyroid dependent or non–parathyroid dependent. Disorders of the parathyroid gland that result in hypercalcemia include primary and tertiary hyperparathyroidism, familial hypocalciuric hypercalcemia, and lithium-induced hypercalcemia. Multiple non–parathyroid dependent hypercalcemic conditions exist (Table 6-5).

Table 6-5. Hypercalcemia: causes, signs, and symptoms

Causes
Endocrine
    Hyperparathyroidism (primary, tertiary)
    Hyperthyroidism
    Multiple endocrine neoplasia syndromes
    Acromegaly
    Pheochromocytoma
    Adrenal insufficiency
Malignancy
    Squamous cell cancers (i.e., lung)
    Pancreatic cancer
    Hypernephroma
    Myeloma
    Breast cancer
    Lymphoma/leukemia (rare)
Granulomatous disease
    Sarcoidosis
    Histoplasmosis
    Coccidioidomycosis
    Tuberculosis
Drugs
    Iatrogenic administration
    Theophylline
    Lithium
    Thiazides
    Vitamin D
    Antacids (calcium containing)
    Vitamin A
Acquired immunodeficiency syndrome
Renal diseases (various)
Familial/genetic causes (various)
Immobilization
Signs and symptoms
Gastrointestinal
    Nausea/vomiting
    Anorexia
    Constipation
    Pancreatitis
    Peptic ulcers
Hemodynamic
    Catechol resistance
    Dehydration
    Hypertension
    Electrocardiogram/conduction changes
    Digitalis sensitivity
    Dysrhythmias
Central nervous system
    Seizures
    Disorientation/psychosis
    Memory loss
    Sedation/lethargy/coma
Renal
    Polyuria
    Nephrolithiasis
    Oliguric failure (late)
Osteopenia/osteoporosis
Weakness/atrophy/fatigability

Normally, four parathyroid glands are found in the lower neck. PTH is secreted in response to low calcium levels detected by the parathyroid gland calcium-sensing receptor. Dysfunction of the calcium sensor results in familial hypocalciuric hypercalcemia with hypercalcemia, and hypocalciuria but minimal elevations in PTH. Recognition of this condition is important because no clinical sequelae appear to result from the hypercalcemia and no treatment is necessary. Inappropriate or autonomous secretion of PTH in the setting of hypercalcemia is first-degree hyperparathyroidism. In 80% of cases, first-degree hyperparathyroidism is due to adenomatous enlargement of a single parathyroid gland; in 5% of cases double adenomas are present. Four-gland hyperplasia is seen in 1% to 10% of cases of hyperparathyroidism, often as part of a multiple endocrine neoplasia (MEN) syndrome. Oversecretion of PTH associated with hypercalcemia occurring in chronic renal failure is called *tertiary hyperparathyroidism*. This is a state of severe four-gland hyperplasia that is not adequately responsive to plasma calcium concentration. Rarely (in fewer than 1% of cases), hyperparathyroidism is due to a parathyroid carcinoma. Hypercalcemia of malignancy is usually associated with destructive bone lesions or secretion of a PTH-like tumor peptide (PTH-RP).

Treatment of hypercalcemia is directed toward the cause. Serum calcium levels greater than 14 mg per dL are life-threatening and should be managed aggressively with rehydration followed by saline diuresis and intravenous administration of bisphosphonate (pamidronate disodium), calcitonin, or mithramycin. High-dose glucocorticoids may be used.

Interview and History

Inherited parathyroid disease occurs in 95% of patients with MEN type I and in 5% to 20% of patients with MEN type II (see Multiple Endocrine Neoplasia, below). Hyperparathyroidism associated with other endocrine diseases or a family history of endocrine diseases should raise the suspicion of a possible MEN syndrome. Depending on the degree of calcium elevation, hypercalcemia can be associated with cognitive deficits ranging from minimal memory loss to confusion to coma. Other signs and symptoms include constipation, excess stomach acid secretion, ulcer symptoms, polyuria, and renal stones. Hypercalcemia from parathyroid disease is associated with bone loss and osteoporosis.

Physical Examination

Hypercalcemia often has no physical signs. The patient should be assessed for hypertension, hyporeflexia, and muscle weakness or atrophy. The patient's ability to protect the airway should be assessed if mental status is depressed. Evidence of volume depletion from anorexia, pancreatitis, renal tubular dysfunction, or vomiting should be sought.

Diagnostic Testing

Key to determining the cause of hypercalcemia is estimating biologically active calcium (total calcium plus albumin) or ionized calcium levels. Abnormal globulin levels or elevated albumin levels result in elevations of total calcium without an increase in the free, biologically active fraction. Once hypercalcemia is confirmed, use of interfering medications should be considered. These include calcium-containing antacids; hydrochlorothiazide diuretics, which reduce renal calcium excretion; and lithium, which causes four-gland parathyroid hyperplasia. Appropriate laboratory studies include PTH level, alkaline phosphatase level, 25-hydroxyvitamin D level, 1,25 dihydroxyvitamin D level, serum phosphorus level, and a 24-hour urine collection to test for creatinine and calcium. Renal function and electrolyte levels should be evaluated and an ECG obtained to assess the possibility of rhythm disturbances. Shortening of the QT interval is characteristic of hypercalcemia.

Preoperative Medication and Instructions

Mild to moderate hypercalcemia (total calcium less than 12 mg per dL) generally does not require specific treatment. However, hypercalcemia often results in polyuria and dehydration. Preoperative volume replenishment may be indicated. Moderate hypercalcemia (total calcium 12 to 14 mg per dL) can be treated with saline hydration, oral administration of furosemide, and adequate salt and water intake. Electrolyte levels should be checked during therapy. Critical hypercalcemia (total calcium greater than 14 mg per dL) is life-threatening and is treated with combinations of vigorous saline hydration, furosemide diuresis, calcitonin, pamidronate disodium, dexamethasone, and mithramycin.

Implications for Perioperative and Anesthetic Management

Volume status should be assessed and adjusted as necessary. Verapamil hydrochloride should be available to treat supraventricular dysrhythmias associated with hypercalcemia. Surgical treatment of first-degree hyperparathyroidism often involves identifying and obtaining biopsies of all four parathyroid glands to rule out hyperplasia. Even if a single adenoma is removed, the surgical disruption of the remaining glands can result in temporary hypocalcemia. The hypocalcemia typically occurs within hours of the surgery but may be delayed for several days. A calcium level (total calcium plus albumin or ionized calcium) should be obtained several hours after surgery and the next morning. Simultaneous measurements of phosphorus levels should be obtained because hypoparathyroidism is associated with reduced renal phosphorus excretion and elevation in serum phosphorus. Postoperative hypocalcemia is permanent in fewer than 10% of patients after parathyroid or thyroid surgery.

PITUITARY-ADRENAL CONDITIONS

Corticotropin-releasing hormone (CRH) from the hypothalamus regulates the production of adrenocorticotropic hormone (ACTH) by the anterior pituitary gland. ACTH controls the production of the glucocorticoid cortisol from the adrenal cortex. Cortisol production is essential for stress responses, hemodynamic stability, and temperature regulation. The average basal adrenal cortisol secretion is 30 mg per day. During maximal stress, adrenal cortisol output may increase tenfold, up to 300 mg per day. A key feature of hypothalamic-pituitary-adrenal physiology is negative feedback suppression of pituitary ACTH release by high levels of endogenous or exogenous glucocorticoids. Long-term glucocorticoid therapy is common for asthma, rheumatoid arthritis, and other inflammatory conditions, and for immune suppression in transplant patients. Thus, many patients are at risk for suppression of their endogenous hypothalamic-pituitary-adrenal axis. The adrenal cortex produces a second steroid hormone, aldosterone, that is under the control of potassium levels and the renin-angiotensin system. Aldosterone increases the reabsorption of sodium from the renal distal tubule and the excretion of potassium. This hormone is central to normal fluid and electrolyte balance. Primary adrenal insufficiency (hemorrhage, tumor, infection) results in loss of both aldosterone and cortisol. Aldosterone secretion is preserved in secondary adrenal insufficiency from exogenous steroid therapy.

Adrenal Cortical Hormone Excess

A pituitary tumor producing ACTH, leading to elevated glucocorticoid production, is traditionally defined as *Cushing's disease*. Ectopic ACTH or CRH production from lung tumors or other neoplasms and primary adrenal neoplasms may result in glucocorticoid oversecretion. *Cushing's syndrome* is the constellation of signs and symptoms of abnormally elevated adrenal glucocorticoid production. It can be mimicked by prolonged high-dose therapeutic glucocorticoid administration. Signs and symptoms of hypercortisolemia include proximal muscle weakness; early fatigue; hypertension; emotional lability; abnormal central fat deposition, especially in the face, between the scapulae, and in the abdomen; mobilization of connective tissues leading to easy bruisability; cutaneous striae; osteoporosis; acne; and virilization in women. Major manifestations relevant to anesthesia are hypertension, obesity, myopathy, and glucose intolerance or frank DM.

Mineralocorticoid excess may result from adrenal aldosteronoma or hyperplasia. Excess mineralocorticoids result in sodium and water retention. Patients exhibit diastolic hypertension, which can cause left ventricular hypertrophy. Potassium wasting produces ECG abnormalities, muscle weakness, and fatigue.

Adrenal Insufficiency

Adrenal insufficiency follows suppression of the hypothalamic-pituitary-adrenal axis or destruction of the adrenal or the pituitary gland. Patients often present with hypotension, fever, and abdominal pain, which resolve with glucocorticoid treatment. Abnormalities in fluid balance and electrolyte levels, fatigue, weakness, and hypotension should be anticipated in adrenal insufficiency. The risk of adrenal hemorrhage is increased in patients on anticoagulation therapy and in the elderly. Intrathoracic or intraabdominal surgery and hypotension predispose patients to adrenal hemorrhage. Infectious causes of adrenal gland destruction include tuberculosis and *Cryptococcus*, *Mycobacterium avium-intracellulare*, and cytomegalovirus infections. Thus, patients with acquired immunodeficiency syndrome should be considered at risk for adrenal insufficiency. Pituitary apoplexy with adrenal insufficiency occurs in patients in the setting of an initially asymptomatic pituitary adenoma. Postpartum hemorrhage is associated with pituitary apoplexy resulting in adrenal insufficiency.

Long-Term Steroid Therapy

In general, patients receiving alternate-day therapy with low-dose steroids (prednisone or equivalent, less than 10 mg every other day for adults) exhibit normal adrenal responses during stress, so that "stress-dose" steroid supplementation is not necessary for minor procedures. Steroid supplementation may be advisable for major procedures. Patients receiving long-term steroid therapy (prednisone or equivalent, more than 5 mg per day for adults) for more than 2 weeks should be considered at risk for adrenal insufficiency during stress. The risk of adrenal insufficiency remains for up to 1 year after the cessation of high-dose steroid therapy. Because perioperative adrenal insufficiency or an addisonian crisis has an extremely high risk of major morbidity or mortality, prophylactic glucocorticoid therapy is probably indicated in most cases in which a risk of adrenal suppression is present. See Chapter 15 for guidelines on perioperative steroid administration.

Interview and History

Abnormalities in the hypothalamic-pituitary-adrenal system are most commonly encountered in patients undergoing long-term treatment with glucocorticoids for other medical conditions. The status of these conditions, such as asthma, inflammatory bowel disease, arthritis, or other steroid-responsive disorders, should be evaluated as needed. Important data include the duration and dosage of steroid therapy, and systemic consequences of glucocorticoid excess (hypertension, myopathy, osteoporosis, DM). Documentation of the patient's medical regimen to control the consequences of glucocorticoid excess is important.

Patients treated for mineralocorticoid or glucocorticoid deficiency should have their medical regimens carefully documented. Recent changes in medication or in symptoms may warrant referral back to the primary physician for evaluation before elective surgery.

Physical Examination

The examination of the patient with hypothalamic-pituitary-adrenal system disorders should include recording of vital signs, particularly the blood pressure with orthostatic signs. Body habitus should be noted because obesity is common in conditions of glucocorticoid excess, whereas asthenia and hyperpigmentation are features of adrenal insufficiency. An assessment of skin and connective tissue integrity aids in planning regional anesthetic approaches and vascular access. Evaluation of the oropharynx may reveal oral thrush, which is common in patients treated with steroids and may complicate airway management. Postponement of elective procedures may be indicated while the infection is treated.

Diagnostic Testing

Measurements of electrolyte and glucose levels are indicated because they are commonly abnormal in hypothalamic-pituitary-adrenal disorders. Coagulation studies and a platelet count are useful in diagnosing the cause of bleeding, particularly in patients presenting with a history of bruisability, as in Cushing's syndrome. A patient with a history of hypertension should be evaluated with an ECG and a chest radiograph (CXR) to assess the possibility of cardiac hypertrophy or dilatation. The results of these tests may indicate the need for an echocardiogram or other cardiac evaluation.

Preoperative Medication and Instructions

In addition to giving patients the routine preoperative instructions, they should be told to continue their glucocorticoid or mineralocorticoid replacement therapy, antihypertension, and cardiac regimens until surgery. Patients with glucose intolerance should have their hypoglycemic regimens adjusted as discussed above.

Implications for Perioperative and Anesthetic Management

Hypovolemia should be anticipated in patients with adrenal insufficiency. The need for carefully titrated volume support may warrant additional monitoring. Invasive monitoring may be indicated for hyperadrenal patients with refractory hypertension. The potential need for invasive monitoring should be considered during the preoperative evaluation and discussed with the patient. Uncorrected electrolyte abnormalities can predispose patients to perioperative dysrhythmias. These should be corrected if possible. Anticipation of dysrhythmias facilitates preparation for intraoperative management. Preexisting myopathy should be recognized because of the possibility of increased sensitivity to muscle relaxants and respiratory insufficiency postoperatively. Glucocorticoid supplementation should be ordered as described in Chapter 15.

OTHER PITUITARY GLAND DISORDERS

In addition to ACTH, the anterior pituitary gland secretes several other trophic hormones. Anterior pituitary cells secreting growth hormone, TSH, luteinizing hormone, and prolactin are regulated by the hypothalamus. Acromegaly associated with excess growth hormone is of principal concern for the anesthesiologist. Adrenal or thyroid deficiency secondary to pituitary dysfunction is possible.

The posterior pituitary gland secretes antidiuretic hormone (ADH), also known as *vasopressin*. This peptide hormone controls the excretion of water by the kidney. Diabetes insipidus (DI) is copious dilute urine formation (more than 1 L per hour) because of ADH deficiency with the potential for hypernatremia and intravascular volume depletion. This condition may be seen after head injury or pituitary surgery. Inappropriate ADH secretion results in hyponatremia, possibly with volume overload.

Interview and History

The possible presence and implications of an intracranial neoplasm must be evaluated in patients presenting with pituitary dysfunction. Past anesthetic history, particularly general anesthesia and airway management history, is essential for the patient with acromegaly. Tongue enlargement and soft tissue hypertrophy in the hypopharynx may complicate mask ventilation, laryngoscopy, and intubation. In addition, acromegalic patients are prone to coronary atherosclerosis and congestive heart failure and should have a careful evaluation for heart disease. DM is associated with acromegaly and should be evaluated and managed as described above. The medical regimen, such as the use of the synthetic ADH analog desmopressin acetate in patients with DI, should be documented.

Physical Examination

The acromegalic patient may present with abnormal facies, enlarged tongue, and hypertrophy of the epiglottis. The airway and cardiovascular system should be carefully inspected. DI patients should be examined specifically to estimate volume status (orthostatic signs).

Diagnostic Testing

Because acromegalic patients are prone to DM, a baseline glucose level should be obtained. A baseline ECG is indicated. Sodium levels should be determined in patients with DI or the syndrome of inappropriate antidiuretic hormone secretion.

Preoperative Medication and Instructions

Patients with DI should continue their hormone therapy. Desmopressin acetate (a chemically modified vasopressin) can be administered by injection (intravenously or subcutaneously), tube insufflation, or nasal spray, or by mouth. The usual dose of injected desmopressin acetate is 0.25 to 0.5 mL (1 to 2 mg) twice daily. The usual dose of desmopressin acetate by nasal spray is 1 to 2 actuations (10 to 20 mg) twice daily. The dose by rhinal tube insufflation is 0.1 to 0.2 mL (10 to 20 mg) twice daily. For oral use, desmopressin acetate is administered in a dosage of 0.1 to 0.2 mg, one to three times per day, for a daily dose of 0.1 to 0.8 mg. The patient's thirst, weight, estimated volume status, and serum osmolality are used to determine the dose of desmopressin acetate.

The hypoglycemic regimen for acromegalic patients should be managed as described above. Acromegalic patients should be alerted to the possibility of intubation while awake and possible postoperative intubation, as well as the chance that a surgical airway will be required. Extra monitoring may be useful in the presence of cardiac disease.

Implications for Perioperative and Anesthetic Management

As indicated above, the acromegalic patient presents the possibility of a challenging airway. Volume status issues are the principal concerns with disorders of the posterior pituitary. Central pressure monitoring and measurement of urine output with an indwelling catheter may be indicated. Desmopressin acetate must be available for patients with DI.

CARCINOID TUMORS

Carcinoid tumors are neuroendocrine neoplasms most commonly found in the gastrointestinal tract, the pancreas, or pulmonary bronchi. Foregut tumors may metastasize to the liver and lymph nodes, among other sites. The clinical presentation of carcinoid tumors depends on the location of the primary tumor, the extent of local invasion, the spread of metastases, and the secretion of hormones. Although serotonin is the principal secretory product of carcinoid tumors, a variety of other biologically active monoamines and neuroendocrine peptides can be released. High levels of these biologically active secretory products may result in *carcinoid syndrome*, a constellation of episodic flushing, hypotension, hypertension, wheezing, and diarrhea. Other potential endocrine effects include hypercalcemia from diarrhea-induced dehydration and Cushing's syndrome with proximal myopathy attributable to tumor co-secretion of CRH. Right-sided cardiac valvular lesions can result from long-standing carcinoid syndrome. Tricuspid insufficiency and pulmonary stenosis can lead to right sided congestive heart failure. Left-sided valvular disease is less common. The diagnostic hallmark of carcinoid syndrome is excessive urinary excretion of the serotonin metabolite 5-hydroxyindoleacetic acid.

Interview and History

The majority of patients (95%) does not present with features of carcinoid syndrome; instead, they experience gastrointestinal symptoms such as nausea, bleeding, or abdominal pain. In patients whose tumors actively secrete hormones, any history of hypotension or wheezing should be elicited, because stress, catecholamines, the induction of anesthesia, or surgical manipulation of the primary tumor or a metastasis may precipitate a carcinoid crisis with refractory hemodynamic or pulmonary sequelae. A history of frequent or protracted bouts of diarrhea suggests the possibility of fluid and electrolyte abnormalities. The patient's nutritional status should be assessed, because gastrointestinal pathology or the avid uptake of tryptophan (the precursor for serotonin) by tumor cells can lead to malnutrition.

The history helps determine the extent of metabolic evaluations and studies to identify metastases. The precise nature of the planned surgical procedure (bronchoscopy, liver resection, bowel resection, etc.) should be identified to ensure that adequate resources, such as blood products, are available.

Physical Examination

The general physical status should be assessed because of the potential for malnutrition (see Chapter 16). Diarrhea may compromise volume status. An estimation of the preoperative fluid status can be obtained by the examination, including assessment of vital signs and any orthostatic changes. Because bronchospasm is a component of the carcinoid syndrome, a lung examination is essential during the preoperative evaluation. The chest examination should include auscultation for cardiac murmurs, especially a murmur suggesting tricuspid valve insufficiency, and a search for signs of right-sided congestive heart failure. Cutaneous manifestations include facial flushing and persistent erythema and telagiectasia.

Diagnostic Testing

In addition to the studies undertaken for diagnosis, patients should have an ECG to determine the presence of supraventricular dysrhythmias and a CXR to identify intercurrent pulmonary processes. The levels of serum glucose, electrolytes, and albumin should be measured, because abnormalities of these parameters occur in carcinoid syndrome.

Preoperative Medication and Instructions

Along with providing routine preoperative instructions, the clinician should consider pretreating patients at risk for carcinoid crises with H_1 and H_2 histamine antagonists. Patients receiving octreotide acetate, a somatostatin analog that reduces the release of mediators from tumor cells, should continue this medication until surgery. Sedation to reduce stress-related release of carcinoid mediators may be beneficial. Depending on the severity of the patient's carcinoid syndrome, presurgical hospitalization for fluid management, monitoring, and premedication may be indicated.

Implications for Perioperative and Anesthetic Management

For the patient undergoing a procedure for carcinoid, the anesthesiologist must appreciate the nature and implications of the planned surgery (i.e., bronchoscopy or pulmonary, bowel, or liver resection). Patients undergoing bowel surgery may have a bowel preparation with hypovolemia or electrolyte disturbances. Preparation to manage carcinoid crisis should include ensuring the availability of bronchodilators (methylxanthines, glucocorticoids), direct-acting vasopressors, and large doses of octreotide acetate. Beta-adrenergic agonists are best avoided because of their propensity to provoke or to worsen exacerbations of carcinoid syndrome. Adequate vascular access for monitoring and for drug and fluid therapy should be discussed with the patient and established in advance of an acute need. Specific pharmacotherapy includes H_1 and H_2 histamine receptor blockers, ketanserin (serotonin receptor antagonist), droperidol, phenylephrine, and octreotide acetate. A general guideline is that anesthetic agents associated with the release of histamine (morphine, curare) or catecholamines (ketamine hydrochloride) should be avoided. The use of regional anesthesia as the primary or adjunctive technique should be considered.

PHEOCHROMOCYTOMA

Pheochromocytomas are tumors of chromaffin cells. The biological effects are due largely to secretion of epinephrine and norepinephrine, but mediators, including dopamine and several peptide hormones, may contribute to the clinical presentation of the tumor. Ninety percent of tumors are found in the adrenal medulla. Extraadrenal locations, including the chest, bladder, and sympathetic chain, are possible. The lesion is solitary in the majority of cases (80% to 90%). Pheochromocytomas may be found in association with other disorders, including MEN (see Multiple Endocrine Neoplasia below) and a variety of neurologic conditions. The diagnosis is established by measuring elevated levels of catecholamines or their metabolic products in the urine.

Interview and History

The presenting feature of pheochromocytoma is typically severe, sustained, or paroxysmal hypertension. A hypertensive crisis may occur with headache, palpitations, pallor, feelings of apprehension, and excessive diaphoresis. Once pheochromocytoma is diagnosed, outpatient therapy is initiated to establish alpha-adrenergic receptor blockade (usually with phenoxybenzamine hydrochloride but sometimes with prazosin hydrochloride). This may require days to weeks. Occasionally, patients are managed by catecholamine depletion with alpha-menthyltyrosine. The patient probably will be admitted for preoperative management to optimize fluid balance and alpha-blockade and to establish beta-adrenergic blockade. The details and the efficacy of the medical regimen used to prepare patients should be ascertained. Achieving maximal alpha-blockade before beta-adrenergic blockade is established is important. Initiating beta-blockade without adequately establishing alpha-blockade may worsen hypertension.

In addition to the usual data, information about specific factors precipitating a crisis should be obtained. Also, the location(s) of the tumor, association with other conditions such as MEN II, and end organ consequences of catecholamine release and hypertension should be elicited. Key data include a history of angina, myocardial infarction, congestive heart failure, or dysrhythmias, because sustained high levels of catecholamines predispose to cardiomyopathy and ischemia.

Physical Examination

Essential information includes assessment of heart rate and blood pressure with orthostatic signs, because patients are often dehydrated. Signs of cardiac enlargement or congestive heart failure should be sought. Body temperature elevations can result from enhanced metabolic rate and decreased heat dissipation. Cannulation sites for invasive monitoring (central venous and intraarterial pressures) and regional anesthesia sites (epidural, spinal) should be inspected to facilitate planning. Extreme caution is mandatory during examination of the abdomen. Simple palpation of a pheochromocytoma may precipitate a hypertensive crisis.

Diagnostic Testing

An ECG is essential to evaluate heart rate, rhythm, and conduction disturbances and to assess for myocardial ischemia or infarction. Echocardiography may be useful to evaluate ventricular function, because catecholamine excess can cause cardiomyopathy. The CXR is important to rule out pulmonary edema and cardiomegaly. The efficacy of the hydration regimen can be assessed by serial hematocrit determinations as intravascular volume is replenished. Electrolyte levels, blood urea nitrogen, and creatinine clearance are important because vasoconstriction compromises renal perfusion. Occasionally, rhabdomyolysis can result in myoglobinuric renal damage. Hyperglycemia is seen in many patients.

Preoperative Medication and Instructions

Patients should continue their α-blockers and β-blockers and other routine medications until surgery. The patient should be advised to expect the placement of cannulae for invasive monitoring, and the use of regional combined with general anesthesia should be discussed.

Implications for Perioperative and Anesthetic Management

Invasive monitoring of the patient undergoing resection of a pheochromocytoma, including central venous pressure measurement, is indicated. Preparation for large volume resuscitation or management of depressed cardiac function is essential. Vasoactive agents, including vasodilators, vasopressors, and β-blockers, should be available. Catecholamine release is common with manipulation of the tumor and may cause sudden, severe hypertension. After resection of the tumor, hypovolemic patients may exhibit profound hypotension.

Several medications commonly administered in the perioperative period may have adverse effects. Opioids, histamine, and indirect sympathomimetic agents can release catecholamines from tumors. Succinylcholine chloride may cause the release of catechols by increasing intraabdominal pressure. Ketamine hydrochloride, halothane, and the vagolytic action of pancuronium bromide potentiate the effects of catecholamines. Cautious administration of medications is advisable when treating patients with known or suspected pheochromocytoma. Of note, the release of catecholamines from pheochromocytomas is not under neural control, so that psychological stress usually does not initiate a crisis.

The perioperative differential diagnosis of a pheochromocytoma crisis includes thyroid storm and malignant hyperthermia.

MULTIPLE ENDOCRINE NEOPLASIA

MEN comprises three syndromes defined by characteristic combinations of endocrinopathies or disease associations: MEN type I, MEN type IIa, and MEN type IIb (Table 6-6). Confusion with the nomenclature arises because MEN type IIb has been called MEN type III. The MEN syndromes result from genetic lesions. Identification of the particular type of MEN syndrome is important because management may differ, depending on the combination of endocrinopathies.

A complicating feature in the diagnosis and management of MEN is the patient-to-patient variation in the clinical expression of the different features of a particular MEN type. Some patients with MEN type I have hyperplasia, but others have adenomas or carcinomas of endocrine organs such as parathyroid glands. These tumors may have varying degrees of endocrine activity. Hypersecretion of different islet hormones (insulin, glucagon, gastrin, vasoactive intestinal polypeptide,

Table 6-6. Characteristics of multiple endocrine neoplasia (MEN) syndromes

MEN type I (Werner's syndrome)	MEN type IIa (Sipple's syndrome)	MEN type IIb (also known as *MEN type III*)
Neoplastic tissue	**Neoplastic tissue**	**Neoplastic tissue**
Parathyroid adenoma	Medullary thyroid carcinoma	Medullary thyroid carcinoma
Pituitary adenoma	Pheochromocytoma	Pheochromocytoma
Pancreatic islet cell	Parathyroid adenoma	Mucosal neuroma
Carcinoid (rare)	**Other features**	Intestinal ganglio-neuromatosis
Meningioma (rare)	Cutaneous lichen amyloidosis (rare)	**Other features**
Lipoma (rare)	Hirschsprung's disease (rare)	Skeletal deformities/ marfanoid habitus

pancreatic polypeptide) produces different clinical presentations. MEN type I syndromes may evolve slowly over decades, and the clinical features depend on the stage of progression at the time of diagnosis. A clinical presentation may have more than one cause. For example, a patient with an ACTH-producing pituitary adenoma may have Cushing's syndrome. But Cushing's syndrome may be attributable to a carcinoid tumor that secretes CRH. In patients with MEN type II (a or b), pheochromocytoma may or may not be clinically manifested, and the clinical effects of medullary thyroid cancers are variable. Additional hereditary polyendocrinopathy syndromes do not fit the MEN subtype classification. These include several "overlap" syndromes and von Hippel–Lindau disease, which have their own characteristic constellations of endocrine dysfunctions.

Interview and History

Because of the variable presentation of the different components of the MEN syndromes, determining which features are clinically significant is important. Thus, in patients with MEN type I, features of hypercalcemia (see Table 6-5), Zollinger-Ellison syndrome (ulcer disease of the upper gastrointestinal tract, increased gastric acid secretion, and non–islet cell tumors of the pancreas), insulinoma, watery diarrhea syndrome, or pituitary dysfunction should be evaluated. In patients with MEN type II, the classical features of pheochromocytoma, calcitonin hypersecretion from medullary thyroid tumors, or hypercalcemia (rare in type IIb) should be sought along with evidence of known variants of MEN type II manifested as Hirschsprung's disease, multiple mucosal neuromas, and so on. If the history suggests the possibility of an inherited MEN type II syndrome, the presence of pheochromocytoma must be excluded before surgery.

Physical Examination

The examination should be guided by the features of the patient's individual expression of the MEN subtype. Thus, evidence of acromegaly from growth hormone–secreting tumors, hypertension from pheochromocytomas, or dehydration from diarrhea-causing tumors should be sought.

Diagnostic Testing

Ideally, evaluation of a MEN syndrome would have identified treatable disturbances before the time of surgery, with resultant attempts at medical management. In patients with a history of a particular manifestation of their MEN syndrome, however, the status of the condition should be determined. Measurement of levels of electrolytes, calcium, magnesium, phosphorous, and glucose may be necessary along with an assessment of renal function. Cardiac testing (ECG, echocardiography, CXR) may be indicated.

Preoperative Medication and Instructions

Other than continuance of the patient's routine medications, no special instructions or preoperative medications are necessary for patients with MEN type I. Patients with Zollinger-Ellison syndrome should continue H_2 receptor antagonists or omeprazole. Patients with insulinoma may be at risk for hypoglycemia while fasting if intravenous glucose is not provided. If octreotide acetate is used to control manifestations of carcinoid tumors, it should be continued. Patients with pheochromocytoma as a manifestation of MEN type II should be medicated and instructed as described above.

Implications for Perioperative and Anesthetic Management

Specific details of perioperative management for patients with MEN syndromes depend on the constellation of clinical features and their status at the time of anesthesia and surgery. The management issues should not be significantly different from those described for patients presenting with isolated endocrinopathies as discussed in previous sections.

PORPHYRIAS

The porphyrias are a collection of conditions resulting from abnormal biosynthesis of heme. Genetic defects in key enzymes lead to the accumulation of heme precursors, which results in photosensitivity, abdominal pain, neuropathy, or mental disturbances, depending on the type of porphyria. The porphyrias are ecogenic disorders; that is, environmental or physiologic factors act in concert with genetic lesions to produce overt signs and symptoms.

The porphyrias are classified into two broad categories depending on the site and nature of the enzyme defect: the hepatic porphyrias and the erythropoietic porphyrias (Table 6-7). The erythropoietic porphyrias are associated with photosensitivity but not with neurologic deficits. The hepatic porphyrias are characterized by combinations of photosensitivity and neurologic involvement. Neurologic involvement in the hepatic porphyrias can include autonomic nervous system dysfunction. Signs of sympathetic activation include tachycardia, sweating, and hypertension. Patients may exhibit orthostatic hypotension. Anxiety, nausea, vomiting, and abdominal pain are prominent presenting features.

Interview and History

At the preanesthetic interview, the subtype of porphyria should be identified. Three of the subtypes—acute intermittent porphyria, variegate porphyria, and hereditary coproporphyria—have been termed *inducible porphyrias* because they are associated with the precipitation of crises by anesthetic agents. The patient's usual clinical manifestations should be defined. Particu-

Table 6-7. Classification of human porphyrias

Type	Photosensitivity	Neurovisceral manifestations
Hepatic porphyrias		
δ-Aminolevulinic acid dehydratase deficiency	–	+
Acute intermittent porphyria	–	+
Hereditary copropor-phyria	+	+
Variegate porphyria	+	+
Porphyria cutanea tarda	+	–
Erythropoietic porphyrias		
X-linked sideroblastic anemia	–	–
Congenital erythro-poietic porphyria	+	–
Erythropoietic proto-porphyria	+	–

larly pertinent data include evidence of CNS or autonomic dysfunction and cutaneous manifestations. Of note, some of the motor neurologic defects from an acute exacerbation may take months or years to resolve.

Elevated steroid hormone levels and use of synthetic sex steroids are associated with acute exacerbations of porphyria. The likelihood of an exacerbation may vary during the female reproductive cycle. Exacerbations may be more frequent during pregnancy. The possibility of pregnancy should be specifically ascertained.

Physical Examination

Examination of the patient with porphyria-associated neurologic deficits should include assessment of vital signs with orthostatic blood pressure measurements, and identification of motor or sensory defects sometimes associated with the hepatic porphyrias. Skin lesions from photosensitivity should be identified.

Diagnostic Testing

Ideally, the porphyria subtype affecting a patient is identified in advance of the perioperative period. Diagnostic testing includes measurement of the levels of major metabolites in blood or urine and DNA analysis. Because the clinical features of the different porphyrias vary, an understanding of the subtype of porphyria is important for perioperative planning.

Laboratory determinations should include a hematocrit and measurement of electrolyte levels. Hyponatremia, hypokalemia, and evidence of impaired renal function should be excluded.

Table 6-8. Common perioperative drugs implicated in precipitating attacks of porphyria

Chloramphenicol	Valproic acid	Pentazocine	Ergots
	Carbamazepine	hydrochloride	
	Phenytoin	Etomidate	
		Benzodiazepines	
		Barbiturates	

Preoperative Medication and Instructions

Patients should continue routine medications and follow routine preoperative instructions. Some medications used in the preoperative period can precipitate attacks of porphyria and probably should be avoided (Table 6-8), although opinions vary, and whether or not all of the agents are problematic in all subtypes of porphyria is uncertain. Patients should not receive benzodiazepines or barbiturates for preoperative sedation.

Implications for Perioperative and Anesthetic Management

Certain common anesthetic agents, including barbiturates, etomidate, and benzodiazepines, should be avoided in patients with porphyria. All opioids (except pentazocine hydrochloride), all potent inhalation anesthetics, nitrous oxide, all muscle relaxants, anticholinergics, anticholinesterases, droperidol, phenothiazines, and local anesthetics are likely to be safe. Ketamine hydrochloride and propofol may be used. Although sex steroids are associated with exacerbations, glucocorticoids appear to be safe. The clinician should be aware of the possibility that general anesthesia can mask an acute attack of porphyria. Regional anesthetic procedures may be complicated by the presence of skin lesions overlying insertion points. In the patient with skin lesions, positioning may require particular care. Medicolegal concerns, however, may deter the clinician from administering a regional anesthetic in patients at risk for neurologic complications of the underlying disease. Of note, dehydration and starvation may precipitate attacks. Patients often present with volume depletion after an exacerbation manifesting with abdominal pain, nausea, vomiting, or diarrhea. Patients with photosensitivity may react to operating room lighting, and alternative light sources or shielding of the patient may be required.

CASE STUDY

A 60-year-old woman is scheduled for an elective urogynecologic procedure the next day. Her medical history includes stress incontinence after four vaginal deliveries and mild asthma, which is presently quiescent off medications. One year ago she presented to her primary care physician with a history of sweating, palpitations, and weight loss. A diagnosis of Graves' disease was made, and the patient was placed on methimazole with control of all symptoms with the exception of persistent Graves' ophthalmopathy. Six weeks before the date of surgery, testing revealed normalization of thyroid hormone levels. The antithyroid medication was stopped.

The patient is thin and alert, with prominent ophthalmopathy (proptosis and stare) and a large goiter. She is diaphoretic, her heart rate is 120 beats per minute, heart rhythm is regular, and the supine blood pressure is normal. The ECG demonstrates sinus tachycardia but no other abnormalities.

The anesthesiologist conducting the interview is concerned that the patient has a recrudescence of her Graves' disease with manifestations of thyrotoxicosis (weight loss, tachycardia, diaphoresis) after cessation of her antithyroid medications. The evaluation is expanded to include orthostatic signs, and a substantial drop in blood pressure is noted with standing. In addition, thyroid function studies (TSH, total T_4, free T_4 index, total T_3), and an electrolyte panel are ordered. Because intraoperative implications in a thyrotoxic state would include intravascular volume depletion, hypermetabolism, tachycardia, relative adrenal insufficiency, and the risk of overt thyroid storm, the anesthesiologist contacts the surgeon to recommend postponement of the procedure and referral back to the primary care physician or an endocrinologist for management of the thyroid condition. He recommends a trial of calcium channel blockers to control the patient's tachycardia, given a history of asthma.

DISCUSSION

The patient has a documented history of Graves' disease, which was initially managed with the antithyroid agent methimazole. Methimazole blocks the formation of T_4 and T_3 but does not cure Graves' disease. Thus, stopping the antithyroid medication permitted a reactivation of the condition. The anesthesiologist in the preoperative clinic recognized signs of hyperthyroidism in this patient, including tachycardia, diaphoresis, dehydration and intravascular volume depletion, and ophthalmopathy. Graves' patients are often very refractory to pharmacologic control of tachycardia. Beta-adrenergic blockade is usually the treatment of choice. Asthma is a relative contraindication to this type of therapy, however, so that calcium channel blockade was recommended as an alternative.

In this situation, the elective surgical procedure can be safely postponed until stabilization of the endocrine condition. Should urgent surgery be required in a patient with untreated or undertreated thyrotoxicosis, a regimen of propylthiouracil, iodine, and beta-adrenergic blockers, combined with steroid and fluid replacement, is indicated. The patient should be prepared for the urgent procedure with guidance from an endocrinologist. Consideration should be given to aggressive monitoring and possible postoperative care in an intensive care unit.

ACKNOWLEDGMENT

The authors thank Dr. Mark Dershwitz for helpful discussion in the preparation of the section on the porphyrias.

BIBLIOGRAPHY

Adam R. The patient with multiple endocrine neoplasia. In: Frost EAM, ed. *Preanesthetic assessment 3*. Boston: Birkhauser, 1991:57–73.

Badola RP. The patient with carcinoid syndrome. In: Frost EAM, ed. *Preanesthetic assessment 4*. Boston: Birkhauser, 1994:12–25.

Cheng EY, Kay J, eds. *Manual of anesthesia and the medically compromised patient*. Philadelphia: JB Lippincott Co, 1990.

Fauci AS, Braunwald E, Isselbacher KJ, et al., eds. *Harrison's principles of internal medicine,* 14th ed. New York, McGraw-Hill, 1998.

Gavin LA. Perioperative management of the diabetic patient. *Endocrinol Metab Clin North Am* 1992;21:457–475.

Patt RB. The patient with pheochromocytoma. In: Frost EAM, ed. *Preanesthetic assessment 1*. Boston: Birkhauser, 1988:92–99.

Stoelting RK, Dierdorf SF, eds. *Anesthesia and coexisting disease*, 3rd ed. New York: Churchill Livingstone, 1993.

Wilson JD, Foster SW, Kronenberg HM, Larsen PR, eds. *Williams textbook of endocrinology,* 9th ed. Philadelphia: WB Saunders, 1998.

Hematologic Issues

Stanley P. Sady and BobbieJean Sweitzer

Many hematologic abnormalities are asymptomatic but may lead to significant perioperative morbidity if not recognized or treated. This chapter describes the preoperative evaluation and preparation of patients with **anemia, hemoglobin disorders** (e.g., **sickle cell disease, thalassemia**), **inherited coagulopathies** [e.g., **hemophilia, von Willebrand's disease** (vWD)], and **acquired coagulopathies** (e.g., **drug-induced coagulopathy, vitamin K deficiency**). The use of **aspirin** (acetylsalicylic acid) and other **nonsteroidal antiinflammatory drugs** (NSAIDs), **anticoagulants**, and **thrombolytic therapy** in patients undergoing surgery are discussed. The etiology and pathophysiology of these conditions are presented with major emphasis on the history and physical examination. Efficacy and economy are stressed in the use of laboratory tests for diagnosis and monitoring.

ANEMIA

Anemia is a reduction below the lower limits of normal (fifth percentile) in the concentration of hemoglobin (Hgb) or red blood cells (RBCs) not explained by the state of hydration. Hgb lower than 11.7 g per dL and hematocrit lower than 35% for women older than 18 years; Hgb lower than 13.2 and hematocrit lower than 39% for men 18 to 65 years; and Hgb lower than 12.6 and hematocrit lower than 37% for men older than 65 are considered the lower limits of normal. The following information should be elicited when a low Hgb or hematocrit value is obtained: (a) Is the decreased Hgb/hematocrit due to a decrease in RBC mass or an increase in plasma volume (e.g., due to pregnancy, oliguric renal failure, congestive heart failure, recumbency chronic disease)? (b) Has the value changed over a short time? A reduction in Hgb of 10% may be the first clue that something is wrong, even if the new value is still normal.

Erythropoietin, primarily secreted by the kidney, enhances erythropoiesis by stimulating production of proerythroblasts and release of reticulocytes from bone marrow. The *reticulocyte count* is the percentage of RBCs occurring as reticulocytes (immature RBCs), which is normally 0.5% to 2.5%. The *reticulocyte production index* is the correction of the reticulocyte count in the presence of anemia (total count is spuriously elevated with reduced total RBCs). *Mean corpuscular volume* is the volume occupied by an RBC, *mean corpuscular hemoglobin* is the amount of Hgb in each RBC, and *mean corpuscular hemoglobin concentration* is the percentage of space in the RBC occupied by Hgb.

Anemia is the most common hematologic abnormality in preoperative patients.[1–3] It is not a diagnosis but rather, like fever, an objective sign of the presence of disease.[4,5] A finding of anemia requires a search for and treatment of the underlying cause (e.g., renal insufficiency, drug reaction). It can be a hallmark of many diseases that may affect anesthetic management.[2,4–6] Except for patients with ischemic heart disease and perhaps some patients with sickle cell disease (see Sickle Cell Disease, below), no evidence exists that normovolemic anemia increases perioperative morbidity and mortality.[1,6] For patients with ischemic heart disease, hematocrits lower than 29% or greater than 34% are associated with increased episodes of myocardial ischemia after vascular surgery. No data confirm the hypothesis that treatment of mild or moderate normovolemic anemia in asymptomatic patients undergoing surgery without major blood loss decreases perioperative complications. The underlying cause of the anemia may be of greater importance to the patient's health than its impact on an elective procedure.

No data exist to define a minimum preoperative Hgb for all patients. A carefully controlled outcome study is not available to confirm the validity of any recommendation. Chronic anemia is tolerated better than acute anemia. Patients with cardiopulmonary or vascular disease with flow-restricting lesions have limited ability to compensate for anemia. Suggested guidelines for transfusion must balance the infectious and immunologic risks with the need for oxygen (O_2) delivery.[7] Preoperative treatment should be directed at eradicating the cause of anemia or modification of the underlying disorder.[4,5]

Hgb concentration is not the sole determinant of the symptoms of anemia nor of the urgency to correct the anemia. Healthy patients may tolerate an Hgb level of 6 to 7 g per dL (hematocrit of 20%) because of physiologic compensation, although cardiovascular work is increased.[2,4,5] The symptoms from anemia depend on the Hgb level, the reduction in O_2-carrying capacity of blood, the change in total blood volume, and the rate at which these develop. Symptoms depend on the manifestations of the disorder that resulted in anemia and the capacity of the cardiovascular and pulmonary systems to compensate. The physiologic compensation to maintain O_2 delivery includes increased blood flow to tissues through autoregulation (redistribution), decreased blood viscosity (which lowers systemic vascular resistance and increases venous return), and increased cardiac output (tachycardia, increased contractility). A rightward shift occurs in the O_2 dissociation curve from increased 2,3-diphosphoglycerate, which facilitates unloading of O_2 at the cellular level.

Understanding the pathogenesis of the anemia is crucial for effective treatment. Iron-deficiency anemia, anemia of chronic disease, and thalassemia are the most prevalent anemias in the United States.[4–6] One should assume that bleeding is the cause of anemia until proven otherwise because of the possible need for urgent intervention in such cases.

Several classifications have been used for anemia. A combined morphologic and kinetic approach is presented here. The morphologic approach is based on characteristic changes in the size and Hgb content of RBCs in the various types of anemia. These changes are detected by computing RBC indices (mean corpuscular volume, mean corpuscular hemoglobin, mean corpuscular hemoglobin concentration) and are confirmed by direct observation of RBCs on the stained blood film. The kinetic classification assumes that the number of RBCs is the result of a dynamic equilibrium between production and destruction. The reticulocyte count and the reticulocyte production index suggest whether problems exist with RBC production (low reticulocyte production index) or survival (high reticulocyte production index).

The search for the cause of anemia should be systematic and include history taking, physical examination, and collection of basic laboratory data. The anemia may have multiple causes and may require hematologic consultation and adjuvant laboratory tests. The cause for most anemias is determined from a careful history and physical examination.[2–5]

History and Physical Examination

The focus of the history and physical examination depends on whether the clinician suspects anemia, a laboratory value indicates an unexpected anemia, or the patient has a known anemia. A patient with a known anemia should be questioned about the onset, previous Hgb values, symptoms, and treatment.

The history taking should elicit information regarding the onset (insidious or acute) and duration of symptoms. Specific symptoms caused by anemia are related to tissue hypoxia (fatigue, angina, dyspnea) and cardiovascular compensation (palpitations, tachycardia). Pain, especially bone pain, occurs with myeloproliferative disorders, cancer, and sickle cell disease. Symptoms suggestive of an underlying disease (e.g., chronic renal failure, infection, an endocrinopathy, malignancy) should be sought.

The most recent date of a normal hematologic examination and response to previous surgery are helpful. Other hints such as a history of acceptance or rejection as a volunteer blood donor or previous iron, folic acid, or vitamin B_{12} therapy are useful. Has the patient had diarrhea, black or bloody bowel movements, hemoptysis, fever, abnormal urine color, changes in body weight, or edema? For women, evaluation should include menstrual history and number of pregnancies and abortions. The family history may reveal Hgb or bleeding disorders. The social history should include information regarding occupation, household customs, hobbies, diet, and exposure to chemicals. The use of prescription and nonprescription drugs should be determined.

Pallor of the skin, conjunctiva, and lips should be noted. The skin and mucus membranes should be inspected for bleeding, petechiae, or purpura. Sternal tenderness can occur in myeloproliferative disorders, myeloma, and acute leukemia. Heart murmurs may occur from increased cardiac output and decreased blood viscosity, which causes turbulence. Palpation for lymph nodes, liver, and spleen should be performed. A pelvic and rectal examination are not usually carried out in a preoperative clinical examination but can be performed to detect bleeding and masses.

Diagnostic Testing

Initial studies include a complete blood cell count (CBC), reticulocyte count, and examination of the peripheral blood smear. The CBC includes an RBC count, Hgb, hematocrit, mean corpuscular volume, mean corpuscular hemoglobin, mean corpuscular hemoglobin concentration, and platelet count. Tests for occult blood in the urine and stool should be performed. Adjuvant laboratory tests include an erythrocyte sedimentation rate; urinalysis; blood urea nitrogen (BUN) level; creatinine; bilirubin level; iron level; total iron-binding capacity; and levels of ferritin, B_{12}, and folate. For example, if a patient has hypochromic microcytic or normocytic anemia, ferritin and iron levels and total iron-binding capacity may diagnose iron deficiency. Vitamin B_{12} and folate levels are indicated for macrocytic anemia in a suspected alcoholic.

An abbreviated laboratory evaluation of anemia is shown in Table 7-1. Consultation with a hematologist may be required for a more thorough assessment. The goal is to make the correct diagnosis with practical and economic efficiency.

Testing in patients with anemia who are likely to need a transfusion include a *type and screen (T&S)* or *type and cross match (T&CM)*.[7] *Typing* involves testing the patient's RBCs for ABO and Rh blood groups. The ABO group is determined by using anti-A and anti-B reagents against the patient's RBCs ("front") and by reverse-typing the patient's serum against A and B reagent cells ("back"). *Screening* for unexpected antibodies is done by incubating the serum with selected reagent RBCs using an anti–human globulin technique (Coombs' test). Typing takes 5 to 10 minutes and screening takes 45 minutes. A positive screen necessitates identification of the unexpected antibody, which can take several hours. A cross match involves incubating the donor's blood with the patient's serum to verify *in vitro* compatibility. It is performed as a short incubation (5 to 10 minutes) to verify ABO compatibility in patients without antibodies or as a long incubation (45 minutes or longer) for patients with clinically significant antibodies. A cross match should be ordered only if a high likelihood exists of transfusing RBCs and is performed only on T&S results less than 72 hours old. Each hospital should have *maximum surgical blood-ordering schedules* that list surgical procedures with the recommended number of cross-matched units of blood and procedures for which a T&S is appropriate.

Preoperative Anesthetic Management

The decreased O_2-carrying capacity that occurs with anemia is the primary perioperative concern. If surgery is performed in the presence of anemia, one should minimize changes that interfere further with O_2 delivery,[2] including: (a) decreases in cardiac output, (b) a leftward shift of the oxyhemoglobin dissociation curve caused by respiratory alkalosis from iatrogenic hyperventilation or hypothermia, and (c) increases in O_2 consumption from shivering or elevated body temperatures.

There are no specific preoperative recommendations for patients with anemia, except those who have or are likely to have sickle cell anemia (see Sickle Cell Disease, below) or ischemic heart disease.[1]

The decision to transfuse preoperatively to a specific Hgb level must be individualized, with consideration given to several factors. These include the cause and duration of the anemia; the intravascular volume, type, and urgency of the operative procedure; anticipated blood loss; and coexisting diseases, especially cardiac, pulmonary, cerebrovascular, and

Table 7-1. Algorithm for the laboratory evaluation of anemia

RPI <2.5 (hypoproliferative process)
MCV <80 fL: hypochromic, microcytic
  Defects in hemoglobin synthesis
  Iron-deficiency anemia (low serum ferritin)
  Hemoglobinopathy (thalassemia)
  Chronic diseases
  Myelodysplastic syndromes
  Porphyrias
  Sideroblastic anemia
MCV 80–100 fL: normochromic
  Early iron-deficiency anemia
  Sudden massive blood loss
  Marrow failure syndromes
  Hemoglobinopathy (sickle cell disease)
  Hemolysis
  Chronic diseases
  (Note: Many microcytic and macrocytic anemias in the early stages
    may present with a normal MCV.)
MCV >100 fL: macrocytic
  Megaloblastic
      Defects in DNA synthesis (vitamin B_{12}, folate deficiency)
      Drug induced (e.g., by chemotherapeutics, anticonvulsants,
        oral contraceptives)
      Myelodysplastic syndromes
  Nonmegaloblastic
      Alcohol
      Membrane cholesterol defects secondary to liver disease or
        hypothyroidism
      Cold agglutinin disease
RPI >2.5
Hemolytic
  Extrinsic cause of RBC destruction (usually acquired)
      Splenomegaly
      Autoimmune hemolytic anemia
  Intrinsic; inherent defect in RBC (usually hereditary)
      Enzymatic defects
          Glucose-6-phosphate dehydrogenase deficiency
          Pyruvate kinase deficiency
      Membrane defects
          Hereditary spherocytosis
      Hemoglobinopathies, including thalassemia
Bleeding disorder
  Acute blood loss
  RBC sequestration in spleen

MCV, mean corpuscular volume; RBC, red blood cell; RPI, reticulocyte production index.
Reprinted with permission from Lee GR, Bithell TC, Foerster J, et al., eds. *Wintrobe's clinical hematology*, 9th ed. Philadelphia: Lea & Febiger, 1993.

peripheral vascular disease. A consensus statement for RBC transfusion guidelines states that the "transfusion of RBCs is rarely indicated when the Hgb concentration is >10 g per dL and almost always indicated when <6 g per dL. The decision to transfuse when the Hgb is between these two levels (6 to 10 g per dL) should be based on the patient's risk for complications of inadequate oxygenation."[7]

Erythropoietin therapy can be used to avoid RBC transfusion, especially for those patients whose initial hematocrit is 33% to 39% and whose surgical blood losses are anticipated to be 1,000 to 3,000 mL.[8] A weekly subcutaneous dose of erythropoietin is given for 4 weeks before surgery, starting at 100 units per kg and increasing to 600 units per kg, if necessary, to produce evidence of increased reticulocytosis. The combination of preoperative erythropoietin therapy and use of autologous blood (normovolemic hemodilution, autotransfusion) may be most effective.[8]

Hemoglobin Disorders

Quantitative (thalassemia) or qualitative (sickle cell) disorders of Hgb caused by DNA mutations result in hypochromic microcytic (thalssemia) and normocytic (sickle cell) anemias.[9] Diagnosis is made with Hgb electrophoresis. More than 300 types of hemoglobinopathies are described in the literature,[2,4,5] but most are quite rare. The most common in the United States is sickle cell disease. Hemoglobinopathies occur in heterozygous and homozygous forms.[4] In the heterozygous form, RBCs contain both normal adult Hgb (Hgb A) and the variant Hgb. Manifestations of the heterozygous state are rarely of clinical significance, and thus patients are said to have the *trait* for that abnormality (e.g., sickle cell trait). Hgb A is absent in the homozygous state; patients have clinical manifestations of variable severity and are said to have anemia (e.g., sickle cell anemia). Patients may have disease from combinations of variant Hgb types or a variant Hgb and a thalassemia gene (e.g., Hgb S–thalassemia).

Thalassemia syndromes are quantitative abnormalities of globin synthesis (inadequate production of normal globin). The α, β, γ, and σ globin chains are synthesized at different rates in the RBC under the control of individual gene loci.[2] The major types of Hgb (A, A_2, F) result when two pairs of globin chains combine with heme.

Sickle Cell Disease

Hgb S is a variant Hgb produced by substitution of valine for glutamic acid in position 6 of the β chain due to a defect on chromosome 11. The polymerization of deoxygenated Hgb S results in a distorted RBC.[10] If the proportion of Hgb S is high enough, the solubility is altered, which leads to precipitation of Hgb in the RBC. Sickle cell disease[2] results in a more rigid RBC, with greater adhesiveness to endothelium, a shorter half-life (10 to 20 days versus 120 days normally), an increased viscosity of blood, and a more rapid release of O_2 (rightward shift of the Hgb dissociation curve: $P_{50} = 31$ mm Hg versus 26 mm Hg normally). Sickled RBCs occlude vascular beds and trigger thrombosis and infarction. Tissues with a limited O_2 supply as a result of stagnant or limited collateral blood flow or high metabolic demand are at particular risk for vasoocclusion and infarction. The potential for a sickled cell to initiate a vasoocclusive event depends primarily on whether the rate of polymer formation is within the RBCs' capillary transit time.[10] Anything that retards RBCs in the microcirculation increases the risk of vasoocclusion in sickle cell disease.

The proportions of Hgb S, Hgb F, and Hgb A_2 that occur in sickle cell disease alter the clinical presentation of the patient (Table 7-2). Acute crises can occur during the perioperative period and are of three types: vasoocclusive crisis, aplastic crisis, and splenic sequestration. Vasoocclusive crises are episodes of abrupt vascular occlusion causing microinfarcts. Severe pain can occur almost anywhere in the body. Treatment consists of O_2 administration, hydration, analgesia and, rarely, transfusion. One manifestation of acute vasoocclusive crisis is the acute chest syndrome, characterized by cough, fever, chest pain, infiltrates on chest radiograph (CXR), and hypoxemia. The clinical picture is a cycle of pulmonary vasoocclusion causing hypoxemia, which leads to progressive pulmonary sickling and worsened hypoxemia. Transfusion is often necessary.

Aplastic crisis is a temporary cessation in erythropoiesis, usually caused by human parvovirus B19 and occurring typically in children. Manifestations are those of severe anemia. It is usually transient (lasting a few days) and self-limited, but transfusion may be necessary.

Splenic sequestration is the pooling of blood in the spleen with a rapid fall in vascular volume. It occurs in children younger than

Table 7-2. Common hemoglobin (Hgb) S variants

	Hgb SS: sickle cell anemia	Hgb SC: sickle cell–Hgb C disease	Hgb SA: sickle cell trait
Hgb (g/dL)	7–8	9–12	13–15
Hgb S (%)	70–80	45–50	30–40
Frequency in African Americans (%)	0.2	0.3	8–10
Life expectancy	30 yr	Slightly reduced	Normal
Propensity for sickling ($++++$, highest; $+$, lowest)	$++++$	$++$	$+$
Pao$_2$ for irreversible sickling	40–45 mm Hg	?	20–25 mm Hg

Pao$_2$, partial pressure of oxygen, arterial.
Data from Roizen M. Anesthetic implications of concurrent diseases. In: Miller RD, ed. *Anesthesia*, 4th ed. New York: Churchill Livingstone, 1994:980–986; Murray DJ. Evaluation of the patient with anemia and coagulation disorders. In: Rogers MC, Tinker JH, Covino BG, Longnecker DE, eds. *Principles and practice of anesthesiology*. St. Louis: Mosby–Year Book, 1993:341–356; and Goodwin SR. Perioperative implications of hemoglobinopathies. *Anesth Analg* 1998;Mar[Suppl]:39–44.

6 years and leads to hypovolemic shock and peripheral circulatory failure, and may be rapidly progressive and fatal. Prompt transfusion is required and splenectomy is completely effective.

No definitive treatment exists for sickle cell diseases, but prevention of crises is key.[4,5,10–12] Conditions that increase O_2 demand, such as fever, increased metabolic rate, infection, shivering, and pain, can lead to crises. Decreased or sluggish blood flow from dehydration, hypothermia, vasoconstriction, hypotension, and stagnant circulation (e.g., from use of tourniquets) should be avoided. Hyperviscosity can be prevented by lowering the mean corpuscular hemoglobin concentration to decrease the polymerization of Hgb S. This can be done by maintaining appropriate vascular volume and inducing hyponatremia, which causes osmotic swelling of RBCs (meticulous laboratory monitoring is required). Antiplatelet drugs (aspirin and other NSAIDs) prevent increased adhesiveness of RBCs. Decreased O_2 binding to Hgb, as occurs with hypoxemia and acidosis, increases sickling. Simple or exchange transfusion with normal adult Hgb (AA) to dilute Hgb S and decrease blood viscosity is an option (see Preoperative Anesthetic Management, below). Hydroxyurea is used to increase Hgb F production. Bone marrow transplantation as a cure is being investigated.

Glucose-6-Phosphate Dehydrogenase Deficiency

Glucose-6-phosphate dehydrogenase (G6PD) deficiency[5,6] is a disorder with a sex-linked recessive mode of inheritance and is present in 10% of African American men. It results in hemolysis of RBCs with resulting anemia. Patients with this disorder may have increased hemolysis with drugs that require G6PD for detoxification.

History and Physical Examination

Preoperative questioning regarding previous and current status of the disease is essential.[2,6,13] Sickle cell disease or variants should be considered in the evaluation of every African American patient. Almost all children born in the United States are screened for sickle cell disease as newborns. The history and physical examination can distinguish between disease, which has major organ involvement of the cardiovascular, pulmonary, renal, and central nervous systems, and sickle cell trait, which has no major clinical manifestations. Anemia and mild jaundice are almost always present with disease but not with trait.[2,4,5] Information about previous surgeries, complications, and treatment is invaluable in preparation for anesthesia.

Anemia or hemochromatosis from multiple transfusions can affect various systems. Patients may have delayed growth and development and frequent infections, which are the leading cause of death. Skeletal involvement includes infarcts with fishmouth vertebrae, aseptic necrosis of the femoral head, osteomyelitis (from *Salmonella* infection) and ankle ulcers. Thrombosis, coma, convulsions, visual disturbances, retinal and vitreous hemorrhages, and strokes may occur. Patients may develop congestive heart failure and cardiomegaly from chronic hypoxia, hemochromatosis, and anemia. Increased intrapulmonary shunting, pulmonary infarction, and the acute chest syndrome (see Sickle Cell

Disease, above) may be seen. Jaundice, unconjugated hyperbilirubinemia from hemolysis, bile cholelithiasis, and splenic infarcts (asplenia) may occur by adolescence. Renal medullary infarcts, papillary necrosis, and priapism are common. G6PD-deficiency patients may be jaundiced but otherwise are relatively normal.

Diagnostic Testing

Some authors recommend use of a rapid screening test for Hgb S for at-risk populations (e.g., African Americans, those of Mediterranean descent) before surgery.[2] The test uses oxidant solutions to determine an RBC sickling tendency. A positive test confirms the presence of Hgb S but does not differentiate among SA (trait) with minimal symptoms, SS (disease), or Hgb S–thalassemia. The test is sensitive but nonspecific. A positive result in a patient with a history of appropriate symptoms likely represents a homozygous state or a variant that may require special preoperative preparation. Hgb electrophoresis is the definitive test for determining the types and proportions of Hgb. Some authors contend that preoperative screening is not useful[13] because it may not alter the anesthetic plan. Prevention of intraoperative hypoxia, hypotension, and acidosis are desirable goals in all patients.

Preoperatively, sickle cell and G6PD-deficiency patients need an Hgb determination. Additional tests may be required if the history and physical examination suggests systemic effects. These may include but are not limited to an electrocardiogram (ECG); CXR; measurement of the levels of bilirubin, serum glutamic oxaloacetic transaminase, serum glutamic pyruvic transaminase, alkaline phosphatase, albumin, BUN, glucose, and creatinine; and measurement of prothrombin time (PT).

Preoperative Anesthetic Management

Patients with sickle cell disease may be less likely to experience problems during regional or general anesthesia than in their normal daily activities.[2] A decrease in O_2 consumption and increased inspired O_2 concentration and blood flow to many tissues during anesthesia should decrease the likelihood of sickling. Splanchnic and renal blood flow decrease during anesthesia and surgery, however, particularly during an abdominal procedure.

Preventive measures include delivery of supplemental O_2, provision of adequate hydration and analgesia, use of sterile techniques to avoid infection, and careful sedation that avoids depression of ventilation with resultant hypoxia and respiratory acidosis. Temperature should be controlled because fever increases the rate of gel formation by Hgb S and hypothermia produces peripheral vasoconstriction.

The use of preoperative transfusion in sickle cell patients is controversial.[1,4–6,9,10,12,14,15] Some authors suggest limiting exchange transfusion to crisis situations.[1] If the reason for surgery is related to an acute complication of sickle cell disease (e.g., priapism, abdominal pain), the threshold for performing transfusion may be lower. Other authors believe that prophylactic transfusion is not necessary, except possibly for those undergoing vitreoretinal surgery.[9] Transfusion usually can be avoided for short, minor procedures that require brief anesthesia (placement of myringotomy tubes, some dental procedures). Tonsillectomy and adenoidectomy, however, appear to carry an appreciable risk of complications in children with sickle cell disease.

The specific transfusion technique used—simple or partial exchange—is not as critical as the hematologic end point. The method of transfusion used depends largely on the clinical urgency and time available. When sufficient opportunity exists, repeated simple transfusions over 2 to 4 weeks are used. In a sickle cell patient weighing 70 kg with an Hgb level of 6 to 7 g per dL, the transfusion of one packed RBC unit should increase the level of Hgb A by 10% to 15% or more.[2] When RBC transfusion is repeated two or three times, the population of sickled Hgb decreases to less than 40%. This benefit lasts for weeks because of the longer life span of normal RBCs compared to sickle cells. When urgent surgery is required, a single volume-exchange transfusion of 60 to 70 mL per kg is satisfactory. A patient with an Hgb level of less than 8 g per dL can probably be managed with simple transfusion, whereas a patient with a higher initial Hgb level may require exchange transfusion to avoid polycythemia. Transfusion to a preoperative Hgb level of 10 to 13 g per dL and Hgb S level of less than 30% to 40% is indicated for procedures requiring prolonged general anesthesia and procedures in which low regional blood flow is anticipated. Cardiac, orthopedic, or neurosurgical procedures involving critical anatomic sites are of special concern.

A patient with sickle cell disease who requires cardiopulmonary bypass needs exchange or simple transfusion to reduce Hgb S to less than 40% preoperatively. During cardiopulmonary bypass, the level of Hgb S decreases further as a result of dilution. Hypothermia is associated with vasoconstriction, decreased blood flow and metabolic rate, and an increased solubility of Hgb S. The increased solubility of Hgb S prevents precipitation and, with the decreased viscosity from hemodilution, the likelihood that sickling will lead to vasoocclusion is markedly decreased during cardiopulmonary bypass. Deep hypothermic arrest may merit special considerations. Autotransfusion has been used successfully when transfusion to lower Hgb S level was performed before anesthesia. Cardiopulmonary bypass carries no risk with sickle cell trait because sickling occurs only with a PO_2 of 20 to 25 mm Hg.

The transfusion goal in the compound heterozygous sickle syndromes (e.g., Hgb S–thalassemia) is to have 30% to 40% or fewer sickleable cells.[9] In these syndromes, all RBCs contain Hgb S and are capable of sickling under certain physiologic conditions. Therefore, the focus should be not on the percentage of Hgb S but rather on the percentage of RBCs that are sickleable. A value of 30% sickleable cells corresponds to approximately 15% Hgb S.

Most authors conclude that no specific anesthetic method is preferable for patients with sickle cell disease. Retrospective review of patient records led authors to conclude that, at most, a 0.5% mortality rate could be attributed to the interaction between sickle cell anemia and an anesthetic agent.[1] Conflicting statements have been made regarding the use of inhaled anes-thetics in sickle cell disease. Some authors have reported that inhaled anesthetics accelerate precipitation of Hgb S *in vitro*; the clinical significance of this is unknown.[14] Others have stated that the use of halothane enhances Hgb S solubility and theo-retically could decrease sickling.[2] Others have reported that the number of circulating sickle cells may decrease during and immediately after general anesthesia, regardless of the drugs used.[6]

Regional anesthesia may produce compensatory vasoconstric-tion and decrease O_2 delivery to nonblocked areas, increasing the risk of sickling and infarction. However, circulatory stasis can be prevented with adequate hydration. Rates of postoperative pain-ful crisis were found to be higher with regional anesthesia than with local or general anesthesia in the Cooperative Study of Sickle Cell Disease.[11,12] Epidural anesthesia has been used to treat painful vasoocclusive crises. The anesthetic technique used is probably less important than meticulous attention to preven-tive measures discussed above.[1,15]

The use of a tourniquet during surgery in patients with sickle cell disease or sickle cell trait is controversial. No definitive stud-ies have been done, but common sense suggests avoiding a tour-niquet or limiting its use to short periods.

To prevent increased hemolysis in patients with G6PD defi-ciency, one should avoid sulfa drugs, quinidine sulfate, prilocaine, antipyretic drugs, nonnarcotic analgesics, vitamin K analogs, and perhaps sodium nitroprusside.[4–6]

Thalassemia

Thalassemia is the most prevalent of all known genetic dis-eases.[4,5,9] More than 100 thalassemia mutations have been identi-fied. Thalassemia syndromes are common in Southeast Asia, India, and the Middle East, and in people of African descent. Globin structures are normal, but because of gene deletion, the rate of synthesis of either the α Hgb chain (α-thalassemia) or β Hgb chain (β-thalassemia) is reduced. In thalassemia, RBCs are more susceptible than normal to oxidative stress because of uncombined globin chains, increased amounts of nonheme iron, and relatively low concentrations of Hgb.[9]

α-Thalassemia

Two copies of the gene that codes for the α-globin chain are located on chromosome 16. The α-thalassemias occur because of inadequate α-globin production. The relative excess of non-α chains causes protein aggregation into insoluble inclusions in the maturing RBC. This leads to premature destruction of maturing erythroblasts (ineffective erythropoiesis), low intra-cellular Hgb (hypochromia), and lysis of defective RBCs in the spleen (hemolysis). The clinical manifestations depend on the number of deleted α-genes. Patients with *silent* α-thalassemia from deletion of one globin chain do not have anemia and are asymptomatic. The α-thalassemia *trait* is characterized by dele-tions of two α-globin chains producing only a mild hypochromic microcytic anemia, and patients are asymptomatic. *Hgb H* results from three α-globin deletions, leading to moderately severe anemia, prominent microcytosis, and mild to moderate hemolysis. These patients have a shortened lifespan and have severe symptoms from the anemia. Hydrops fetalis is a lethal intrauterine disease resulting from complete deletion of the α-globin chains.

β-Thalassemia

The β chains are coded by two β-globin genes on chromosome 11. β-Thalassemia is caused by an excess of α chains, which denature developing RBCs, leading to their premature death in the marrow or shortened survival in the circulation. Symptoms depend on the type of β-thalassemia. *Thalassemia minor (trait)* is asymptomatic; symptoms in *thalassemia intermedia* are severe, but the patient is not transfusion dependent; in *thalassemia major* (*Cooley's anemia,* characterized by total absence of β chains), the patient is transfusion dependent.

History and Physical Examination

Patients with thalassemia may have facial deformities, including malar enlargement, which occur from erythropoietin-stimulated ineffective erythropoiesis, and marked expansion of the bone marrow because of the genetic inability to produce useful Hgb. If a patient is transfusion dependent, careful preoperative evaluation of hepatic, cardiac, and endocrine function is warranted because of iron toxicity (hemochromatosis). Cardiomyopathy, congestive heart failure, conduction defects, and arrhythmias may occur, especially after repeated blood transfusions with resultant hemochromatosis. Congestive heart failure also develops from severe anemia and an expanded plasma volume resulting from shunting of a large fraction of the cardiac output through hypertrophied marrow cavities and an enlarged liver and spleen. Hepatic dysfunction occurs because of fibrosis and cirrhosis from hemochromatosis. Delayed growth and maturation, and pancreatic insufficiency with glucose intolerance are possible.

Diagnostic Testing

Thalassemia is characterized by hypochromic microcytic anemia. A peripheral blood smear reveals RBCs of various shapes, possibly target cells and nucleated RBCs. Hgb electrophoresis assists in the diagnosis. Preoperatively, a hematocrit is necessary. Additional tests may be required if the history and physical examination suggest systemic effects. These tests may include but are not limited to an ECG, CXR, measurement of serum glutamic oxaloacetic transaminase, serum glutamic pyruvic transaminase, alkaline phosphatase, albumin, bilirubin, BUN, creatinine, and glucose levels, and measurement of PT.

Preoperative Anesthetic Management

Anesthetic considerations depend on the severity of the ane-mia.[2,15] See the subsection Preoperative Anesthetic Management under Anemia (above). If the patient is transfusion dependent, the effects of hemochromatosis and the likelihood of cardiomyopathy and hepatic dysfunction should be considered. The use of deferoxamine mesylate, an iron chelator, has no implications for anesthesia. If facial deformities are present, fiberoptic intubation should be considered.

ERYTHROCYTOSIS (POLYCYTHEMIA)

A patient with a hematocrit of more than 50% has an absolute (primary or secondary) or relative erythrocytosis. *Relative* erythrocytosis results from a reduction in plasma volume, is usually chronic, and is seen in middle-aged, obese, hypertensive men.[5,6,16] Diuretic therapy for treatment of hypertension may contribute to the plasma volume deficit.

Primary erythrocytosis (polycythemia vera) is a neoplastic stem cell disorder characterized by increased RBC mass, splenomegaly, thrombocytosis, and leukocytosis.[1,5,6,16] *Secondary* erythrocytosis results from a physiologically appropriate response to tissue hypoxia or inappropriate increases in erythropoietin production with certain renal and hepatic disorders. Causes of tissue hypoxia include high altitude, presence of high-affinity Hgb, cardiopulmonary disease, obesity-hypoventilation syndrome, obstructive sleep apnea, and presence of carboxyhemoglobin from smoking. Renal cysts; hydronephrosis; and tumors of the kidney, liver, and posterior fossa have been reported to increase erythropoietin production.

The increased blood viscosity and decreased O_2 delivery that accompany erythrocytosis are thought to partly explain the central nervous system (CNS) symptoms (transient ischemic attacks, decreased level of consciousness) and retinal, cardiac, and peripheral vascular symptoms seen. Patients with uncontrolled polycythemia vera have a very high surgical morbidity and mortality, mostly due to thromboembolic events.[1,4–6,16] In these patients, a high platelet count may further increase the risk.[16] The platelet count at which such risk is increased is not known.

History and Physical Examination

The history should elicit information regarding any history of smoking, sleep or pulmonary disorders, exercise intolerance, obesity, or cyanotic congenital heart disease, and previous hematocrit values. Inquiries should be made about a personal or family history of kidney or liver disease (e.g., tumors, cysts) and familial erythrocytosis. Patients should be questioned about symptoms of hyperviscosity, such as headache, dizziness, visual disturbances, fatigue, paresthesia, transient ischemic attacks, and decreased mental acuity.[5] Previous thromboembolic events should be explored.

Examination should concentrate on the general overall appearance (obesity, fatigued look, cyanosis), evidence of cardiopulmonary disease (see Chapters 3 and 4), CNS deficits, and splenomegaly.

Diagnostic Testing

A very high hematocrit (60% or higher for men, 57% or higher for women) is almost always indicative of a primary or secondary erythrocytosis and is not due to decreased plasma volume. In such cases, a diagnosis of polycythemia vera is supported by the presence of leukocytosis, thrombocytosis, or splenomegaly. Specialized studies, including assessment of serum carboxyhemoglobin and erythropoietin levels, urinalysis, sleep studies, and renal and liver imaging may be needed to differentiate among the secondary causes of erythrocytosis.[5] Preoperatively, these patients need a CBC and additional studies as suggested by the history and physical examination, including a CXR, ECG, and measurement of arterial blood gases, BUN, and creatinine levels.

Preoperative Anesthetic Management

In polycythemia vera, phlebotomy should be performed to decrease the hematocrit to less than 45% before elective surgery. In secondary erythrocytosis for which it is physiologically appropriate, the benefits of decreasing blood viscosity with phlebotomy must be balanced against the risk of decreased O_2-carrying capacity. In secondary erythrocytosis, the hematocrit goal is 50% to 60%.

Phlebotomy should be performed with removal of 350 to 500 mL of blood daily until the target hematocrit is reached. This may be modified to 200 to 300 mL per day in elderly patients or those with cardiac disease. The emergent situation requires that plasma transfusion follow phlebotomy to quickly lower the hematocrit without causing hypovolemia. Blood viscosity can be decreased by intravenous infusion of crystalloid solution or low-molecular-weight dextran.[6]

COAGULOPATHIES

Damage to the vascular endothelium initiates three phases of hemostasis: primary hemostasis, coagulation, and fibrinolysis. Primary hemostasis, which occurs within seconds of vascular injury, involves the interaction of blood vessels and platelets resulting in a platelet plug. Coagulation reinforces the plug with a fibrin clot through the interaction of clotting factors (coagulants). Finally, fibrinolysis liquefies the clot to restore blood flow. Thus, hemostasis stops bleeding and restores blood flow in the healed vessel. Understanding the normal coagulation response to tissue injury is important in approaching perioperative bleeding problems. A brief summary of the coagulation system is given below. Complex details of hemostasis are provided in the references.[3–5,17]

Blood vessel breakage exposes subendothelial cells. Platelets adhere to subendothelial elements through highly specific receptor-ligand interactions and release stored substances such as von Wille-brand factor (vWF), fibrinogen, and adenosine diphosphate (ADP). This induces nearby platelets to aggregate, become activated, and release their contents. Other substances released by platelets, such as thromboxane A_2, produce intense vasoconstriction, decreasing blood flow. Endothelial cells secrete endothelin, a pow-erful vasoconstrictor, and endothelium-derived relaxing factor, now known as *nitric oxide*, a powerful vasodilator and inhibitor of platelet aggregation.

Fibroblasts release tissue factor, which, along with the classic extrinsic system of coagulation, act to generate a localized clot. The classic intrinsic system of coagulation is initiated by contact activation of factor XII (Hageman factor), which is less important physiologically because patients deficient in factor XII do not have bleeding diatheses.

Coagulation is modulated by dilution of procoagulants in flow-ing blood; removal of particulate matter and activated factors by the reticuloendothelial system, especially the liver; and antago-nism of activated procoagulants by inhibitors. Tissue plasmino-gen activators (t-PAs), released from damaged vessel walls, convert plasminogen to plasmin, which lyses fibrin clots, fibrino-gen, and other procoagulants.

Coagulopathies are disruptions of normal hemostatic func-tion. Coagulopathies commonly involve multiple sites and are spontaneous, whereas a structural lesion is typically local, induced mechanically or otherwise. A method to diagnose bleed-ing divides hemostatic problems into those involving platelets, coagulation factors or, by exclusion, blood vessels. This is largely a laboratory question, but clinical clues can help differ-entiate them. Bleeding due to a platelet problem is often diffi-cult to stop but, once stopped, does not resume. Platelet disorders cause petechiae and bleeding from mucous mem-branes (nosebleeds, gastrointestinal bleeding, menorrhagia, hematuria). In bleeding related to coagulation factors (deficien-cies of factors VIII and IX), initially the bleeding stops due to a platelet plug, but bleeding resumes and causes hematomas and hemarthroses.

Coagulopathies can be inherited or acquired. An inherited coagulopathy is usually present from infancy and a family history exists. Acquired disorders typically begin in adult life and are associated with an underlying disease, negative history on previ-ous challenges (e.g., major surgery without transfusion require-ments),[17] and no family history.

Platelet Disorders

Platelet disorders can be quantitative (thrombocytopenia) or qualitative. Qualitative platelet disorders are either inherited or acquired. Inherited qualitative platelet disorders, with the excep-tion of vWD (also classified as an inherited coagulation disorder because it is caused by a deficiency of a plasma factor; see von Willebrand's Disease, below), are rare. More common are acquired platelet disorders, usually associated with drug use or medical conditions (renal and liver diseases). Drugs (e.g., aspirin, phenylbutazone, NSAIDs, alcohol, dextran, antibiotics) can inter-fere with platelet receptors or membrane function by interfering with prostaglandin synthesis or by inhibiting phosphodiesterase activity.[18] Volatile anesthetics and nitrous oxide (*in vitro*) produce a dose-related decrease in ADP-induced platelet aggregation, of unclear clinical significance.[6]

Thrombocytopenia

Thrombocytopenia is defined as a platelet count of less than 150,000 per cubic millimeter.[4,5,18] The cause of thrombocytopenia is decreased production, sequestration, or increased destruction of platelets. Decreased production may be due to neoplasms, aplastic anemia, or toxins such as chemotherapy. Sequestration may occur from hypersplenism and is usually accompanied by anemia and leukopenia. Portal hypertension from cirrhosis can cause splenomegaly and increased sequestration of platelets. Increased destruction can be nonimmune or immune mediated and may occur from infection, idiopathic thrombocytopenic purpura (ITP), disseminated intravascular coagulation (DIC), or thrombus formation on catheters.

The cause should be determined and corrected because thrombocytopenia poses a risk of bleeding that is inversely related to the platelet count (Table 7-3). For a given platelet count, the risk of bleeding is increased when anemia, fever, infection, or a platelet function defect (e.g., use of aspirin or NSAIDs) coexist. In consumptive disorders caused by drugs, discontinuation of the drug should lead to a normal platelet count within 5 to 10 days. If thrombocytopenia is caused by DIC, treatment should be directed at the underlying disease.

Table 7-3. Risk of bleeding in relation to platelet count

Platelet count (number per mm^3)	Comments
>100,000	Excessive bleeding, even with severe trauma, is rare.
50,000–100,000	Usually adequate hemostasis for most operative procedures (except perhaps cardiac surgery and neurosurgery).
20,000–50,000	Trauma or surgery may precipitate excessive bleeding.
10,000–20,000	Spontaneous cutaneous or mucosal surface bleeding is common.
<10,000	Major spontaneous bleeding into genitourinary tract or central nervous system may occur.

Data from Roizen M. Anesthetic implications of concurrent diseases. In: Miller RD, ed. *Anesthesia*, 4th ed. New York: Churchill Livingstone, 1994:980–986; Murray DJ. Evaluation of the patient with anemia and coagulation disorders. In: Rogers MC, Tinker JH, Covino BG, Longnecker DE, eds. *Principles and practice of anesthesiology*. St. Louis: Mosby–Year Book, 1993:341–356; Stoelting RK, Dierdorf SF. *Anesthesia and co-existing disease*, 3rd ed. New York: Churchill Livingstone, 1993; and Murray DJ. Monitoring of hemostasis. In: Rogers MC, Tinker JH, Covino BG, Longnecker DE, eds. *Principles and practice of anesthesiology*. St. Louis: Mosby–Year Book, 1993:846–862.

Use of heparin can cause a clinical syndrome of immune complex–mediated thrombocytopenia, thrombosis, or both, known as *heparin-induced thrombocytopenia* (HIT) or heparin-associated thrombocytopenia.[19] HIT typically develops 7 to 14 days after the initiation of heparin but may occur within a day in patients previously exposed to heparin. Severe thrombocytopenia may develop, but bleeding rarely occurs in patients who have not had surgery. Two types of HIT are seen. Type I is mild and asymptomatic; type II causes severe thrombocytopenia and is more likely to cause thrombotic complications. Type I HIT often resolves despite continued heparin therapy and is thought to represent an exaggerated form of the normal platelet aggregatory response to heparin. Type II HIT resolves only after heparin is stopped. The mechanism for HIT is not completely understood but appears to involve immune-mediated platelet activation. HIT is diagnosed by the serotonin release assay (available only in specialized research settings), less sensitive but widely used platelet aggregation studies, and enzyme-linked immunosorbent assay.

Treatment of HIT is immediate discontinuation of heparin. Alternative anticoagulants include the heparinoid drug danaparoid sodium, as well as hirudin or platelet inhibitors such as iloprost and aspirin. Low-molecular-weight heparin (LMWH) is contraindicated.

Idiopathic (Autoimmune) Thrombocytopenic Purpura

Idiopathic (autoimmune) thrombocytopenic purpura (ITP/ATP) in adults is usually a chronic disorder of insidious onset.[4,5,20–22] It is characterized by a reduced platelet count, increased peripheral destruction of platelets, and augmented platelet production. Autoantibodies are produced against platelets and possibly against megakaryocytes, which leads to the phagocytic destruction of these cells. Purpura and hemorrhage occur if the platelet count reaches a critical level, usually below 30,000 per cubic millimeter. In adults, spontaneous remissions are usually remissions of purpura only. The acute form of ITP is mostly limited to children with viral infections. A chronic form occurs in patients 20 to 40 years of age. Chronic ITP is an insidious disease in which easy bruising and petechiae are initial symptoms. The presenting complaint may be menorrhagia or epistaxis. Bleeding is predominantly dermal and mucosal. The diagnosis of ITP is based solely on clinical criteria because platelet antibody studies and bone marrow aspiration are of uncertain value. The history, physical examination, and peripheral blood smear can exclude most alternatives.

In pregnant patients, ITP may be complicated by the transfer of antiplatelet antibodies across the placenta, with resultant neonatal thrombocytopenia, purpura, and hemorrhage. Fifty percent of mothers with ITP give birth to children with transient thrombocytopenia (lasting weeks to months). Pregnancy usually does not affect the course of ITP. The current recommendations are that delivery should be managed according to standard obstetric practice, with a cesarean section performed only for obstetric indications. Some physicians recommend percutaneous umbilical blood sampling near term or fetal scalp vein sampling during labor to support a decision for cesarean section should severe thrombocytopenia be found in the fetus.

The treatment of chronic ITP is palliative, not curative, and is directed toward the inactivation or removal of the major site of platelet destruction and antiplatelet antibody production, the spleen. Corticosteroids prevent sequestration of antibody-coated platelets by the spleen and probably impair antibody production. Gamma globulin or platelet transfusions are used in urgent situations.

Thrombocytosis

Thrombocytosis, defined as a platelet count of more than 500,000 per cubic millimeter, may be primary (a myeloproliferative disorder with increased platelet production independent of normal regulatory control) or secondary (associated with iron deficiency or neoplastic, chronic inflammatory, and postoperative states). Epinephrine increases from the stress of surgery mobilize platelets from the spleen and lung.[5] The platelet count usually returns to normal with treatment of the underlying disorder. Patients with polycythemia vera [see Erythrocytosis (Polycythemia), above] and essential thrombocythemia (primary thrombocytosis)[5,6] have an increased risk of thrombotic or bleeding events, respectively. Individuals may have both thrombosis and hemorrhage. The risk of thrombosis and hemorrhage seems to be increased in older patients and those with prior thrombotic or hemorrhagic events. Use of aspirin may worsen the hemorrhagic tendency in these patients. No specific platelet count is predictive of hemorrhage or thrombosis. The most common sites of hemorrhage are mucosal surfaces; the most common thrombotic events are mesenteric and deep venous thrombosis, pulmonary embolism, and cerebral, coronary, and peripheral arterial occlusions. Thromboembolic events are rare in patients with secondary thrombocytosis or chronic myelogenous leukemia.

History and Physical Examination

The history should focus on drug use or toxin exposure, recent blood transfusions, infection, malnutrition, and bone pain. One should inquire specifically about circumstances surrounding bleeding complications and any episodes of thrombosis. Examination may reveal ecchymosis, petechiae, lymphadenopathy, hepatosplenomegaly, and signs of liver disease (see Chapter 9).

Diagnostic Testing

Laboratory studies in patients with platelet disorders include a platelet count and further studies dictated by findings of the history and physical examination.

Preoperative Anesthetic Management

If a treatable cause is found, surgery should be delayed until therapy is successful. If bleeding occurs, surgery is needed in the interim, or no therapy is available, then platelet transfusions are appropriate.

Circulating platelet numbers and function are the main determinants of the safety of regional blockade in patients with thrombocytopenia. Recommendations regarding minimal acceptable platelet counts abound, but little evidence exists to support the use of one value over another. Not only the absolute value of the platelet count but the rate of change over time should be considered. The anesthesiologist must consider the risks versus benefits of regional anesthesia in patients with thrombocytopenia. Preoperative transfusion should be planned as close to surgery as possible because of the decreased survival of transfused platelets. The amount of transfused platelets depends on the current platelet count and goal. One unit of platelets increases the platelet count by 5,000 to 10,000 per cubic millimeter in the average adult.[7] If regional anesthesia is highly desirable, then platelets are infused as the block is performed. If thrombocytopenia is diagnosed preoperatively, then elective surgery should be delayed. The choice of anesthetic technique in parturient women with ITP depends on several factors. The proposed method of delivery, gestational age, associated or coincident obstetric complications, coagulation status, history of recent hemorrhage, and other significant medical history influence the type of anesthesia used. Recommendations for patients with thrombocytosis include lowering platelets to the normal range with plateletpheresis or chemotherapy in those patients who are older, have coexisting vascular disease, or have had prior thrombotic or hemorrhagic events.

The approach for the patient with HIT who requires anticoagulation for surgery (e.g., cardiac or vascular surgery) includes (a) delaying surgery until the laboratory tests for HIT become negative, (b) using platelet inhibitors (aspirin, dipyridamole, iloprost) with heparin, and (c) using an alternative anticoagulant (see Thrombocytopenia, above). Clinical experience with the use of alternative anticoagulants in patients with HIT who require anticoagulation during surgery is limited.

Hereditary Coagulation Disorders

Hereditary coagulation disorders may be encountered in surgical patients. Frequently, consultation with a hematologist is required for effective perioperative management.

Hemophilia

Hemophilia patients include those with deficiencies of factor VIII, factor IX, or factor XI.[2-5] These patients have a prolonged partial thromboplastin time (PTT) and a normal PT. Even mild trauma experienced in daily life causes bleeding in these patients. Bleeding occurs deep in tissues and often is severe enough to require urgent fasciotomy of extremities or craniotomy for a rapidly expanding hematoma.[2] Recurrent hemarthrosis may require corrective or palliative procedures due to destructive changes in joints. Approximately 50% of operations in hemophiliacs are orthopedic.[3]

Factor VIII deficiency, or hemophilia A, is X-linked recessive and therefore occurs almost exclusively in males. The incidence of hemophilia A is 1 in 10,000, and it accounts for 85% of patients with hemophilia. The severity of the bleeding varies from kindred to kindred, but within a given family the clinical severity is relatively constant (i.e., relatives are likely to be affected similarly).[4]

The severity of bleeding relates directly to the degree of factor VIII deficiency. Few manifestations occur with 20% of normal coagulant activity. Unfortunately, the majority of hemophiliacs have a severe form of the disease with less than 1% of normal activity. Before December 1992, lyophilized factor VIII concentrates, made from pooled plasma samples from as many as 20,000 donors, were contaminated with hepatitis B and C and human immunodeficiency virus (HIV). Now, recombinant factor VIII is used.

Factor IX deficiency (Christmas disease), or hemophilia B, accounts for 14% of cases of hemophilia. The inheritance pattern and clinical features are indistinguishable from those of hemophilia A. Factor XI deficiency (hemophilia C) accounts for 1% of cases of hemophilia. The inheritance pattern is autosomal recessive and bleeding is less severe than with hemophilia A or B. Hemophilia C is most common in people of Jewish descent. It is not always associated with clinical bleeding and may not require treatment of the patient before or during surgery. Factor XII deficiency is especially common among patients of Asian descent but is not associated with an increased risk of bleeding, and treatment is not indicated.

von Willebrand's Disease

vWD is caused by qualitative and quantitative deficiencies in factor VIII. Factor VIII and vWF circulate as a complex. The disease has an autosomal dominant (types 1 and 2) and recessive (type 3) mode of inheritance and affects both genders.[4–6] It is the most common congenital bleeding disorder, with an incidence of 1%. Severe (homozygous) vWD is much rarer, with an incidence similar to that of hemophilia A. In the majority of cases, vWD is identified as a result of bleeding episodes in childhood. Use of aspirin in vWD markedly increases hemostatic defects. Clinically significant vWD is almost always associated with a prolonged PTT (normal PT), although mild cases may have a normal PTT. Levels of vWF increase during acute reactions, which can mask the laboratory diagnosis. If the patient experiences only mild bleeding and frequent bruising, this deficiency may be unsuspected. A von Willebrand panel includes a test for ristocetin cofactor (a functional assay for vWF, the presence of which leads to platelet aggregation when the antibiotic ristocetin is added), a test for vWF antigen (an immunologic test), and a factor VIII activity level. Many forms of vWD exist because of quantitative and qualitative differences in the vWF produced (Table 7-4). The distinction of various subtypes is essential for determining appropriate therapy.

Acquired Coagulation Disorders

Vitamin K Deficiency

Vitamin K deficiency leads to deficiencies of factors II, VII, IX, and X, and proteins C and S. It can occur from malnutrition, intestinal malabsorption, obstructive jaundice, and antibiotic-induced elimination of intestinal flora necessary for the synthesis of vitamin K. It is characterized by a prolonged PT and a normal PTT.

Table 7-4. Types of von Willebrand's disease

Type	Characteristics	Treatment
1	80% of cases; quantitative defect	Desmopressin*
2A	Abnormal multimer pattern; quantitative and qualitative defect	Desmopressin*
2B	Rare; abnormal multimer pattern; quantitative and qualitative defect, autosomal dominant	Desmopressin* may produce thrombocytopenia
2M	Qualitative defect; normal multimer pattern	Desmopressin*
2N	Qualitative defect; vWF levels are normal; only factor VIII is reduced	Desmopressin* effect may be too short-lived
3	Rare; low to nondetectable levels of vWF	Desmopressin* usually not effective

vWF, von Willebrand factor.
*Desmopressin acetate. With type 2B or when desmopressin acetate is not effective, vWF-containing factor VIII concentrates or cryoprecipitate may be used instead.

Drug-Induced Coagulopathy

Heparin (see the section Heparin, below) is inactivated in the liver and excreted by the kidneys and has a prolonged anticoagulant effect in hepatorenal disease. Heparin overdose is manifested as subcutaneous hemorrhages and deep tissue hematomas. Protamine sulfate, in an intravenous dose of 1 mg per 100 units of heparin, antagonizes the effect of heparin by neutralizing the acidic charge on the heparin molecule. Protamine sulfate may produce adverse cardiopulmonary reactions, especially hypotension if given rapidly, as well as anaphylactic and anaphylactoid reactions, and pulmonary vasoconstriction through complement activation.

Overdose of warfarin (warfarin sodium; see Warfarin, below) can occur from an incorrect dose of warfarin or administration of an agent that potentiates warfarin. The list of drugs that potentiate warfarin is extensive[4] and includes aspirin, other NSAIDs, cimetidine, tricyclic antidepressants, and antibiotics (other fluoroquinolones such as ciprofloxacin). Warfarin overdose results in ecchymoses, mucosal hemorrhage, and subserosal bleeding in the gastrointestinal tract. Fresh frozen plasma is given to restore procoagulant levels to 30% of normal and is monitored using the PT and the international normalized ratio (INR; see Prothrombin Time and Partial Thromboplastin Time, below). Vitamin K may be given in the same dose and time course as for vitamin K deficiency.

Administration of thrombolytics (e.g., streptokinase, urokinase, recombinant t-PA; see Antiplatelet Drugs and Thrombolytic Agents, below) in full therapeutic doses can cause bleeding with increases in the PTT and decreases in fibrinogen.[4]

Massive Blood Transfusion

Massive blood transfusion is defined as replacement of more than one blood volume within several hours.[7] Patients who have received many units of blood may have deficient clotting manifested by diffuse microvascular bleeding or oozing from the mucosae, wounds, and puncture sites. Massive blood transfusion may be accompanied by acidosis, DIC, hypothermia, and hemolytic transfusion reaction, which complicate the diagnosis of a coagulopathy. The most common cause of deficient clotting after massive blood transfusion is lack of functioning platelets, but *prophylactic* administration of platelets or fresh frozen plasma is not recommended.

Disseminated Intravascular Coagulation

DIC is characterized by uncontrolled activation of the coagulation system, with consumption of platelets and procoagulants. DIC occurs with many disorders, including obstetric complications (abruptio placentae, amniotic fluid embolus), infections, neoplasms, hemolytic reactions, vasculitis, hypoxia, hypoperfusion states, massive tissue injury, anaphylaxis, snake bites, and drug reactions.[3-5] The pathophysiology is poorly understood. Triggers act on the processes of platelet adhesion and aggregation and the contact-activated (intrinsic) and tissue-activated (extrinsic) pathways of coagulation. Normal compensatory processes are overwhelmed. The result is bleeding, shock, and vascular occlusion in various organs.

Other Coagulation Disorders

A variety of obstetric diseases, such as preeclampsia/eclampsia, abruptio placentae, amniotic fluid embolism, and the HELLP syndrome (*h*emolysis, *e*levated *l*iver enzymes, *l*ow *p*latelets) are associated with acute and chronic coagulation disorders.[18]

History and Physical Examination

Preoperative questions pertaining to coagulopathies should be part of the usual history taking.[2,3,6] Does the patient have a history of excessive blood loss with other surgeries (circumcision, tonsillectomy, adenoidectomy), umbilical cord separation, childbirth, dental extraction, menstruation, or venipuncture? Has excessive or abnormal bleeding and bruising occurred in response to nonsurgical trauma such as brushing or flossing the teeth? Has the patient had epistaxis, hematuria, or melena? Inquiry should be made about the use of antiplatelet agents or anticoagulants (aspirin, NSAIDs, warfarin). One should look for conditions associated with bleeding disorders, such as uremia, malignancy, liver disease, alcoholism, glomerulonephritis, and collagen vascular diseases (vasculitis, systemic lupus erythematosis). Does the patient have relatives with bleeding disorders? If the patient has a known bleeding disorder, what blood component or drugs have been used to manage bleeding in the past?

Patients with hemophilia may have hepatitis, cirrhosis, or HIV infection from prior blood or factor VIII transfusions. This is not an issue for patients who have received only recombinant factor VIII.

Petechiae suggest thrombocytopenia, abnormal platelet function, or defects in vascular wall integrity. Ecchymoses indicate subcutaneous bleeding associated with a procoagulant deficiency. Hemarthrosis or deep bleeding into skeletal muscles is more likely caused by a procoagulant deficiency than thrombocytopenia or a defect in platelet function. Jaundice suggests liver dysfunction. Hepatosplenomegaly suggests liver or spleen abnormalities.

Diagnostic Testing

The vast majority of patients presenting for surgery does not have bleeding disorders. No routine coagulation screening should be performed for patients who are not on anticoagulants and who have no history suggestive of a coagulopathy.[10,17] For such patients, preoperative laboratory assessment of hemostasis rarely, if ever, adds additional information that would predict blood loss, alter an anesthetic or surgical plan, or contribute to medical care.[18] Instead, the history and physical examination should be sufficient to identify those few patients who have a bleeding disorder. An unexpected abnormality in the PT or PTT in an asymptomatic surgical patient undergoing a minor procedure rarely results in adverse events. The clinical value of assessing the PT before surgery has been challenged, because all unsuspected causes of a prolonged PT with a normal PTT are extremely uncommon.

Preoperative coagulation testing (Fig. 7-1) should be efficient and economical. Patients with a personal or family history of bleeding, whether presenting for minor or major surgery, merit a complete evaluation: PT, PTT, platelet count, and further testing as needed to identify a specific coagulopathy.

Diagnosing a coagulation defect before surgery is important to facilitate the differential diagnosis of intraoperative bleeding.[6] Diagnosis and treatment of congenital and acquired coagulopathies during a major surgical procedure associated with pathologic blood loss are difficult and often lethal.[2] Complicated diagnostic tests and therapies may be required.

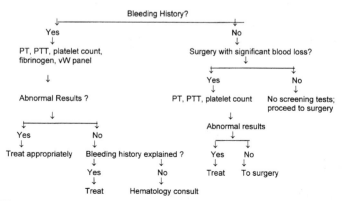

Fig. 7-1. Algorithm for preoperative coagulation testing. (PT, prothrombin time; PTT, partial thromboplastin time; vW, von Willebrand.)

The diagnosis of DIC is made by laboratory studies with clinical evidence of major organ dysfunction (CNS and pulmonary, renal, and hepatic systems). Laboratory findings in DIC are variable but include increased PT and fibrin degradation products, decreased fibrinogen level and platelet count, and shortened or variable prolongation in the PTT.

A few circumstances may exist that merit coagulation testing in the absence of symptoms or history of bleeding. Operative procedures associated with very large blood loss, such as orthopedic trauma, aortic and major vascular procedures, liver resection, and acute burn grafts, probably merit determination of a preoperative coagulation profile, which frequently serves as a reference for later tests of coagulation. Other circumstances requiring coagulation testing include the use of cardiopulmonary bypass and procedures involving systemic anticoagulation with warfarin or intravenous heparin (see Anticoagulants, Antiplatelet Drugs, and Thrombolytics, below).

Laboratory tests of coagulation as described below are useful in the following conditions:[6] (a) the history and physical examination suggest the possibility of a coagulation disorder, (b) the patient is on anticoagulant therapy, (c) a coexisting disease that may alter coagulation (e.g., liver or renal disease) is present, and (d) the surgery may alter coagulation (cardiopulmonary bypass, liver transplantation).

Prothrombin Time and Partial Thromboplastin Time

PT reflects the activity of the extrinsic (factor VII) and common (factors I, II, V, and X) pathways. Tissue thromboplastin and calcium are added to the patient's plasma, and the time to form a clot is measured. A normal PT is 10 to 12 seconds. A problem with PT measurement is that different types of thromboplastin reagents exist that have varying sensitivities to factor deficiencies.

The INR is a calculated value derived from testing each thromboplastin against an international standard thromboplastin; it thus standardizes the PT so that results are comparable across laboratories. Depending on the reagents used, for a PT of 1.3 to 1.5 times normal, the INR is 2 to 3, and for a PT of 1.5 to 2.0 times normal, the INR is 3.0 to 4.5. The INR applies only to patients on warfarin.

PTT reflects the activity of the intrinsic and common pathways, except factor XIII. Partial thromboplastin, an extract of rabbit brain phospholipid, is added to the patient's plasma as a substitute for platelet phospholipid. Activated partial thromboplastin time (aPTT) is a PTT modified by surface-activating factors XI and XII before the addition of partial thromboplastin.

Table 7-5. Differential diagnosis of prolongation of prothrombin time (PT) and/or partial thromboplastin time (PTT)

PT	PTT	Deficient factor
↑	Normal	VII*
Normal	↑	VIII, IX, XI, XII
↑	↑	II, V, X*

↑, increased.
*Hereditary deficiency of this factor is extremely uncommon.

Surface activation occurs *in vivo* by contact with negatively charged substances (collagen, connective tissue, endotoxin) and *in vitro* by diatomaceous earth (celite, kaolin) or a surface activator (crushed glass). The aPTT gives shorter and more consistent results than the PTT and normally is 25 to 35 seconds. Laboratories usually report the aPTT as the PTT. The terms are used interchangeably in this text.

The PT and PTT may be useful in uncovering coagulation factor deficiencies (Table 7-5). With single-factor deficiencies, the PT or PTT is prolonged when coagulation factor activity is less than 30% of normal.[18] With single-factor deficiencies, coagulation factor activity of 30% or more of normal provides effective perioperative hemostasis. Higher factor levels may be required if multiple factors are deficient, such as in liver disease. With multiple-factor deficiencies, when coagulation factor activity is less than 50% to 60%, the PT or PTT may be prolonged. Specific inhibitors to factors VIII and IX exist that can be detected by prolongation of PTT.

Deficiencies of factor VIII (hemophilia A), factor IX (hemophilia B), and factor XI (hemophilia C) prolong the PTT but yield a normal PT. Heparin prolongs the PTT. Causes for prolongation of the PT include warfarin therapy and vitamin K deficiency (the latter can prolong the PTT if severe enough). Liver disease and DIC prolong both PT and PTT. However, abnormalities in PT or PTT are unlikely to be the first indication of unexpected liver disease or DIC. Unsuspected warfarin or heparin therapy is extremely rare. Lupus anticoagulant may prolong the PTT.

Platelet Count

A platelet count is the most important preoperative coagulation test. Adequate platelet levels (see Thrombocytopenia, above) are extremely important for normal hemostasis during surgery (see Table 7-3).

Bleeding Time

The template bleeding time or Ivy's bleeding time was once thought to be an *in vivo* indicator of platelet function. Bleeding time is now known to be neither reliable nor an effective predictor of bleeding during surgery.[2,3,5,23] The bleeding time is usually normal if platelet counts are higher than 100,000 per cubic millimeter and is inversely related to platelet count.[5,18] Abnormal bleeding times have been found with disorders not associated with platelet dysfunction such as anemia, systemic lupus erythematosus, vitamin K deficiency of the newborn, amyloidosis, congenital heart disease, and in the presence of factor VIII inhibitors.[3,23] It may be used as part of laboratory screening for vWD and during surgery for patients with severe forms of vWD.[5] However, the data supporting its use even in these situations are unclear.

Fibrinogen Level

Fibrinogen is an acute-phase reactant. Normal fibrinogen levels are 160 to 350 mg per dL; levels less than 100 mg per dL may be inadequate to produce a clot.[3,18] The fibrinogen level is often decreased in DIC. Congenital fibrinogen deficiency, which may cause mild spontaneous bleeding, is extremely rare. When the fibrinogen level is increased, typically other acute-phase reactants are increased as well. In such circumstances, heparin may be less effective because heparin binds to and is neutralized by many acute-phase reactants (known as *heparin resistance*).

Activated Clotting Time

Measurement of activated clotting time (ACT) evaluates the intrinsic and common pathways of coagulation.[17] In this test, fresh whole blood is added to a test tube that contains an activator of factors XI and XII, such as diatomaceous earth. A normal time for clotting is 90 to 120 seconds. The ACT is a convenient method to monitor heparin's anticoagulant effect because it increases linearly with increasing doses of heparin. Frequently, the ACT is measured during cardiopulmonary bypass. It is far less sensitive than the PTT for detecting factor deficiencies, however.

Preoperative Anesthetic Management

For patients with hemophilia A, the level of factor VIII should be increased to nearly 100% before elective surgery, such as a dental extraction, and then maintained above 50% for 10 to 14 days.[4,6] However, major surgery is feasible with only 30% of factor VIII activity. Multiple formulas exist for calculating requirements for factor VIII. Generally, administration of 1 IU per kg raises the factor VIII level 2%. In addition, the fibrinolytic inhibitor ε-aminocaproic acid (Amicar) can be given as an intravenous bolus of 100 mg per kg and continued orally at 100 mg per kg every 6 hours. Tranexamic acid, another fibrinolytic inhibitor, has also been used, especially before dental procedures.

Intramuscular injections should be avoided whenever possible in hemophiliac patients because of the risk of uncontrolled bleeding. Spinal or epidural anesthesia should be avoided in patients with hemophilia, except perhaps in those patients with mild hemophilia without symptoms and a normal PTT. Usually, peripheral nerve blocks are contraindicated. Certainly, these are risk-versus-benefit decisions that must consider factors such as comorbid disease or difficulty in intubation.

Management principles for hemophilia B are the same as for hemophilia A. Fresh frozen plasma or factor IX concentrates can be used. The level of factor IX should be 50% or higher before major surgery; 1 IU per kg of factor IX increases the plasma level by 1%. Infusion of factor IX concentrate every 24 hours maintains adequate plasma levels.

Desmopressin [desmopressin acetate, or 1-desamino-8-D-arginine vasopressin (DDAVP)] is useful in patients with hemophilia A and vWD type 1. Desmopressin increases endothelial cell release of factor VIII, vWF, and plasminogen activator. An intravenous dose of 0.3 μg per kg in 50 mL of saline can produce a prompt threefold to fourfold increase in vWF activity. Desmopressin should be given slowly (over 15 to 30 minutes) to avoid hypotension, flushing, tachycardia, and headache. The goal is to raise vWF to 80 to 100 U per dL, replace abnormal vWF, and raise levels of factor VIII. Administration of desmopressin results in considerable variation in vWF levels. The response pattern in individual patients can be determined by infusing desmopressin and following the change in factor VIII and vWF. A nasal spray of desmopressin delivering a dose of 150 μg into each nostril may be useful in patients with vWD. Desmopressin probably should not be used more frequently than every 48 hours because tachyphylaxis may occur due to depletion of endothelial stores. Epsilon-aminocaproic acid (4 g orally every 4 hours) or tranexamic acid (1.5 g orally every 8 hours) should be given to counteract the release of plasminogen activator by desmopressin.

If cryoprecipitate is needed, ten bags of cryoprecipitate, consisting of 1,000 to 1,200 units of factor VIII, are infused, and response is monitored by measuring a ristocetin cofactor activity level. The goal is to increase the ristocetin cofactor activity level to more than 50%. Treatment is repeated every 12 hours until clinical bleeding is controlled. Many factor VIII concentrates do not provide effective therapy for vWD because they do not contain vWF. Humate-P has been approved by the U.S. Food and Drug Administration for use in vWD patients.

Administration of desmopressin may be dangerous for patients with type 2B vWD because an increase in abnormal vWF may cause increased binding to platelets, resulting in removal of platelets and thrombocytopenia. Abnormal vWF can be replaced with normal vWF using cryoprecipitate or factor VIII concentrates that contain vWF. The fibrinolytic inhibitor ε-aminocaproic acid may be used, especially in circumstances in which local fibrinolysis can be expected, such as dental extraction.

Treatment of vitamin K deficiency is determined by the urgency of the situation. Use of fresh frozen plasma (3 units) is rapidly effective, but the vitamin K analog phytonadione, given at a dose of 0.5 to 1.0 mg subcutaneously or intravenously, requires 6 to 24 hours to achieve correction. The PT should be checked 6 or more hours after vitamin K is given.

To reverse the effects of thrombolytics, cryoprecipitate is given to increase fibrinogen levels to 100 mg per dL along with 2 units of fresh frozen plasma to replace factor V and other procoagulants, and 6 units of platelets because of impairment in platelet adhesion and aggregation. Further steps include giving ε-aminocaproic acid.

Replacement of blood products (after massive blood transfusion) should be based on laboratory tests, including PT, PTT, and platelet and fibrinogen levels. Prompt replacement of intravascular volume and avoidance or correction of hypothermia are the best means to prevent a coagulopathy.[2,3,7]

Treatment of DIC is directed at correcting the underlying disorder and providing hemodynamic support. If emergency surgery is necessary, administration of platelets, fresh frozen plasma, and cryoprecipitate as indicated by laboratory guidance may be beneficial.[3,6] Treatment with heparin is controversial.

HYPERCOAGULABLE STATES

Causes of hypercoagulable states include resistance to activated protein C, deficiencies of antithrombin III (AT-III) and proteins C and S, hyperhomocystinemia, antiphospholipid syndrome, Trousseau's syndrome, dysfibrinogenemia, abnormalities of fibrinolysis, certain drugs (e.g., oral contraceptives), lupus anticoagulant, and anticardiolipin antibody.[5]

Resistance to activated protein C has been identified as a major cause of venous thrombosis.[5] It is caused by a specific mutation (factor V Leiden) that results from a single nucleotide substitution. In the heterozygous state, it has a prevalence of 3% to 5% in the white population, is autosomal dominant, and is by far the most common congenital hypercoagulable condition. Patients usually present with deep venous thrombosis or pulmonary embolism.

Use of oral contraceptives increases the risk of thromboembolism. This risk is compounded by other factors such as smoking. Use of oral contraceptives is associated with a twofold to fourfold risk of postoperative thromboembolic complications.

AT-III is a naturally occurring anticoagulant that binds to thrombin, inactivating it. Heterozygous congenital AT-III deficiency is uncommon and homozygous deficiency has not been reported. Acquired AT-III deficiency occurs in patients being treated with heparin; in patients with severe liver disease, nephrotic syndrome, DIC, sepsis, preeclampsia, or fatty liver of pregnancy; and after surgery.[3]

Protein C is a vitamin K–dependent anticoagulant that inhibits factors Va and VIIIa. Protein C deficiency does not cause abnormalities in routine coagulation tests. Protein C deficiency may be inherited; may be acquired by patients with liver disease, DIC, or adult respiratory distress syndrome; or may occur postoperatively, postpartum, or after hemodialysis. Protein S, also a vitamin K–dependent anticoagulant, acts as a cofactor in the protein C–catalyzed inactivation of factors Va and VIIIa.

The mechanism by which lupus anticoagulant, anticardiolipin antibody, and the antiphospholipid syndrome cause a hypercoagulable state is unknown.[5] Elevated levels of homocysteine cause vascular damage, which leads to arterial and venous thrombosis. Homozygous homocystinuria is rare, but the heterozygous state may be present in 2% or more of the population.

Trousseau's syndrome is the association of cancer with an increased propensity to develop migratory recurrent thromboembolism. The pathophysiology may be a chronic subclinical form of DIC. The cancer is usually a solid tumor of the pancreas, colon, lung, or breast and may be occult.

History and Physical Examination

Recurrent thrombosis, thrombosis in atypical sites in otherwise healthy patients, or a family history of such suggest an underlying hypercoagulable state. Lupus anticoagulant, anticardiolipin antibody, and antiphospholipid syndrome are associated with autoimmune diseases. Clinical signs, although unreliable in the diagnosis of deep venous thrombosis, include pain, tenderness, erythematous palpable subcutaneous cords, and brawny skin changes of venous stasis. One should always specifically inquire about oral contraceptive use because many patients do not consider these medications as "drugs."

Diagnostic Testing

If the history and physical examination suggest an underlying hypercoagulable state, levels of protein C, protein S, and AT-III can be measured, an assay for activated protein C resistance can be performed, and an antiphospholipid antibody panel (lupus anticoagulant, anticardiolipin antibody) can be obtained. Consultation with a hematologist is required in this circumstance. Lupus anticoagulant may or may not prolong the PTT. Its presence may increase the risk of thrombosis, but it is not associated with an increased risk of bleeding unless the antiphospholipid antibody causes significant thrombocytopenia or hypoprothrombinemia (low factor II) and consequently a prolonged PT. Except in the rarest circumstances, the lupus anticoagulant prolongs the PT only if it also prolongs the PTT.

Preoperative Anesthetic Management

Patients with deficiencies of proteins C and S and AT-III, and symptomatic resistance to activated protein C should be transfused with fresh frozen plasma to raise the level of the deficient or abnormal regulatory factor to normal before surgery. For AT-III deficiency, long-term treatment is with warfarin and acute correction is with administration of AT-III in specific concentrates (which is expensive) or administration of 2 units of fresh frozen plasma. Plasma AT-III activity usually increases 1% to 2% for each unit per kilogram of AT-III concentrate administered.[5] Depending on the baseline value, 20 to 50 U per kg increases the AT-III level to 100%, the preoperative goal. One should assess plasma AT-III activity and repeat infusions every 24 hours for 7 days after surgery. Regional anesthesia is not contraindicated in these patients.[6]

If feasible, use of oral contraceptives should be discontinued 2 to 4 weeks before elective surgery. This is especially important if the surgery is of a type associated with an increased risk of thromboembolism (e.g., joint replacement) and during and after prolonged immobilization.

Patients with the lupus anticoagulant, anticardiolipin antibody, or antiphospholipid syndrome should be treated with intravenous heparin followed by warfarin. Before surgery, heparin is substituted for warfarin per the usual protocol (see next section).

ANTICOAGULANTS, ANTIPLATELET DRUGS, AND THROMBOLYTICS

Many patients are taking medications that alter the coagulation system, affect surgical hemostasis and regional anesthesia techniques, and increase bleeding from tissue trauma. This section describes the mechanisms of action of anticoagulants, antiplatelet drugs (aspirin, other NSAIDs), and thrombolytics. Common uses of these drugs are given, along with methods for monitoring their effects and preoperative anesthetic implications of their use.

Warfarin

Warfarin sodium (Coumadin) depletes vitamin K–dependent factors II, VII, IX, and X, and proteins C and S. Its reaches maximal blood concentrations in 90 minutes, has a half-life of 24 to 48 hours, and has excellent bioavailability.[2] Patients fully anticoagulated with warfarin usually have an INR (see Prothrombin Time and Partial Thromboplastin Time, above) of 2.0 to 3.0. The only exception is patients with mechanical prosthetic heart valves, for whom an INR of 2.5 to 3.5 is recommended. After warfarin is stopped, approximately 4 days are required for the INR to reach 1.5, which is considered acceptable for surgery and regional anesthesia.[24] More time may be required when the INR is maintained above 3.0. Considerable variability is seen in the response to oral anticoagulation therapy, and the PT (INR) should be monitored regularly.

The concurrent use of other medications, including aspirin, other NSAIDs, and heparin, probably increases the risk of bleeding for patients on warfarin and does so without influencing the PT (INR). Many medications interact with warfarin, either as antagonists (barbiturates, corticosteroids, haloperidol, phenytoin) or as potentiators (amiodarone hydrochloride, broad-spectrum antibiotics, cimetidine, indomethacin, phenytoin, quinidine, salicylates, tricyclic antidepressants).[4,5] Warfarin is used in the treatment of thromboembolism and in patients with valvular disease, prosthetic heart valves, ventricular mural thrombi (in the setting of acute myocardial infarction or dilated cardiomyopathy), and atrial fibrillation.[3]

Heparin

Heparin sodium (unfractionated) is a glycosaminoglycan that binds to AT-III, causing a conformational change in AT-III that accelerates its interaction with thrombin and factor Xa by a thousandfold. Unfractionated heparin is a heterogenous mixture of polysaccharide chains with molecular weights of 3,000 to 30,000 daltons. Heparin has an immediate onset and a half-life of 90 to 120 minutes. For patients being treated with heparin, a PTT of 1.5 to 2.0 times normal is associated with adequate anticoagulation and the lowest risk of bleeding. Minidose or low-dose heparin is used for prophylaxis of thromboembolism. Intravenous heparin in full anticoagulant doses is used to treat thromboembolism. The concurrent use of aspirin or other NSAIDs may increase the risk of bleeding complications for patients receiving heparin. Use of warfarin with standard heparin is very likely to increase the risk of bleeding.

Low-dose, subcutaneous heparin is given at 5,000 units every 8 to 12 hours. The maximum anticoagulant effect occurs within 50 minutes and returns to baseline within 4 to 6 hours. The PTT typically remains in the normal range and usually is not monitored, but wide variation in response has been reported.

Low-Molecular-Weight Heparin

LMWHs are fragments of unfractionated heparin produced by controlled enzymatic or chemical depolymerization that yields chains with a mean molecular weight of 5,000 daltons. Both unfractionated heparin and LMWH exert their anticoagulant activity in the same manner—that is, by binding to AT-III and accelerating its interaction with thrombin. LMWHs have greater activity against factor Xa than against thrombin, unlike unfractionated heparin, which has equivalent activity against factor Xa and thrombin. LMWH exhibits a dose-dependent antithrombotic effect assessed by measuring the anti–factor Xa activity level.[15,25] Peak anti–factor Xa activity occurs 3 to 4 hours after a subcutaneous injection of LMWH. Anti–factor Xa levels are two to four times higher than those seen with unfractionated heparin and increase further with renal failure. Monitoring of anti–factor Xa levels is not routinely done because it is not predictive of bleeding risk. Monitoring of PTT is not useful.

The advantages of LMWH compared with unfractionated heparin include a higher and more predictable bioavailability after subcutaneous administration, lesser effects on platelet function, and a longer biological half-life, which makes one injection per day sufficient for most patients. Concomitant administration of medications affecting hemostasis, such as antiplatelet drugs, unfractionated heparin, or dextran, carries an additional risk of hemorrhagic complications, including spinal hematoma.

Antiplatelet Drugs and Thrombolytic Agents

Antiplatelet drugs include aspirin, other NSAIDs, ticlopidine hydrochloride (Ticlid), and dipyridamole (Persantine). They are used in unstable angina, transient ischemic attacks, myocardial infarction, and deep venous thrombosis, and in patients with artificial heart valves and vascular grafts.[4] Aspirin and other NSAIDs work by inhibiting cyclooxygenase and interfering with prostaglandin synthesis. The effects of aspirin are irreversible for the 7-day lifespan of platelets, whereas other NSAIDs reversibly inhibit platelet aggregation. Platelet function should be assumed to be decreased for 1 week with aspirin and for 1 to 3 days with other NSAIDs.

Ticlopidine hydrochloride inhibits platelet aggregation by inhibiting ADP-induced binding of platelets and fibrinogen, and platelet-platelet interactions. The effect is irreversible for the life of the platelets. Dipyridamole inhibits platelet function by a poorly understood mechanism, probably by inhibiting platelet phosphodiesterase.[4]

Thrombolytics (e.g., streptokinase, urokinase, recombinant t-PA) dissolve fibrin clots by activating the endogenous fibrinolytic system. Streptokinase and urokinase have low fibrin selectivity and produce significant degradation of plasma proteins, including fibrinogen. Recombinant t-PA is highly selective, activating only fibrin-bound plasminogen. Thrombolytic therapy is used in the treatment of unstable angina, peripheral arterial occlusions, deep venous thrombosis, pulmonary embolism, and occluded indwelling catheters and arteriovenous shunts.[3] These agents can produce bleeding complications, and reocclusion of treated vessels occurs in a significant number of cases. Clot lysis results in elevated levels of fibrin degradation products, which have an anticoagulant effect by inhibiting platelet aggregation. Patients who receive thrombolytics frequently receive intravenous heparin concurrently.

Diagnostic Testing

Laboratory tests used with anticoagulants, antiplatelet agents, and thrombolytics are presented in Table 7-6. Patients on warfarin and standard intravenous heparin should have a PT and PTT,

Table 7-6. Characteristics of anticoagulants, antiplatelet agents, and thrombolytics

Agent	PT	PTT	Time to peak effect	Time for recovery to normal	Diagnostic testing
Intravenous heparin sodium	↑ or normal	↑↑↑	Minutes	4–6 h	Monitor ACT, PTT
Subcutaneous heparin sodium (low dose): 5,000 units every 8–12 h	Normal	Normal	40–50 min	4–6 h	PTT usually normal
LMWH	Normal	Normal	3–5 h	12+ h	Anti–factor Xa activity not routinely monitored
Warfarin sodium	↑↑↑	↑	4–6 d	4–6 d*	Monitor PT (INR)
Aspirin	Normal	Normal	Hours	5–8 d	Bleeding time not valid
NSAIDs	Normal	Normal	Hours	1–3 d	Bleeding time not valid
Thrombolytics	↑	↑	Minutes	1–2 d	Monitor PTT if also on heparin sodium

↑, clinically insignificant increase; ↑↑↑, clinically significant increase; ACT, activated clotting time; INR, international normalized ratio; LMWH, low-molecular-weight heparin sodium; NSAIDs, nonsteroidal antiinflammatory drugs; PT, prothrombin time; PTT, partial thromboplastin time.
*Less with loading dose.
Modified from Horlocker TT. *Regional anesthesia and coagulation. ASA Refresher Course.* Philadelphia: Lippincott Williams & Wilkins and the American Society of Anesthesiologists, 1998;26:81–94.

respectively, measured before regional anesthesia or surgery. No tests are indicated for patients taking usual doses of aspirin, other NSAIDs, or other antiplatelet drugs who do not have an abnormal bleeding history. Platelet function tests and bleeding time are not useful in monitoring the effect of aspirin or other NSAIDs. Monitoring of thrombolytic therapy is not routinely required.

Preoperative Anesthetic Management

Preoperative evaluation of the coagulation status is important in deciding whether to use regional anesthesia and to help in determining whether intraoperative bleeding is surgical, due to a hemostatic defect, or both.

For patients on long-term warfarin therapy, the goal is to balance the risks of thromboembolism against perioperative bleeding. If the INR is 2.0 to 3.0, the INR should be allowed to fall spontaneously to 1.5 or less by withholding four scheduled doses of warfarin.[24] If the INR is more than 3.0 and the desired surgical goal is less than 1.3, warfarin should be withheld for a longer time. The INR should be measured the day before surgery; if the INR is more than 1.8, a small subcutaneous dose (e.g., 1 mg) of vitamin K should be administered and the INR should be measured in 3 to 6 hours. Alternative prophylaxis should be considered while the INR is less than 2.0. The INR should be rechecked on the day of surgery.

Kearon and Hirsch[24] presented recommendations for preoperative and postoperative anticoagulation for patients with acute and chronic arterial and venous thromboembolism, mechanical heart valves, and nonvalvular atrial fibrillation (see Chapter 4). Preoperative intravenous administration of heparin is not indicated for most patients who are taken off long-term oral anticoagulants. The major exceptions are patients who have had an acute venous or arterial thromboembolism within 1 month before surgery. In those circumstances, surgery for the patient taking warfarin is best managed by substituting intravenous heparin for 2 to 3 days. Heparin should be given preoperatively while the INR is less than 2.0 and should be stopped 6 hours before surgery.

Elective surgery should be postponed for the first month after an episode of venous or arterial thromboembolism. Patients who have been on anticoagulation therapy for longer than 1 month after a venous or arterial thromboembolism do not need to be admitted to the hospital for heparin therapy before surgery. A patient who has been receiving anticoagulant therapy for less than 2 weeks after a pulmonary embolism or a proximal deep venous thrombosis should have a vena caval filter inserted. The same also applies to a patient who has a high risk of bleeding from heparin. Reversal of warfarin therapy for emergency surgery may be accomplished by administering 10 to 15 mg of vitamin K (intravenously or subcutaneously), which may be effective in 3 to 6 hours. Administration of 5 to 8 mL per kg of fresh frozen plasma may be used for more rapid reversal.

Regional anesthesia and surgery should be postponed for at least 24 hours after administration of a thrombolytic. Puncture of compressible vessels should be avoided for 10 days after administration of thrombolytic drugs. Coagulation tests are not useful in these situations. See Acquired Coagulation Disorders, above, for reversal therapy of thrombolytic agents.

COAGULOPATHIES AND REGIONAL ANESTHESIA

The decision to use regional anesthesia for a patient receiving anticoagulants, antiplatelet drugs, or thrombolytics should be made on an individual basis, with the small but definite risk of spinal, epidural, or peripheral hematoma weighed against the benefits of regional anesthesia. Except in extraordinary circumstances, the risk of hematoma outweighs the potential benefits of regional anesthesia in patients with known coagulopathies or significant thrombocytopenia, those who have received thrombolytics within the previous 24 hours, and fully anticoagulated patients.

The patient's coagulation status should be normal at the time of spinal or epidural anesthesia, and the level of anticoagulation must be carefully monitored while an epidural catheter is in place.[26] After central neuraxial block, risk factors for bleeding include use of anticoagulant drugs, presence of coagulopathies, and occurrence of a bloody or difficult tap. The risk is greater for epidural than for spinal anesthesia[26,27] because the epidural space has a prominent venous plexus. A hematoma is a potentially devastating complication of spinal or epidural anesthesia. The risk of a hematoma after central neuraxial anesthesia has been estimated to be 1:150,000 after epidural anesthesia and 1:220,000 after spinal anesthesia.[26,27] The risk that bleeding will cause cord compression and paraplegia after neuraxial blockade may be as low as 1:1,000,000. Anticoagulation therapy is associated with 25% of spontaneous spinal hematomas. Guidelines are available that can be followed to decrease the risk of spinal hemorrhagic complications.[27] Foremost is to avoid the use of regional anesthetic techniques in patients with coagulopathies. PT, PTT, and platelet levels should be normal when regional anesthesia is used.

Several studies have demonstrated the relative safety of central neural block and subsequent administration of subcutaneous unfractionated low-dose heparin. Spinal hematomas are rare in patients who undergo major conduction blocks while receiving low-dose heparin.[26,27] The risk of neuraxial bleeding may be reduced by delay of the heparin injection until after the block has been instituted and may be increased in debilitated patients or after prolonged therapy. During minidose prophylaxis, no contraindication exists to the use of neuraxial techniques.[25]

Intravenous heparin can be used in patients with a central neuraxial continuous catheter *after* placement of the catheter. Factors increasing the risk of spinal hematoma in such patients include a preexisting coagulopathy, thrombocytopenia, concomitant aspirin therapy, traumatic or difficult needle placement, heparinization within 1 hour of spinal or epidural puncture, and lack of or inappropriate anticoagulant monitoring. No data exist to support postponement of surgery for 24 hours if a bloody tap occurs. If a decision is made to proceed, however, full discussion with the surgeon and careful postoperative neurologic monitoring are warranted. Patients fully anticoagulated with continuous intravenous administration of heparin should have the infusion discontinued 4 to 6 hours before needle or catheter placement, unless early normalization is verified by a PTT. Reversal of heparin effect should be carried out if necessary. Complications occurring during the regional anesthesia require thorough documentation and reasonable follow-up.

The higher incidence of spinal hematoma after use of LMWH in the United States than in Europe may be a result of the difference in dose and dosage schedules.[26] The recommended dose of one LMWH, enoxaparin sodium, is 40 mg once daily in Europe compared with 30 mg every 12 hours in the United States. Decisions about postoperative analgesia and thromboprophylaxis with LMWH should be made preoperatively. Regional anesthesia should be done at least 10 to 12 hours after the last LMWH dose. Patients receiving high doses of LMWH (e.g., enoxaparin sodium 1 mg per kg twice daily) require longer delays (24 hours). LMWH administration should be delayed for at least 2 hours after spinal or epidural anesthesia is performed or an indwelling catheter is removed. Indwelling catheters should be removed before initiation of LMWH thromboprophylaxis. Catheter removal should be delayed at least 10 to 12 hours after a dose of LMWH. The presence of blood during needle placement warrants an additional delay (24 hours) in initiating postoperative thromboprophylaxis. It does not require postponement of surgery. A single-dose spinal anesthetic may be the safest neuraxial technique for patients receiving preoperative LMWHs.

Guidelines have been formulated for performing neuraxial blocks in patients receiving oral anticoagulants.[25] Spinal or epidural anesthesia followed by anticoagulation with warfarin is probably safe.[26] For patients on long-term oral anticoagulation therapy, warfarin should be stopped for at least 4 days, and the PT (INR) should be measured before central neuraxial block. If the INR is normally maintained above 3.0, then warfarin should be withheld for a longer period. A PT of less than 14.0 (INR below 1.3) is appropriate for performance of regional anesthesia. When patients receive an initial dose of warfarin just before surgery, the PT (INR) should be checked before central neuraxial block if the first dose was given 24 hours or more earlier, or if a second dose has been administered.

Antiplatelet drugs (aspirin, other NSAIDs), by themselves, appear to present no added risk of spinal hematoma in patients undergoing neuraxial blockade.[25,26] One case of spontaneous epidural hematoma (in the absence of anesthesia) has been reported in a patient with a history of aspirin ingestion. Evidence exists that blood loss is increased in patients receiving 1.2 to 3.6 g of aspirin per day and undergoing total hip replacement.[6] The risk of spinal hematoma in patients receiving ticlopidine hydrochloride or tirofiban hydrochloride M-hydrate is unknown. No relation exists between the use of antiplatelet medications and the occurrence of bloody taps producing clinically significant collections of blood within the spinal canal.

Patients do not need any coagulation tests before regional anesthesia if they have a normal bleeding history and are only taking aspirin, other NSAIDs, ticlopidine hydrochloride, or tirofiban hydrochloride M-hydrate. Although these drugs present an added threat to patients who have coagulopathies (hemophilia, vWD, treatment with warfarin or heparin), use of these drugs should not increase the risk of hematomas in patients with otherwise normal hemostatic function.[18]

The risk of spinal hematoma in patients who receive thrombolytic therapy is less well defined.[26] Two cases of spinal hematoma in patients with indwelling catheters who received thrombolytic agents have been reported in the literature. Patients receiving or about to receive thrombolytic drugs should not undergo spinal or epidural anesthesia. For what length of time neuraxial or peripheral nerve blocks should be avoided after discontinuation of these drugs is not clear. In those patients who have received regional anesthesia near the time of fibrinolytic or thrombolytic therapy, close neurologic monitoring should be carried out. Furthermore, in these cases, neuraxial infusions should be limited to drugs minimizing sensory and motor blockade (opioids, very low dose local anesthetics). Patients who receive heparin with thrombolytic drugs are at high risk of bleeding during spinal or epidural anesthesia.[25]

Sufficient data and experience are not available to determine if the risk of neuraxial hematoma is increased when neuraxial techniques are combined with full anticoagulation in cardiopulmonary bypass procedures.[28] Intrathecal and epidural opioids, and epidural local anesthetics have been used in patients undergoing cardiopulmonary bypass. A single-shot spinal anesthetic may be the safest neuraxial technique in such patients.

CASE STUDY

A 16-year-old girl is scheduled for embolization with anesthesia because conservative measures to control her nosebleed have failed. She denies previous surgeries or significant medical illnesses. She denies pregnancy. Her last menstrual period was 2 weeks ago, and she mentions that she has very heavy periods. She uses aspirin about once a week for "tension headaches"; her last aspirin use was the previous day. On further questioning about bleeding abnormalities, she admits to "bruising easily" and to having to return to the dentist for "extra packing" after a tooth extraction a year earlier. The patient denies any family history of bleeding disorders.

Blood pressure is 100/60 mm Hg and heart rate is 92 beats per minute while lying down; blood pressure is 84/56 mm Hg and heart rate is 113 beats per minute while standing. Her weight is 50 kg. Examination reveals an anxious, pale female with nasal packing in place and ecchymoses on her upper extremities at intravenous line insertion and blood-drawing sites. She has a few resolving ecchymoses on her lower extremities. The rest of the examination is normal. She has no hepatosplenomegaly.

Suspecting a possible coagulopathy, the anesthesiologist orders a hematocrit, PT, PTT, and platelet count. The hematocrit is 31.3 g per dL, and the other values are normal. Still suspicious, the anesthesiologist consults a hematologist, who diagnoses type 1 vWD. The patient is given a 500 mL saline bolus and 15 units of desmopressin in 50 mL of saline. During the infusion, the patient complains of a headache and her blood pressure drops to 90/50 mm Hg while lying down. The infusion rate is decreased, and her blood pressure returns to baseline. Her nosebleed resolves over the next 24 hours without further intervention. She is discharged home and instructed to avoid aspirin and other NSAIDs and to use desmopressin nasal spray immediately before and during her menstrual periods. She is informed of the surgical and anesthetic implications of her disease and encouraged to obtain a Medic-Alert bracelet (see Chapter 14). She should be followed by a hematologist.

REFERENCES

1. Roizen M. Anesthetic implications of concurrent diseases. In: Miller RD, ed. *Anesthesia*, 4th ed. New York: Churchill Livingstone, 1994:980–986.
2. Murray DJ. Evaluation of the patient with anemia and coagulation disorders. In: Rogers MC, Tinker JH, Covino BG, Longnecker DE, eds. *Principles and practice of anesthesiology*. St. Louis: Mosby–Year Book, 1993:341–356.
3. Petrovich CT. Hemostasis and hemotherapy. In: Barash PG, Cullen BF, Stoelting RK, eds. *Clinical anesthesia*, 3rd ed. Philadelphia: Lippincott–Raven Publishers, 1996:189–217.
4. Lee GR, Bithell TC, Foerster J, et al., eds. *Wintrobe's clinical hematology*, 9th ed. Philadelphia: Lea & Febiger, 1993.
5. Ruberstein E, Federman DD, eds. *Scientific American medicine*. New York: Scientific Medicine, 1997. Hematology I–VI.

6. Stoelting RK, Dierdorf SF. *Anesthesia and co-existing disease*, 3rd ed. New York: Churchill Livingstone, 1993.
7. American Society of Anesthesiologists, Committee on Transfusion Medicine. *Questions and answers about transfusion practices*, 3rd ed. Park Ridge, IL: American Society of Anesthesiologists, 1998.
8. Goodnough LT, Monk TG, Andriole GL. Erythropoietin therapy. *N Engl J Med* 1997;336:933–938.
9. Sharon BL. Transfusion medicine I: transfusion therapy in congenital hemolytic anemias. *Hematol Oncol Clin North Am* 1994; 8:1053–1086.
10. Bunn HF. Pathogenesis and treatment of sickle cell disease. *N Engl J Med* 1997;337:762–769.
11. Koshy M, Weiner SJ, Miller ST, et al. Surgery and anesthesia in sickle cell disease. Cooperative Study of Sickle Cell Diseases. *Blood* 1995;86:3676–3684.
12. Vichinsky EP, Haberkern CM, Neumayr L, et al., and the Preoperative Transfusion in Sickle Cell Disease Study Group. A comparison of conservative and aggressive transfusion regimens in the perioperative management of sickle cell disease. *N Engl J Med* 1995;333:206–213.
13. Scott-Conner CEH, Brunson CD. The pathophysiology of the sickle hemoglobinopathies and implications for perioperative management. *Am J Surg* 1994;168:268–274.
14. Dierdorf SF. Anesthesia for patients with rare and coexisting diseases. In: Barash PG, Cullen BF, Stoelting RK, eds. *Clinical anesthesia*, 3rd ed. Philadelphia: Lippincott–Raven Publishers, 1996: 461–487.
15. Goodwin SR. Perioperative implications of hemoglobinopathies. *Anesth Analg* 1998;Mar[Suppl]:39–44.
16. Fellin F, Murphy S. Hematologic problems in the preoperative patient. *Med Clin North Am* 1987;3:477–487.
17. Petrovitch C. *Perioperative evaluation of coagulation. ASA Refresher course.* Philadelphia: Lippincott Williams & Wilkins and the American Society of Anesthesiologists, 1992;20:169–190.
18. Murray DJ. Monitoring of hemostasis. In: Rogers MC, Tinker JH, Covino BG, Longnecker DE, eds. *Principles and practice of anesthesiology*. St. Louis: Mosby–Year Book, 1993:846–862.
19. Slaughter TF, Greenberg CS. Heparin-associated thrombocytopenia and thrombosis. Implications for perioperative management. *Anesthesiology* 1997;87:667–675.
20. Bassell GM, Horbelt DV. Hematologic disease. In: Datta S, ed. *Anesthesia and obstetric management of high risk pregnancy*. Boston: Mosby–Year Book, 1991:348–351.
21. Hauch MA, Bromley B. Autoimmune diseases. In: Datta S, ed. *Anesthesia and obstetric management of high risk pregnancy*. Boston: Mosby–Year Book, 1991:397–399.
22. Karpatkin S. Autoimmune (idiopathic) thrombocytopenic purpura. *Lancet* 1997;349:531–536.
23. Rodgers RPC, Levin J. A critical reappraisal of the bleeding time. *Semin Thromb Hemost* 1990;16:1–20.
24. Kearon C, Hirsh J. Management of anticoagulation before and after elective surgery. *N Engl J Med* 1997;336:1506–1511.
25. Enneking FK, Benzon H. Oral anticoagulation and regional anesthesia: perspective. *Reg Anesth Pain Med* 1998;23(6)[Suppl 2]:140–177.
26. Horlocker TT. *Regional anesthesia and coagulation. ASA Refresher Course.* Philadelphia: Lippincott Williams & Wilkins and the American Society of Anesthesiologists, 1998;26:81–94.
27. Vandermeulen EP, Van Aken H, Vermylen J. Anticoagulants and spinal-epidural anesthesia. *Anesth Analg* 1994;79:1165–1177.
28. Chaney MA. Benefits of neuraxial anesthesia in patients undergoing cardiac surgery [Editorial]. *J Cardiothorac Vasc Anesth* 1997;11:808–809.

Renal Disease

Ricardo Martinez-Ruiz and BobbieJean Sweitzer

Renal failure affects multiple organ systems. An understanding of how renal disease alters normal physiology is imperative for safe administration of anesthesia.

This chapter begins with a section on general considerations followed by a discussion of the etiology and pathophysiology of renal disease. Information regarding what to look for during physical examination and history taking is provided. Recommendations for diagnostic testing and its significance in the preoperative assessment of renal failure patients are presented. Specific anesthetic considerations and a case study conclude the chapter.

GENERAL CONSIDERATIONS

Anesthesiologists are providing care for a growing population of patients with renal dysfunction. Life expectancy of patients with end-stage renal disease (ESRD) has increased because of improvements in renal replacement therapies and transplantation. Five percent of adults in the United States have renal disease. Mortality rate for dialysis patients after major procedures is 5.6%[1] but may approach 57% after emergency cardiac valve replacement.[2] In the surgical population, death is due primarily to septic complications, postoperative bleeding, congestive heart failure, unexplained hypotension, and hyperkalemia. Deaths attributed to bleeding, cardiovascular dysfunction, and hyperkalemia tend to occur within the first 24 hours after surgery.[3] Sepsis usually occurs 2 or more days postoperatively. Hyperkalemia, the most common postoperative complication, occurred in one-third of ESRD patients, and it was the primary reason dialysis was required within 24 hours after surgery in 36% of cases in one series.[3]

Hypotension and the use of nephrotoxic drugs during the perioperative period aggravate preexisting chronic renal insufficiency. The role of anesthesia in contributing to this morbidity and mortality cannot be easily ascertained. Perioperative morbidity and mortality may be reduced by understanding the underlying disease, identifying those patients at risk, and optimizing the anesthetic management to prevent further complications.

ETIOLOGY AND PATHOPHYSIOLOGY

Renal dysfunction can be divided into acute renal failure (ARF), chronic renal failure (CRF), and acute superimposed on chronic renal failure.[4] When total glomerular filtration rate (GFR) is 35% to 50% of normal, overall renal function is sufficient to keep the patient symptom free.[5] Blood urea nitrogen

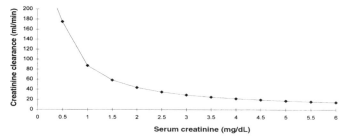

Fig. 8-1. Calculated creatinine clearance versus serum creatinine level in a 70-kg, 50-year-old man. This graph shows how deceiving the nonlinear relationship between creatinine clearance and serum creatinine levels can be. Small changes in serum creatinine level may represent a precipitous drop in renal function, yet still be within normal range. Plot was generated using the following formula:

$$\text{Creatinine clearance (mL/min)} = \frac{(140 - \text{age}) \times \text{body weight in kg}}{72 \times \text{serum creatinine}}$$

(Reprinted with permission from Cockcroft DW, Gault MH. Prediction of creatinine clearance from serum creatinine. *Nephron* 1976;16:31–41.)

(BUN) and serum creatinine levels may be normal or slightly elevated. A nonlinear relationship exists between creatinine clearance, a surrogate for GFR, and serum creatinine (Fig. 8-1). Small changes in serum creatinine may represent a significant loss of function. This is the reason a serum creatinine level is an inaccurate measure of renal function. When GFR is 20% to 35% of normal, azotemia occurs and initial manifestations of renal insufficiency appear.[5] With further loss of nephron mass (GFR less than 20% of normal), the patient develops overt renal failure.

Acute Renal Failure

ARF is characterized by a rapid decline in GFR, retention of nitrogenous waste products, and perturbations of electrolytes, acid-base homeostasis, and extracellular fluid volume.[6] ARF is present in 1% of patients on hospital admission, 5% of patients during hospitalization, and 30% of patients admitted to intensive care units.[6,7] Oliguria (urine output less than 400 mL in 24 hours) is a frequent but not necessarily constant feature (50%). ARF is usually asymptomatic and is diagnosed when biochemical screening of patients reveals a recent increase in BUN and creatinine concentrations. It may complicate a wide range of diseases, which for purposes of diagnosis and management are divided into three categories (Table 8-1)[7]: (a) conditions that cause renal hypoperfusion (prerenal ARF), (b) those that directly involve the renal parenchyma (intrinsic ARF), and (c) conditions that result in urinary tract obstruction (postrenal ARF).

Table 8-1. Common causes of acute renal failure

Prerenal (55%)
 Hypovolemia
 Congestive heart failure
Renal (40%)
 Acute tubular necrosis secondary to ischemia
 Toxins (aminoglycosides and radiocontrast agents)
 Nephritis
 Heme pigments
Postrenal (5%)
 Benign prostatic hypertrophy
 Cancer of prostate or cervix
 Neurogenic bladder

The kidney is relatively unique among major organs in its ability to recover from almost complete loss of function. Nevertheless, ARF is a predictor for major in-hospital morbidity and mortality, in large part due to the serious nature of the illness that precipitated the ARF.

Prerenal Acute Renal Failure

Decreases in intravascular volume or reductions in cardiac output decrease perfusion to the kidneys, resulting in an accumulation of nitrogen waste products (azotemia). Prerenal azotemia is rapidly reversible if the underlying cause is corrected. Precipitating factors in the outpatient setting include vomiting, diarrhea, poor fluid intake, fever, use of diuretics, and congestive heart failure. Elderly patients are particularly susceptible to prerenal azotemia because of their predisposition to hypovolemia and the high prevalence of renal artery atherosclerotic disease among this population.[7] The use of angiotensin-converting enzyme (ACE) inhibitors in combination with diuretics can cause prerenal azotemia in patients with large-vessel or small-vessel renal vascular disease.[7] The use of nonsteroidal antiinflammatory drugs (NSAIDs) can precipitate prerenal azotemia in patients with diminished renal perfusion by deranging intrarenal hemodynamics.[6] Drugs such as cyclosporine and tacrolimus produce vasoconstriction of small renal vessels and can cause prerenal ARF.[7] Despite adequate volume status, disease states that compromise renal perfusion, such as congestive heart failure, liver dysfunction, or septic shock, produce prerenal azotemia. In surgical patients, prerenal azotemia is a common cause of renal dysfunction.

Intrinsic Acute Renal Failure

Damage to renal tissue in ARF is primarily ischemic or toxic in nature. Prerenal azotemia may lead to ischemic tubular necrosis when blood flow is sufficiently compromised to result in the death of tubular cells. Although most cases of ischemic ARF are reversible if the underlying cause is corrected, irreversible cortical necrosis can occur if the ischemia is severe.[7] Exposure to toxins such as aminoglycoside antibiotics and radiocontrast agents is the second most common cause of ARF.[6] Other implicated toxins are heme pigments and chemotherapeutic agents (e.g., cisplatin). Ischemia and toxins often combine to cause ARF in severely ill patients with sepsis, hematologic cancers, or acquired immunodeficiency syndrome (AIDS).[7] Cholesterol embolism during cardiopulmonary bypass, aortic surgery, or manipulation of catheters through the aorta is a frequent cause of renal dysfunction.

Other causes of intrinsic ARF include damage to renal interstitium or the glomerulus. Renal failure due to acute interstitial nephritis is most often caused by an allergic reaction to a drug.[7] It is usually reversible after withdrawal of the offending medication. Corticosteroids may aid in the recovery of renal function during acute interstitial nephritis, but their role remains controversial because controlled studies are lacking.[7]

Patients with glomerulonephritis can present with subacute or acute renal failure. Identifying a cause through serologic assay or immunopathologic examination of the kidney is important, because prompt use of immunosuppressive agents, plasma exchange, or both may be indicated to reduce life-threatening complications and decrease the incidence of ESRD.[7]

Acute nephritic syndrome is characterized by an abrupt onset of hematuria, reduction in GFR, red blood cell (RBC) casts, mild proteinuria, hypertension, edema, and azotemia. It is caused by diffuse inflammatory changes in the glomerulus and has multiple causes (e.g., poststreptococcal glomerulonephritis, Goodpasture's syndrome).

Postrenal Acute Renal Failure

Postrenal ARF occurs when the urinary outflow tract is obstructed. Obstruction can be either mechanical (prostatic hypertrophy, cancer of the prostate or cervix, retroperitoneal disorders) or functional (as occurs with a neurogenic bladder).[7] Less frequent postrenal causes of ARF are bilateral renal calculi, papillary necrosis, blood clots, bladder carcinoma, fungal infection, retroperitoneal fibrosis, colorectal tumors, and other malignant conditions. Intratubular obstruction can be caused by the presence of various crystals (uric acid, calcium oxalate), use of acyclovir, sulfonamide, or methotrexate sodium, and the presence of myeloma light chains.[7] Postrenal causes need to be diagnosed quickly, because recovery of renal function is inversely related to the duration of obstruction.[6]

Chronic Renal Failure

Progressive and irreversible destruction of nephron mass eventually leads to CRF. Surviving nephrons compensate for the reduction of renal mass, which leads to structural and functional hypertrophy. This compensatory hypertrophy is due to adaptive hyperfiltration mediated by increases in glomerular capillary pressures and flows. Eventually these changes become maladaptive and predispose to sclerosis of the residual glomerular population.[5]

The most common causes of CRF are diabetes mellitus, hypertensive nephrosclerosis, chronic glomerulonephritis, chronic interstitial nephritis, analgesic nephropathy, and polycystic kidney disease. Possibly because of aggressive treatment of glomerulonephritis, diabetes mellitus and hypertension are now the leading causes of CRF.

Diabetes mellitus affects the kidney in many ways (termed *diabetic nephropathy*) and results in mild proteinuria, nephrotic syndrome, progressive renal failure (decline in GFR), and hypertension. Glomerular lesions cause the majority of abnormal clinical findings. Mortality of diabetic patients on dialysis is three times higher than that of nondiabetic patients. Hypertension exposes the renal circulation to elevated intraluminal pressures, causing arteriolar lesions resulting in nephrosclerosis and chronic renal insufficiency.

Polycystic kidney disease is autosomal dominant in 90% of cases and is responsible for 10% of ESRD in the United States. It is the most common hereditary tubule disorder, and 50% of patients have ESRD by age 60. The kidneys are markedly enlarged with multiple cysts. Gross hematuria is common, nephrolithiasis occurs in 15% to 20% of cases, and hypertension is frequent. Extrarenal manifestations are common. Hepatic cysts are present in 50% to 70% of patients, are usually asymptomatic, and do not affect liver function. Intracranial aneurysms occur in 10% of patients, and mitral valve prolapse is present in 25%.

Nephrotic syndrome is a predictable complex that follows a severe prolonged increase in glomerular permeability of proteins.[8] Common causes of nephrotic syndrome include diabetic glomerulosclerosis and membranous glomerulopathy. The main feature is proteinuria (3.5 g per day per 1.73 m^2) and hypoalbuminemia (less than 3 g per dL). Generalized edema and hyperlipidemia are frequently present. Arterial and venous thromboembolism and infectious complications are common. Specific attention to volume status is critical because hypovolemia may lead to ARF.

Uremia is the clinical syndrome that results from profound loss of renal function. It includes anemia, malnutrition, defective energy use, and impaired metabolism of carbohydrates, fats, and proteins. As renal reserve is diminished in CRF, sudden stresses such as infections, dehydration, or toxin exposure may produce overt uremia in a previously compensated patient.[5] Although the cause of the syndrome remains unknown, the term *uremia* was originally adopted because of the presumption that the abnormalities resulted from retention of BUN and other end products of metabolism normally excreted in the urine.

Every organ system in the body is affected by the impact of a reduction in nephron mass. Fluid retention in uremia often results in congestive heart failure or pulmonary edema. This pulmonary edema is usually a low-pressure, high-permeability type with normal cardiac filling pressures. The excess lung water is seen radiologically in a classic butterfly-wing distribution. This low-pressure pulmonary edema and cardiopulmonary abnormalities associated with circulatory overload usually resolve with vigorous dialysis.[9] In addition to providing dialysis, congestive heart failure should be treated as indicated for patients without ESRD except that diuretics should not be used. Patients on digoxin and hemodialysis pose a diagnostic challenge if digoxin toxicity is suspected. Protein-bound digoxin-like immunoreactive substances in the serum of dialysis patients interfere with measurements of digoxin. Clinical findings of digoxin toxicity (see Chapter 4) assume greater importance in this situation.

Patients with ESRD and patients managed long term with dialysis have a high incidence of accelerated atherosclerosis leading to coronary, cerebral, and peripheral vascular disease. These complications are secondary to hypertension, hyperlipidemia, glucose intolerance, chronically elevated cardiac output, metastatic vascular and myocardial calcification, and possibly impaired myocardial oxygen delivery caused by uremic toxins.[10] Fifty percent of deaths in patients on hemodialysis are due to cardiovascular disease. Symptomatic patients commonly have improvement of functional status and resolution of symptoms with coronary artery bypass grafting. The benefits of angioplasty, however, have been minimal, with a restenosis rate of more than 80% at 6 months. Uremic pericarditis is a rare complication with adequate dialysis therapy.[10] If pericarditis is present, other causes (e.g., viral infection, myocardial infarction) must be ruled out. Intensive dialysis is therapeutic. Administration of systemic anticoagulants should be avoided to minimize the occurrence of hemorrhagic tamponade.[10]

Hypertension is a common complication of ESRD. Dialysis is very effective treatment for hypertension secondary to fluid retention, and use of antihypertensive drugs in this setting is inappropriate. Those patients with preexisting essential hypertension require drug therapy. Rarely, patients may develop accelerated or malignant hypertension, manifested by markedly elevated systolic and diastolic blood pressures, encephalopathy, and seizures. Intravenous administration of sodium nitroprusside, labetalol hydrochloride, or enalaprilat, and control of extracellular fluid volume generally controls the hypertension.

A normocytic normochromic anemia used to be common in patients with CRF. Hemoglobin levels range from normal values in patients receiving erythropoietin to 5 to 9 g per dL in untreated patients. The anemia is multifactorial, but decreased production of erythropoietin is the main cause. Other factors include a decreased half-life of RBCs, increased RBC membrane fragility, hemolysis, and decreased bone marrow production.[9] Increased blood loss secondary to gastrointestinal fluid losses and iron, folic acid, and vitamins B_{12} and B_6 deficiencies plays a lesser role. Currently, with the widespread use of recombinant human erythropoietin (Epogen), patients with CRF may have normal hematocrits. Erythropoietin therapy consists of administration of 50 to 150 U per kg subcutaneously three times a week.

Uremic patients have clinically increased bleeding. Spontaneous bleeding is rare, however, and a specific cause must be ruled out when it occurs. Patients usually have prolonged bleeding times secondary to platelet dysfunction and a decrease in platelet adhesiveness. Bleeding time does not predict surgical bleeding, and its measurement is not recommended (see Chapter 7). Prothrombin time (PT) and partial thromboplastin time (PTT) are usually normal. Platelet counts and thrombopoietic activity are mildly decreased in CRF.

Liver dysfunction from hepatitis (viral, drug related), chronic hepatic venous congestion, and hemosiderosis are common.[9] Rates of infection with hepatitis B (35%) and hepatitis C (30% to 70%) are high from dialysis and blood transfusions.[11] Hepatic dysfunction secondary to chronic hepatic venous congestion is seen in 5% to 10% of patients with CRF.

Gastroesophageal reflux is common, and delayed gastric emptying, hyperacidity, and an increase in gastric volume increase the risk of aspiration with general anesthesia. Gastrointestinal bleeding may occur secondary to gastritis and duodenitis.[9]

Malnutrition (see Chapter 16) may be seen with ESRD because of anorexia, the nephrotic syndrome, nausea, vomiting, and underlying diseases (e.g., AIDS). Cachexia may be masked by edema and increased weight from fluid retention. Hypovolemia is usually due to excessive gastrointestinal fluid losses or overzealous diuretic therapy.

CRF patients have a mild metabolic acidosis, usually with a normal anion gap. If the bicarbonate level is less than 12 to 15 mEq per L, other causes of metabolic acidosis (ketoacidosis, lactic acidosis) should be sought. The presence of an osmolal gap (the difference between the measured and the calculated osmolality) suggests the presence of a low-molecular-weight nephrotoxin, such as ethylene glycol. Hyperkalemia is the most serious and common electrolyte perturbation.[3] Hyperkalemia is usually well tolerated by CRF patients for unknown reasons. Hypokalemia after dialysis is common and should not trigger potassium replacement.[10] Hyponatremia, hyperphosphatemia, and hypocalcemia may be present. The presence of hypercalcemia and hyperuricemia may suggest a malignancy. Elevated creatine kinase levels with a normal creatine kinase-MB fraction occur in 30% of renal failure patients.[10] Also, elevated creatine kinase levels may indicate rhabdomyolysis, with its potential nephrotoxic effects. Albumin levels may be decreased secondary to chronic disease, poor nutritional status, or excessive losses, as in the case of nephrotic syndrome. Triglyceride levels are elevated but cholesterol level is usually normal.

Uremic patients commonly have a mixed sensory and motor neuropathy, especially in the lower extremities. Adequate dialysis improves the symptoms. Altered mental status and seizures may be a manifestation of uremic encephalopathy, but other causes (e.g., intracranial bleeding, dialysis disequilibrium, infections) should be investigated. Uremic seizures are uncommon in this era of dialysis and are a diagnosis of exclusion. Seizures and coma may be a result of brain edema in the setting of malignant hypertension. Dialysis dementia is very rare with removal of aluminum from the dialysate bath and the use of phosphate binders.[10]

Uremic patients have an increased susceptibility to infectious complications because of a depressed immune system. Functional defects in macrophages, neutrophils, and monocytes have been described.[10] Intravenous access is frequently needed, and intravenous access sites provide a port of entry for bacteria.

Renal osteodystrophy is a generic term for secondary hyperparathyroidism and adynamic bone disease. The former is a result of phosphate retention and calcitriol deficiency, which produces an increased bone turnover. The latter is the product of impaired osteoblastic and osteoclastic activity. Metastatic calcification of soft tissues develops when the calcium-phosphate product exceeds 60. Generalized bone decalcification occurs, which makes these patients prone to spontaneous fractures.[5]

Patients on hemodialysis may have a higher rate of depression than is commonly recognized. Many symptoms such as anorexia, failure to thrive, functional impairment, and noncompliance are common to both ESRD and depression.

Acute on Chronic Renal Failure

Patients with acute on chronic renal failure present with an acute deterioration superimposed on an already diminished baseline renal function. They are at high risk for perioperative renal dysfunction, and any insult to the kidneys is magnified. The general approach used for patients with ARF should be followed.

RENAL TRANSPLANTATION

Renal transplantation returns the majority of ESRD patients to a nearly normal lifestyle. Typically, transplant patients are maintained on combinations of prednisone, azathioprine (Imuran), cyclosporine, and possibly antilymphocyte globulins. The major toxic effects of azathioprine is marrow suppression. Immunosuppressed patients have an increased incidence of infection and malignancies. Complications of glucocorticoids include gastrointestinal bleeding, impaired wound healing, and diabetes mellitus. Cyclosporine can cause renal and hepatic toxicity.

HISTORY AND PHYSICAL EXAMINATION

During the preoperative evaluation, the history should focus on the patient's ability to perform exercise and the presence of shortness of breath, angina, paroxysmal nocturnal dyspnea, and orthopnea. This gives the physician information about the patient's cardiovascular conditioning, presence of ischemic heart disease, and potential fluid overload. Jugular venous distention, a displaced apical heart impulse, an S_3 or S_4 heart sound, lung crackles, hepatic congestion, and peripheral edema are signs of congestive heart failure. Patients with nephrotic syndrome present with generalized edema due to severe hypoalbuminemia and low oncotic intravascular pressure that favors fluid transfer into the interstitium.

The patient should be carefully questioned about the presence of chest pain, prior myocardial infarction, level of activity, and the presence of risk factors (smoking, diabetes mellitus, obesity, family history). See Chapter 3 for guidelines for the evaluation of patients with suspected ischemic heart disease. The presence and symmetry of peripheral pulses should be assessed. One should note options for vascular access and the presence of arteriovenous fistulas or central catheters (see Intravenous Access, below).

The clinical presentation of pericarditis in patients with uremia is similar to that seen in nonuremic patients. It may be painless, and a pericardial rub may be heard. Signs of pericardial tamponade include jugular venous distention, pulsus paradoxus (decrease in systolic blood pressure of more than 10 mm Hg during normal inspiration), and shock.

Anemia, when present, produces nonspecific symptoms such as malaise and fatigue or may precipitate angina. A history of bleeding problems should be sought. The patient's skin and mucus membranes should be examined for pallor and evidence of petechiae and ecchymoses. Nausea, vomiting, and recurring episodes of hiccoughs are common in renal failure. These symptoms can complicate the anesthetic induction. Significant nausea and vomiting may result in dehydration. If this is suspected, measurement of orthostatic vital signs is indicated. A history of jaundice suggests hepatitis. Hyperkalemia, mild hyponatremia, and hyperphosphatemia are usually asymptomatic. Hypocalcemia may manifest with paresthesias, cramps, mental status changes, presence of Chvostek's sign (contraction of facial muscles after tapping of the facial nerve) or Trousseau's sign (carpopedal spasm produced by application of a tourniquet or blood pressure cuff to the forearm for 3 minutes). Evidence of malnutrition (loss of muscle mass and weight) should be sought. A history of bone pain and pathologic bone fractures should be elicited. The patient's current weight must be recorded. Obtaining records of the last dialysis with fluid balance calculations and predialysis and postdialysis body weight permits an assessment of fluid status.

The patient's history and physical examination may reveal the cause of renal dysfunction. A history or physical findings of volume depletion or exposure to nephrotoxic medications or angiography provide important diagnostic information and suggest specific interventions. Muscle injury or ischemia may cause rhabdomyolysis resulting in ARF. Acute anuria is seen in postrenal ARF. A rash may accompany allergic interstitial nephritis. Atheroembolic renal failure may be associated with livedo reticularis and signs of embolic phenomena. Bone pain in an elderly patient should suggest multiple myeloma as a cause of ARF. Pulmonary hemorrhage and sinusitis should lead the physician to consider systemic vasculitis with glomerulonephritis.

DIAGNOSTIC TESTING

Patients with renal insufficiency or ESRD who are being evaluated for anesthesia need an ECG; hematocrit; and measurement of electrolyte, BUN, and creatinine levels. Additional findings of the history and physical examination may necessitate a PT, PTT, platelet count, chest radiograph (CXR), urinalysis, albumin level, or chemical stress test (see Chapter 3). BUN and creatinine levels should be used to assess the efficacy of dialysis treatment. Dialysis is expected to reduce BUN levels by 65% from predialysis values.[10]

An ECG should be reviewed for signs of ischemia, left ventricular hypertrophy, a strain pattern, and arrhythmias. The baseline ECG may be abnormal because of metabolic abnormalities. Hyperkalemia manifests as peaked T waves. The indications for stress testing are the same as for patients without renal disease (see Chapter 3). Dipyridamole or dobutamine hydrochloride stress testing may be necessary, however, because renal failure patients perform poorly on exercise testing. In patients with pericarditis, the ECG shows diffuse ST and T wave changes. Small QRS complexes develop as fluid accumulates in the pericardial sac. A high percentage of patients with CRF and hypertension have left ventricular hypertrophy or a dilated cardiomyopathy, which should be evident on the ECG and CXR. A CXR may show signs of cardiomegaly, pericardial effusion, congestive heart failure, or pulmonary edema. ESRD patients on erythropoietin should have normal or near-normal hematocrits. If anemia is present, causes other than ESRD should be explored (see Chapter 7). Routine PT and PTT are not indicated unless there is a history of bleeding.

Assessment of urine indices and urinalysis are rarely indicated in the preoperative evaluation of patients with established renal insufficiency or failure. Urinalysis and determination of urine indices are inexpensive diagnostic screening tests for renal disease. In the case of deteriorating renal function (even in patients with known renal disease), they may provide additional etiologic clues. In the absence of RBCs, heme positivity of urine suggests the presence of myoglo-

Table 8-2. Indices for differential diagnosis between prerenal and renal azotemia

	Prerenal	Renal
Urine osmolality (mOsm/kg)	>500	<350
Urine/plasma osmolality	>1.3	<1.1
Urine sodium (mEq/L)	<20	>40
Urine/plasma urea	>8	<3
Urine/plasma creatinine	>40	<20
Fractional excretion of sodium (FE_{Na})*	<1%	>2%

*FE_{Na} is calculated as follows:

$$FE_{Na} = \frac{U_{Na} \times P_{Cr} \times 100}{P_{Na} \times U_{Cr}}$$

where U_{Na} is urine sodium concentration, P_{Cr} is plasma creatinine concentration, P_{Na} is plasma sodium concentration, U_{Cr} is urine creatinine concentration.

bin or hemoglobin and supports a clinical diagnosis of rhabdomyolysis or a transfusion reaction. The characteristics of casts aid in the evaluation. Pigmented granular casts are typically found in ischemic or toxic ARF, white cell casts in interstitial nephritis, and red cell casts in glomerulonephritis. The presence of eosinophils in urine may suggest allergic interstitial nephritis, although the diagnostic value of a finding of eosinophiluria is limited because it is seen in other causes of ARF (atheroembolism, pyelonephritis). Oxalate crystals are seen with ethylene glycol ingestion.[7]

Measurements of urine osmolality, urinary sodium (U_{Na}) concentration, and fractional excretion of sodium (FE_{Na}) help differentiate between prerenal azotemia in which the reabsorptive capacity of tubular cells and the concentrating ability of the kidney are preserved, and tubular necrosis in which both functions are impaired (Table 8-2). Inability to concentrate the urine is one of the earliest functional defects seen with tubular damage. Patients with oliguria and ARF due to prerenal causes usually have a urine osmolality greater than 500 mOsm per kg, a U_{Na} concentration less than 20 mmol per L, and a FE_{Na} less than 1.0%. In contrast, in patients with tubular necrosis urine osmolality is less than 350 mOsm per kg, the U_{Na} concentration is greater than 40 mmol per L, and FE_{Na} is more than 1.0%. Although the urine indices may allow differentiation of prerenal azotemia from tubular necrosis, they do not completely distinguish the two conditions. Early in the course of certain processes that lead to tubular damage (myoglobinuria, exposure to radiocontrast agents, sepsis, urinary obstruction) the U_{Na} concentration can be low.[7]

Renal ultrasonography is a useful means of diagnosing obstruction, but its sensitivity may be only 80% to 85%. A nondilatated collecting system does not exclude the possibility of obstruction, especially when the condition is acute, when retroperitoneal fibrosis is present, or if the patient is hypovolemic. Ultrasonography can identify stones and determine kidney size, which, if small, suggests chronic renal insufficiency. If the index of suspicion for obstruction is high, antegrade or retrograde contrast studies of the urinary outflow tract may be required to establish the site of obstruction and provide relief.[7]

In general, renal biopsy is not necessary in the evaluation and treatment of patients with ARF. However, when the history, clinical features, and laboratory and radiologic investigations have excluded prerenal and postrenal causes and suggest a diagnosis of primary renal disease other than ischemic or toxin-related ARF, a kidney biopsy may establish the diagnosis and guide therapy.[7]

ANESTHETIC CONSIDERATIONS

Anesthetic management should be tailored to maintain stable renal function during the perioperative period. Conditions that decrease renal perfusion (hypovolemia, hypotension) and the use of nephrotoxic agents (aminoglycosides, radiocontrast agents) should be avoided. The anesthesiologist should identify patients with an increased risk for perioperative renal dysfunction: patients having interruption of renal blood flow secondary to suprarenal aortic cross clamping; patients undergoing cardiopulmonary bypass; patients with preexistent renal dysfunction, especially diabetic patients; and patients with poor myocardial function.

Volume Status

Maintenance of effective intravascular volume is the most important strategy for preserving renal perfusion and preventing renal impairment. The consequences of fluid overload (pulmonary edema, respiratory failure) can easily be reversed, but ischemic renal failure that results from intravascular volume contraction is associated with a high morbidity and mortality.[1] Preoperative fluid deficits that result from fasting (*nil per os* status), bowel preparations, diseases associated with fluid loss such as vomiting or diarrhea, and the osmotic diuretic effects of radiocontrast agents must be corrected. Because intraoperative urine output is not an accurate indicator of renal perfusion, assessment of the adequacy of volume repletion therapy may require placement of a central venous or pulmonary artery catheter. Frequent determinations of central venous pressures, cardiac output, and stroke volume are useful in determining volume status, especially in patients with impaired myocardial function. Volume overload is treated with fluid restriction, diuretics, ultrafiltration, or dialysis.

Albumin supplementation is not indicated in patients with nephrotic syndrome. The kidney promptly filters most of the administered albumin with just a transient increase in oncotic pressure. Patients receiving albumin have been shown to have an increased mortality.[12]

Coronary Artery Disease

Patients with renal insufficiency have an increased risk of perioperative coronary events. Proper risk stratification and management are recommended as in patients without renal failure (see Chapter 3).

Anemia

Anemia from CRF is usually well tolerated. It is not uncommon to have ESRD patients with hematocrits of more than 30% with the use of erythropoietin. Adequate iron and folate supplementation should be assured.

Metabolic Status

The recommendation is that dialysis patients be dialyzed within 24 hours of their surgical procedure. Hyperkalemia is one of the most life-threatening problems encountered perioperatively and can be controlled with dialysis. Other maneuvers include hyperventilation and sodium bicarbonate administration, which produce a pH change with translocation of potassium into the cells. Glucose and insulin infusions move potassium intracellularly. Calcium gluconate directly counteracts hyperkalemic cardiac effects and can be given to prevent or treat arrhythmias. Potassium-binding ion-exchange resins (Kayexalate), given orally, bind potassium in the colon.

Metabolic acidosis is not treated unless serum bicarbonate is less than 15 mmol per L. Other causes of acidosis (i.e., ketoacidosis, lactic acidosis) should be treated appropriately. Replacement may be necessary with bicarbonate orally or intravenously if acidosis is severe. Arterial blood gas levels and the clinical condition should guide therapy.

Hyponatremia is treated with free-water restriction. Hyperphosphatemia is treated by reduction of dietary phosphate intake and use of phosphate-binding antacids (e.g., Amphojel). Hypocalcemia is treated if symptomatic (see History and Physical Examination, above) or when sodium bicarbonate is administered.

Renal Preservation

In certain animal models of nephrotoxic or ischemic ARF, the administration of "renal dose" dopamine hydrochloride (1 to 5 μg per kg per minute) produced increases in renal blood flow and GFR. Most human studies, however, have failed to demonstrate that dopamine hydrochloride administration prevents ARF in high-risk patients or improves renal function or outcome in patients with established ARF.[13] In ARF patients, forced diuresis using furosemide or mannitol may convert an oliguric to a nonoliguric ARF. This will not change prognosis but may help in fluid management.

Pharmacology

The pharmacokinetics of many drugs are altered by renal insufficiency. Changes in volume of distribution and protein binding affect the availability of drugs. Knowledge of the pathways of metabolism and elimination helps in predicting the kinetics of drugs. The effects of dialysis on drug removal should be considered.[14] A summary of anesthetic drug use in renal failure patients is provided in Table 8-3.

Table 8-3. Simplified list of anesthetic pharmacologic considerations in cases of renal insufficiency

Decrease induction drug doses.
Decrease benzodiazepine doses.
Avoid meperidine hydrochloride.
Effects of morphine are potentially prolonged.
Cisatracurium besylate is the nondepolarizing agent of choice.
Succinylcholine chloride is safe when potassium level is <5.5 mEq/L.
Anticholinesterase effects are prolonged.
Use of sevoflurane, especially at low flows, is controversial.

In general, lipid-soluble drugs are poorly ionized and are metabolized by the liver to water-soluble forms before elimination by the kidney.[15] With a few exceptions, the metabolites have little biological activity. Drugs that are highly ionized at physiologic pH tend to be eliminated unchanged by the kidney, and their duration of action may be prolonged by renal dysfunction. Any medication given to a patient with renal insufficiency may display unpredictable pharmacokinetics, with adjustments of dosages dependent on half-life, pathway of elimination, and volume of distribution.

Benzodiazepines, phenothiazines, and butyrophenones are metabolized in the liver to both active and inactive compounds, which are then eliminated by the kidney. Benzodiazepines are 90% to 95% protein bound. Lorazepam (Ativan), in particular, is not recommended for patients with severe renal failure due to its potential for accumulation. Diazepam should be used with caution because of its long half-life and active metabolites. Benzodiazepines are not appreciably removed by dialysis. An alpha-adrenergic blockade with phenothiazine derivatives may accentuate cardiovascular instability, particularly in recently dialyzed patients.

Narcotics are metabolized in the liver but may have a more intense and prolonged effect in patients with renal failure, particularly in hypoalbuminemic patients, because of reduced protein binding. The use of remifentanil hydrochloride is an option when intense narcotic effects are needed but one wants to avoid prolonged sedation. This unique narcotic is ultra–short acting and is metabolized by serum and tissue esterases. Its elimination is independent of renal function.[16]

Renal Function

Patients with normal kidneys experience transient postanesthetic alterations in renal function. These alterations occur despite insignificant changes in blood pressure and cardiac output, which suggests that changes in intrarenal distribution of blood flow are responsible.[17]

All inhalational agents and many induction agents cause myocardial depression, hypotension, and mild to moderate increases in renal vascular resistance, which lead to a decrease in renal blood flow and GFR. Compensatory catecholamine secretion causes redistribution of renal blood flow. Levels of antidiuretic hormone (ADH) do not change during halothane or morphine anesthesia but increase with surgical stimulation. Hydration before the induction of anesthesia attenuates the rise in ADH produced by painful stimuli. Spinal and epidural anesthesia decrease renal blood flow, GFR, and urine output.

When the duration of anesthesia is brief, changes in renal function are reversible. Renal blood flow and GFR return to normal within a few hours. With extensive surgery and prolonged anesthesia, impaired ability to excrete a water load or concentrate urine develops and may last for several days.

Nephrotoxic drugs should be avoided whenever possible in patients with chronic renal insufficiency, transplants, or with an increased risk of developing renal dysfunction.

Bleeding Abnormalities

Dialysis partially corrects platelet dysfunction.[18] The recommendation is that dialysis be performed within 24 hours of the surgical procedure. Additional hemostatic options include use of desmopressin acetate (DDAVP) (0.3 μg per kg administered intravenously over 5 minutes), cryoprecipitate, or conjugated estrogens (0.6 mg per kg administered intravenously). These agents shorten the bleeding time and may decrease blood loss during surgical procedures in dialysis patients. Desmopressin acetate is safe and well tolerated. It increases circulating levels of factor VIII and von Willebrand factor. It decreases perioperative blood loss in patients with CRF and has a more rapid onset of action than estrogen therapy. Unlike cryoprecipitate, it is not associated with infectious risks of human blood product administration.[9] Adequately dialyzed patients do not require prophylactic treatment except perhaps in cases in which bleeding could be disastrous (i.e., neurosurgery) or in which massive blood loss is anticipated (hepatic resection). One should have a low threshold for treating clinically significant bleeding, even in adequately dialyzed patients.

Nutrition

Patients who have nephrotic syndrome or who are malnourished may benefit from postponement of elective procedures while measures are instituted to optimize nutritional status (see Chapter 16).

Regional Anesthesia

The use of regional anesthesia avoids the effects of muscle relaxants, narcotics, and potent volatile anesthetics administered during general anesthesia. In addition, it decreases the risk of aspiration and iatrogenic pulmonary infection. Peripheral nerve blocks are indicated for procedures involving the extremities. Brachial plexus block is the preferred anesthetic for placement of an arteriovenous fistula.[19]

The bleeding tendency associated with uremia could theoretically be a problem with spinal or epidural anesthesia because of the risk of hematoma formation. If the patient is on an adequate dialysis regimen, however, primary platelet function is almost normal. No reports have been published of epidural hematoma formation in this patient population, and regional anesthesia has been used successfully for renal transplantation.[9,20]

The use of regional anesthesia in patients with uremic polyneuropathy is controversial. Most anesthesiologists agree that its use is contraindicated, although some authors differ.[9]

Aspiration Risk

Renal failure patients are considered at high risk for aspiration. The necessity for rapid-sequence intubation should be weighed against the potential hemodynamic changes that can occur.[9] These patients should receive histamine$_2$ antagonists (e.g., ranitidine, hydrochloride), a gastric motility agent (e.g., metoclopramide), and a nonparticulate antacid (e.g., sodium citrate).

Intravenous Access

Renal failure patients have intravenous lines placed frequently, so finding access may be difficult. Placing the intravenous line in the extremity without an arteriovenous fistula or graft is preferable. Arteriovenous fistulas should be protected (not compressed, well padded) and assessed frequently for presence of a thrill, and all efforts should be made to minimize the chances of thrombosis. Some patients have a central catheter for dialysis, which should be accessed only in an emergency. Dialysis catheters are flushed with large quantities of heparin sodium and should be aspirated before use.

In patients with renal insufficiency or conditions that commonly lead to ESRD, arm veins, especially the cephalic veins of the nondominant arm, should not be used for intravenous catheter placement or venipunctures.[21] This is to preserve these vessels for construction of a primary arteriovenous fistula. Likewise, catheterization of subclavian veins is associated with central venous stenosis. Significant stenosis of the subclavian vessels usually prevents use of the entire ipsilateral arm for arteriovenous fistulae. Patients and health care providers must be educated about preserving vascular access for future arteriovenous fistula construction.

Other Considerations

Perioperative steroid coverage may be required if patients have been taking corticosteroids[9] (see Chapter 15). Transplant patients should continue their immunosuppressive therapy.

CASE STUDY

A 49-year-old woman with a history of chronic glomerulonephritis with ESRD requiring hemodialysis three times per week presents for elective laparoscopic cholecystectomy. Her last dialysis was 2 days previously (through her left arm arteriovenous fistula). She has no history of ischemic heart disease and is moderately active. She denies recent episodes of nausea and vomiting and does not produce urine. Her current medications include erythropoietin, ranitidine hydrochloride, oral bicarbonate, and a calcium channel blocker.

Vital signs are blood pressure, 130/90 mm Hg; heart rate, 82 beats per minute; respiratory rate, 16 per minute; and temperature, 37.1°C. Cardiac examination reveals a left-sided S_4, a displaced point of maximum impulse, and no evidence of jugular venous distention. Lungs are clear to auscultation. Her abdomen is tender to palpation in the right upper quadrant with no signs of peritonitis. Her arteriovenous fistula is patent. Laboratory findings include a hematocrit of 32%, potassium level of 5.6 mEq per L, bicarbonate level of 15 mEq per L, BUN level of 80 mg per dL, and creatinine level of 7.5 mg per dL. An ECG is consistent with left ventricular hypertrophy. CXR shows clear lungs.

This is an elective surgery that requires a general anesthetic. Performing surgery 2 days after dialysis with significant metabolic abnormalities as noted is not ideal. The case should be rescheduled so dialysis can be arranged within 24 hours of surgery. Her hematocrit is acceptable. Invasive monitoring is not needed in the setting of surgery with minor blood loss and fluid shifts without signs of sepsis. Because of the potential risk for aspiration secondary to ESRD, a rapid-sequence intubation should be planned. The patient should receive ranitidine hydrochloride, sodium citrate, and metoclopramide. Risk of bleeding should not be increased in this patient who is receiving regular dialysis, because platelet function should be close to normal. Preoperative administration of desmopressin acetate is not necessary for this patient, but the threshold for using this relatively benign intervention should be low if increased bleeding (e.g., oozing in the surgical field) occurs.

REFERENCES

1. Miller CF. Evaluation of the patient with renal disease. In: Rogers M, Covino BG, Tinker JH, eds. *Principles and practice of anesthesiology.* St. Louis: Mosby–Year Book, 1993:299–310.
2. Zamora JL, Bordine JT, Karlberg H, et al. Cardiac surgery in patients with end-stage renal disease. *Ann Thorac Surg* 1986;42: 113–117.
3. Pinson CW, Schuman ES, Gross GF, et al. Surgery in long-term dialysis patients: experience with more than 300 patients. *Am J Surg* 1986;151:567–571.
4. Brenner BM, Mackenzie HS. Disturbances of renal function. In: Fauci AS, Braunwald E, Isselbacher KS, et al., eds. *Harrison's principles of internal medicine*, 14th ed. New York: McGraw-Hill, 1998:1498–1504.
5. Lazarus JM, Brenner BM. Chronic renal failure. In: Fauci AS, Braunwald E, Isselbacher KS, et al., eds. *Harrison's principles of internal medicine*, 14th ed. New York: McGraw-Hill, 1998: 1513–1520.
6. Thadhani R, Pascual M, Bonventre JV. Acute renal failure. *N Engl J Med* 1996;334:1448–1460.

7. Brady HR, Brenner BM. Acute renal failure. In: Fauci AS, Braunwald E, Isselbacher KS, et al., eds. *Harrison's principles of internal medicine*, 14th ed. New York: McGraw-Hill, 1998:1504–1513.

8. Orth SR, Ritz E. The nephrotic syndrome. *N Engl J Med* 1998;338:1201–1211.

9. Weir PHC, Chung FF. Anesthesia for patients with chronic renal disease. *Can Anaesth Soc J* 1984;31:468–480.

10. Ifudu O. Care of patients undergoing hemodialysis. *N Engl J Med* 1998;339:1054–1062.

11. Jankovic N, Cala S, Nadinic B, et al. Hepatitis C and hepatitis B virus infection in hemodialysis patients and staff: a 2 year followup. *Int J Artif Organs* 1994;17:137–140.

12. Cochrane Injuries Group Albumin Reviewers. Human albumin administration in critically ill patients: systemic review of randomised controlled trials. *BMJ* 1998;317:235–240

13. Denton MD, Chertow GM, Brady HR. "Renal-dose" dopamine for the treatment of acute renal failure: scientific rationale, experimental studies and clinical trials. *Kidney Int* 1996;49:4–14.

14. Nancarrow C, Mather LE. Pharmacokinetics in renal failure. *Anaesth Intensive Care* 1983;11:350–359.

15. Lee B, Sapirstein A. Specific considerations with renal disease. In: Hurford WE, Bailin MT, Daviron JK, et al., eds. *Clinical anesthesia procedures of the Massachusetts General Hospital*, 5th edition. Philadelphia: Lippincott–Raven Publishers, 1998:47–64.

16. Hoke JF, Shlugman D, Dershwitz M, et al. Pharmacokinetics and pharmacodynamics of remifentanil in persons with renal failure compared with healthy volunteers. *Anesthesiology* 1997;87:533–541.

17. Sladen RN. Effect of anesthesia and surgery on renal function. *Crit Care Clin* 1987;3:373–393.

18. Remuzzi G, Livio M, Marchiaro G, et al. Bleeding in renal failure: altered platelet function in chronic uremia only partially corrected by hemodialysis. *Nephron* 1978;22:347–353.

19. Solomonson MD, Johnson ME, Ilstrup D. Risk factors in patients having surgery to create an arteriovenous fistula. *Anesth Analg* 1994;79:694–700.

20. Wyant GM. The anaesthetist looks at tissue transplantation: three years' experience with kidney transplants. *Can Anaesth Soc J* 1967;14:255–275.

21. National Kidney Foundation Dialysis Outcomes Quality Initiative. Clinical practice guidelines for vascular access. *Am J Kid Dis* 1997;4[Suppl 3]:S150–S191.

Hepatobiliary Disease

Rae M. Allain and Zenaide M. N. Quezado

Patients with hepatobiliary disease may pose several challenges to the anesthesia care team seeking to provide an effective, safe anesthetic and to avoid perioperative complications. A careful preoperative assessment is crucial to appropriate preparation and management of these patients. This chapter reviews the appropriate assessment and care of patients with **hepatitis**, **cirrhosis**, **cholelithiasis**, and **pancreatitis**, and of those who have undergone **hepatic transplantation**.

DEFINITIONS

Hepatitis is nonspecific inflammation of the liver. The pathophysiology involves direct hepatocellular damage, which may progress to hepatocyte necrosis and loss of liver function. Most commonly, hepatitis is the result of viral infection or exposure to toxins, including alcohol and drugs. Six causal viral agents, labeled hepatitis A, B, C, delta (D), E, and G, have been described as the major causes of clinical cases of hepatitis, but other viral agents, including herpesvirus, coxsackievirus, and Epstein-Barr virus, may produce the clinical syndrome of hepatitis.

Hepatitis A and hepatitis E are similar in that both infections rely on enteric transmission; both produce acute, self-limited disease; and neither exists in a chronic state. The diagnosis of acute hepatitis A is confirmed by the detection of immunoglobulin M (IgM) antibody to hepatitis A virus (IgM anti-HAV) in serum.

Hepatitis B and hepatitis C may exist in acute and chronic forms, usually discernible by history and laboratory tests. Both viruses are transmitted parenterally, but hepatitis B also is capable of transmission via sexual or close physical contact. Fortunately, the widespread introduction of hepatitis B vaccine for the military, the institutionalized population, prisoners, health care workers, and other high-risk groups appears to be diminishing the incidence of hepatitis B infection from occupational exposure. Hepatitis B vaccination is strongly recommended for all health care personnel. Hepatitis B or C infection can lead to chronic hepatitis, cirrhosis, or hepatocellular carcinoma. Acute hepatitis B infection is diagnosed by the detection of IgM antibody to hepatitis B core antigen (IgM anti-HBc). Usually, hepatitis B surface antigen (HB_sAg) and hepatitis B virus DNA (HBV DNA) are detectable in serum during acute infections. Five percent to 10% of adult patients with acute hepatitis B become chronically infected, which is identifiable in the majority by the sustained presence of HB_sAg in serum. Abnormally elevated levels of serum alanine aminotransferase (ALT) and lifelong serum HB_sAg positivity are characteristic of chronic hepatitis B infection, although some people, termed *healthy carriers*, are HB_sAg

213

positive without elevated ALT level or symptoms of liver disease. Individuals who have had an episode of hepatitis B and recover or who have received the vaccine have a positive hepatitis B surface antibody (anti-HBs). Anti-HBs is a long-lived antibody, usually detectable for life. Acute hepatitis C is diagnosed by detection of antibody to hepatitis C virus (anti-HCV) in the clinical setting of hepatitis. Fifty percent to 70% of patients with acute hepatitis C develop chronic hepatitis C, and 90% of these patients have detectable serum levels of anti-HCV. Even when complete clinical recovery occurs, the hepatitis C virus is rarely totally cleared after acute infection. Measurement of serum hepatitis C virus RNA (HCV RNA) shows that 90% of patients remain chronically infected, although some do not have clinical evidence of chronic hepatitis.

Hepatitis D virus is a defective RNA virus reliant on coinfection with hepatitis B virus. Its clinical importance lies in the higher likelihood of fulminant hepatitis during acute hepatitis B infection and a worse clinical course of chronic hepatitis B infection with concurrent hepatitis D carriage. Hepatitis G has been described in a patient with chronic hepatitis C. Whether the parenterally transmissible hepatitis G may exist in a chronic state is not known.

Similar to the viral entities, drugs or toxins may produce acute hepatitis. Alcohol ingestion is a common cause of acute hepatitis. Histologic examination of the liver reveals a cellular injury pattern similar to that in acute viral hepatitis but marked by the presence of proteinaceous, eosinophilic cytoplasmic inclusions, termed *Mallory's bodies*. Repeated bouts of alcoholic hepatitis may lead to progressive liver disease that culminates in alcoholic cirrhosis. In addition to alcohol, many other drugs may cause acute hepatitis, including halothane, isoniazid, acetaminophen, and nitrofurantoin. Environmental and occupational toxins are potential causes of acute hepatitis with possible fulminant hepatic failure.

Cirrhosis is the common end point of a variety of progressive insults to the liver. Histologically, cirrhosis is marked by disruption of the hepatic architecture with formation of fibrous tissue, scarring, and nodular areas of attempted regeneration of liver parenchyma. The important role of the liver in homeostasis is demonstrated by the complex pathophysiology resulting from chronic liver injury and cirrhosis. Fibrosis increases resistance to blood flow through the liver, which results in elevated pressures in the portal vein, termed *portal hypertension*. To divert venous blood around the scarred liver, collateral vascular channels develop wherever portal and systemic circulations are joined by capillaries. These collateral vessels, or portosystemic shunts, may form in the retroperitoneum or in the abdomen, complicating surgical procedures. Most problematic, however, is bleeding from esophageal varices, which may lead to massive upper gastrointestinal tract hemorrhage requiring endoscopic, radiologic, or surgical intervention. Congestion of the portal vein may cause splenomegaly, with resultant splenic sequestration of platelets and peripheral thrombocytopenia. Another sequela of portal hypertension is ascites, the abnormal excessive accumulation of peritoneal fluid. Ascites often results in respiratory compromise (pleural effusion, decreased diaphragmatic excursion) or infection of the peritoneal cavity, termed *spontaneous bacterial peritonitis*.

Some patients with cirrhosis develop the hepatorenal syndrome, a functional renal failure that is poorly understood but characterized by severe renal vasoconstriction and a very high mortality. Diagnosis of hepatorenal syndrome is often difficult, because patients with cirrhosis are at risk of renal failure from other causes, including prerenal azotemia (from overdiuresis or bleeding) or acute tubular necrosis (caused by sepsis or drug toxicity). In addition, urinary indices mimic a prerenal state (see Chapter 8), which makes hepatorenal syndrome a diagnosis of exclusion once hypovolemia and other correctable causes of acute renal failure have been eliminated. Interestingly, kidneys afflicted by hepatorenal syndrome are histologically normal and can be transplanted to others with complete functional recovery. Thus, definitive therapy for hepatorenal syndrome consists of correcting the underlying hepatic dysfunction through liver transplantation. Rarely, patients with cirrhosis may develop hepatopulmonary syndrome, characterized by abnormal pulmonary vasodilatation with ventilation/perfusion mismatch and severe arterial hypoxemia. Finally, neurologic compromise is a common finding in portal hypertension. Failure of the liver to clear intestinally absorbed biogenic amines results in abnormal exposure of the brain to these substances, which is thought to result in hepatic encephalopathy.

The progressive failure of hepatocyte function seen in cirrhosis is important because of the role of the liver as the body's toxin remover. For example, many anesthetic drugs (thiopental sodium, morphine sulfate) are metabolized in the liver before elimination. Impaired hepatocyte number or function may result in prolongation of drug effect in patients with cirrhosis. Also, many proteins that normally bind anesthetic medications (e.g., albumin) are synthesized in diminished amounts by the diseased liver so that a greater amount of drug is present in the unbound, active form. Both of these effects warrant a decrease in the dose of drug administered to the patient with cirrhosis. However, severe cirrhotic liver disease with ascites results in an increase in the volume of distribution of many drugs, which may require an increased dose for equivalent effect. Because the majority of proteins involved in coagulation are synthesized in the liver, cirrhosis is usually associated with coagulopathies. Decreases in the vitamin K–dependent clotting factors (factors II, VII, IX, and X) are reflected by a prolonged prothrombin time (PT) and partial thromboplastin time (PTT). Fibrinogen levels are often decreased, which further impairs clot formation. Also, failure of the liver to clear activated factors may lead to fibrinolysis, measurable by elevated levels of fibrin degradation products. Some patients with cirrhosis may develop disseminated intravascular coagulation, indicated by an elevated level of D-dimer. In addition, thrombocytopenia frequently occurs in cirrhosis because of platelet sequestration by the enlarged spleen seen with portal hypertension. The end result is an overall proclivity for bleeding in patients with cirrhosis.

Cholelithiasis is common, occurring in an estimated 8% of men and 20% of women older than 40 years. When indicated, surgical resection of the gallbladder (cholecystectomy) is performed. The pathophysiology of cholelithiasis is the crystallization of bile components into stones, composed predominantly of cholesterol or pigments. Obstruction of the cystic or common bile duct by gallstones usually results in cholecystitis (acute inflammation of the gallbladder wall), causing pain (biliary colic) and possible bacterial infection. In uncomplicated, acute cholecystitis, medical management with bowel rest, antibiotic administration, gastric decompression, and intravenous fluid resuscitation resolves the process in 75% of patients. The natural history of cholelithiasis, however, is one of recurrent symptoms of biliary colic and cholecystitis in the majority of patients, so that most clinicians recommend elective cholecystectomy after successful treatment of the acute condition. Those patients who develop a complication of cholecystitis, including gangrene, perforation, abscess, enteric fistula, or recurrent sepsis, usually require emergent cholecystectomy.

Pancreatitis is an inflammation of the pancreas and may be acute or chronic. In the United States, acute pancreatitis is most frequently attributable to alcohol ingestion. A secondary cause is gallstone obstruction of the pancreatic duct. Third, a wide variety of drugs may induce pancreatitis. A minority of cases are hereditary or idiopathic. The exact pathophysiology of acute pancreatitis is unknown, but autodigestion of the pancreas by the release of proteolytic enzymes within the pancreas itself is inherent to the disease process. Once released, these proteolytic enzymes cause cell injury and death. Destruction may be mild and the disease self-limited, or extensive with a protracted, necrotizing course. Usually serum amylase and lipase levels are elevated, but lipase elevation is more specific because amylase has nonpancreatic sources. In addition, the trypsinogen level, if available, may be useful in diagnosing pancreatitis because this enzyme is only found in the pancreas. None of these blood tests is reliable for diagnosing pancreatitis in the presence of renal failure, however. Acute pancreatitis may have systemic manifestations—among them, hypotension, anemia, metabolic aberrancies, sepsis, renal dysfunction, and respiratory failure, including acute respiratory distress syndrome. Chronic pancreatitis is characterized by recurrent bouts of acute pancreatitis; alternatively, an indolent, unremitting pattern of pancreatic inflammation may be classified as chronic pancreatitis. The causes of chronic pancreatitis are similar to those of acute pancreatitis, but idiopathic causes play a greater role.

Patients with acute pancreatitis may present to the operating room for surgical débridement of an infected necrotic pancreas or for drainage of a pancreatic abscess. Morbidity and mortality rates are significant; thus, percutaneous radiologically guided drainage procedures are increasingly used for approachable abscesses. For those patients with severe acute pancreatitis caused by gallstones, papillotomy guided by endoscopic retrograde cholangiopancreatography may be a technique necessitating anesthesia. Patients in remission from acute pancreatitis or those with chronic pancreatitis may require operative intervention for drainage of pseudocysts. Pseudocysts are collections of fluid, dead tissue, pancreatic enzymes, and blood that may complicate pancreatitis and require intervention because of chronic pain, intestinal obstruction, infection, or large or increasing size with risk of rupture. Patients with chronic pancreatitis unresponsive to medical management may present for pancreatectomy or Whipple's resection (pancreaticoduodenectomy).

The number of **liver transplants** performed in the United States is increasing annually (4,450 were performed in 1998)

Table 9-1. Adverse effects of immunosuppressive drugs used in liver transplantation

Drug	Potential effect	Indicated preoperative tests
Cyclosporine	Renal toxicity	BUN, creatinine
Tacrolimus	Renal toxicity	BUN, creatinine
Azathioprine (Imuran)	Myelosuppression	CBC
Corticosteroids	Sodium retention	Sodium
	Hypokalemia	Potassium
	Hyperglycemia	Glucose
	Alkalosis	Bicarbonate

BUN, blood urea nitrogen; CBC, complete blood cell count.

because of the greater number of available organs and improved success rates. The epidemiology of end-stage liver disease and the advent of liver transplantation as the only curative therapy suggest that an increasing number of liver transplant recipients will require anesthesia in the future. Thus, the anesthesiologist must be familiar with the special considerations regarding the patient who has undergone liver transplantation. Use of immunosuppressant medications increases a patient's risk for rare opportunistic infections. Cyclosporin may cause nephrotoxicity, hypertension, and accelerated atherosclerotic coronary artery disease. Azathioprine (Imuran) causes myelosuppression. Adverse effects of corticosteroids include gastric ulceration, glucose intolerance, glaucoma, skin atrophy, and poor wound healing. Table 9-1 outlines adverse effects of immunosuppressant medications and indicated preoperative tests.

HISTORY

Hepatobiliary disease causes a wide variety of symptoms. The medical history provides important clues to specific diagnoses. Anesthesiologists should determine if the patient has had **hepatitis** and, if so, questions regarding the causes, therapies, and current status of the disease (resolved, chronic, or progressive to cirrhosis) should follow. Many cases of hepatitis go undiagnosed. A history of jaundice, dark urine, anorexia, nausea and vomiting, and right upper quadrant pain may indicate liver disease. Frequently these symptoms are accompanied by fever, malaise, and pruritus. The cause may be delineated by careful query of travel history, ingestion of potentially contaminated foods, sexual contacts, intravenous drug abuse, alcohol use, history of blood transfusions, and drug or toxin exposure.

Biliary colic and **cholelithiasis** are usually discriminated from hepatitis by the severe, acute nature of the right upper quadrant pain, which is sometimes precipitated by a fatty meal. Accompanying symptoms may include nausea, vomiting, fever, and chills.

The diagnosis of **cirrhosis** should be considered in the patient with known or suspected liver disease who complains of anorexia, fatigue, weakness, increasing abdominal girth, jaundice, or easy bruisability. The patient may notice muscle wasting despite an increase in weight due to salt and fluid retention. Family members may report subtle neurologic findings suggestive of encephalopathy, including forgetfulness, intermittent confusion, sleep disturbances, and personality changes.

Pancreatitis manifests with complaints of severe abdominal pain, localized in the epigastrium, with radiation to the back. Pain is usually accompanied by anorexia, abdominal distention, nausea, and vomiting. Some patients may report diarrhea or steatorrhea and weight loss.

PHYSICAL EXAMINATION

Physical examination of the patient with hepatobiliary disease may reveal a myriad of abdominal and systemic findings. Jaundice and scleral icterus denote bilirubin concentration of more than 3 mg per dL and trigger a long list of diagnostic possibilities. Percussion of the abdomen may reveal hepatomegaly (liver span greater than 12 cm in the midclavicular line). A palpable liver edge may indicate venous congestion, amyloidosis, tumor, or hepatitis. Tenderness of the liver with palpation is a sign of acute hepatitis. This is distinguished from Murphy's sign, a sharp right upper quadrant pain occurring with palpation during inspiration and seen in acute **cholecystitis**.

Evidence of **cirrhosis** may be apparent on physical examination. The patient may be jaundiced, with a distended abdomen, and may have a cachetic appearance. Auscultation of the chest often reveals diminished breath sounds at the bases, suggestive of atelectasis or pleural effusions. Inspection and palpation of the precordium may show an increased apical impulse amplitude, which suggests a hyperdynamic heart. In addition, a systolic flow murmur from increased cardiac output may be present. Abdominal examination may demonstrate a palpable, firm, or nodular liver. Cirrhosis with portal hypertension often causes splenomegaly, with the spleen palpable below the left costal margin. Ascites is diagnosed by abdominal percussion demonstrating shifting dullness in the dependent portions of the abdomen and by evidence of a fluid wave if the quantity of ascites is great. Coagulopathy, which may accompany cirrhosis, may manifest with ecchymoses. Other skin signs of cirrhosis are plentiful, including spider angiomas, palmar erythema, and a circle of dilated veins radiating from the umbilicus, termed *caput medusae*. Table 9-2 is a summary of physical findings.

Physical examination of the patient with **pancreatitis** is significant for absent bowel sounds, abdominal tenderness and rigidity, fever and, if the patient is severely hypovolemic, hypotension and evidence of shock. Frequently, jaundice is present. If a pancreatic pseudocyst exists, it may be palpable in the abdomen.

The patient who has undergone liver transplantation typically has physical findings related to immunosuppressant therapy. Corticosteroid treatment results in a cushingoid appearance, characterized by hirsutism, moon facies, central obesity with limb wasting, and thin, striated skin. Cyclosporin causes hypertension, hirsutism, and gingival hyperplasia.

Table 9-2. Physical signs of cirrhosis

Skin
  Jaundice
  Ecchymoses
  Spider angiomas
  Caput medusae
  Palmar erythema
  Clubbing
Chest
  Tachycardia
  Hyperdynamic precordium
  Systolic flow murmur
  Tachypnea
  Decreased basilar breath sounds
Abdomen
  Distention
  Ascites
  Nodular, palpable liver edge
  Splenomegaly
Musculature
  Wasting/cachexia
Nervous system
  Scleral icterus
  Encephalopathy
  Asterixis
Genitourinary system
  Gynecomastia (males)
  Testicular atrophy

PREOPERATIVE TESTING

Simple laboratory testing of the liver's functional capacity is difficult because of the liver's multifactorial role in physiologic processes. Important liver functions include glucose regulation, synthesis of proteins (clotting factors, plasma proteins), drug and toxin metabolism, and bilirubin formation and excretion. No single test can measure all of these functions, so workup of the patient with hepatobiliary disease frequently involves groups of tests intended to target the various hepatic functions. Preoperative testing for hepatobiliary disease should be performed only if suggested by the patient's history or physical examination. Serum tests to assess liver function should complement information gleaned from the history and physical examination.

Elevations in the hepatic transaminases, aspartate aminotransferase (AST) and ALT, are frequently found in **hepatitis**. Because AST may be of nonhepatic origin, ALT is more specific for hepatocellular injury. The highest levels of AST and ALT are seen in cases of viral, toxic, and ischemic hepatitis. Serum transaminase levels should be determined for any patient suspected of having acute hepatitis by preoperative evaluation. In addition, serologic testing for hepatitis A, B, and C should be performed. If acute hepatitis is suspected, values for lactate dehydrogenase (LDH), bilirubin, alkaline phosphatase, albumin, and PT should be determined. **Alcoholic hepatitis** is associated with serum transaminase levels of less than 300 to 500 IU per L and an AST to ALT ratio greater than 2.

Patients with a history of hepatitis generally fall into two categories: (a) those with resolved hepatitis and (b) those with chronic hepatitis with a variable level of disease. Because hepatitis A has no chronic state, a history of a previous self-limited episode of hepatitis A merits no further workup. However, the patient with chronic hepatitis should have a panel of preoperative tests as outlined above for those with acute hepatitis, including measurement of AST, ALT, LDH, bilirubin, alkaline phosphatase, and albumin levels as well as PT. Serum AST and ALT levels correlate with severity of histologic damage in most forms of hepatitis. In hepatitis C, history, physical examination, and tests of liver synthetic function may be more useful than hepatocellular enzyme determinations in assessing disease severity. Synthetic function of the liver is inferred by measuring the levels of those proteins synthesized only by hepatocytes, including albumin, prothrombin, and fibrinogen. Quantification of HCV RNA, representative of the viral load, may be obtained from reverse transcription techniques. This method can determine the severity of hepatic disease without resorting to a liver biopsy. Noteworthy is the fact that concomitant renal failure results in low serum levels of the aminotransferases, so that AST and ALT levels may not reflect the extent of hepatic injury.

Patients with symptomatic **cholelithiasis** and **cholecystitis** usually present with biliary tract obstruction or stasis, an elevated alkaline phosphatase level, and normal to elevated bilirubin level. Classically, in these conditions, the hyperbilirubinemia is due to conjugated (direct) bilirubin. Cholestasis, however, may be parenchymal or ductal in origin, and fractionation of bilirubin into direct and indirect components usually does not aid differentiation. Alkaline phosphatase levels may be elevated from nonbiliary sources. Specifically, γ-glutamyl transpeptidase and 5'-nucleotidase are elevated in hepatobiliary obstruction. Patients presenting with clinical evidence of cholelithiasis and supportive serum indices should undergo abdominal ultrasonography, a rapid, noninvasive diagnostic study and the procedure of choice for identifying gallstones. Because cholestatic liver disease may impair absorption of vitamin K, PT should be measured preoperatively in patients scheduled for surgery.

The **cirrhotic** patient deserves careful investigation before anesthesia. A cause for the cirrhosis (alcoholism, hepatitis, primary biliary cirrhosis, congestive heart failure) must be sought. Standard tests of hepatobiliary function, including levels of AST, ALT, alkaline phosphatase, LDH, bilirubin, albumin, and globulin, should be obtained. Clotting function should be assessed with a PT and PTT. Because chronic cirrhosis can be associated with a fibrinolytic state, evaluation of fibrinogen level should be considered, especially if other clotting studies are abnormal or the potential for blood loss is great. Given the significant risk of bleeding in cirrhotic surgical patients, a hematocrit is indicated. For all but the most minor procedures, typing and cross matching of blood is desirable. A preoperative white blood cell count should be obtained given the high risk of occult infection, especially spontaneous bacterial peritonitis, in these patients. Because cirrhosis may be complicated by portal hypertension with hypersplenism and splenic sequestration of platelets, a platelet count should be checked to evaluate for thrombocytopenia. Measurement of bleeding time is not generally useful in the workup of these patients. Avid sodium retention associated with ascites or an aggressive diuretic regimen to treat the ascites may result in significant electrolyte abnormalities. Thus, sodium, chloride, potassium, and bicarbonate determinations are indicated. Blood urea nitrogen (BUN) and creatinine levels are important because liver failure may be complicated by the hepatorenal syndrome, characterized by intense renal vasoconstriction, oliguria, azotemia, and renal failure. Glucose determination is warranted because liver failure may cause hypoglycemia. For cirrhotic patients with significant respiratory signs or symptoms (dyspnea, hypoxemia, tachypnea), a chest radiograph (CXR) and evaluation of oxygenation via pulse oximetry or arterial blood gas analysis should be made. Significant hypoxemia in the absence of parenchymal lung disease or a significant effusion on CXR should raise the possibility of hepatopulmonary syndrome. See Table 9-3 for a complete listing of indicated diagnostic tests for the patient with cirrhosis.

Typical surgeries for the patient with pancreatitis include débridement or drainage of necrotic or infected pancreatic and peripancreatic tissue. Under these circumstances, the patient may be gravely ill but with few options other than surgical intervention. Hence, preoperative workup should include assessments of all major organs. Blood tests should include measurement of electrolyte, calcium, phosphate, magnesium, BUN, creatinine, and glucose levels, complete blood count, and PT and PTT. Determination of transaminase, bilirubin, alkaline phosphatase, LDH, triglyceride, and albumin levels is indicated. An electrocardiogram is important because most patients have a sinus tachycardia and many may develop atrial tachydysrhythmias. Because acute pancreatitis is often accompanied by a left pleural effusion, symptoms of respiratory compromise, and even acute respiratory distress syndrome, a CXR should be evaluated. Physical signs and symptoms of significant respiratory compromise indicate the

Table 9-3. Preoperative tests for the patient with cirrhosis

Hepatic	AST, ALT, alkaline phosphatase, LDH, albumin, globulin levels
Hematologic	Hematocrit, PT, PTT, platelet count, ± fibrinogen level
Infectious	White blood cell count
Metabolic	Sodium, chloride, potassium, bicarbonate, glucose levels
Renal	Blood urea nitrogen, creatinine levels
Pulmonary	Chest radiograph, ± pulse oximetry, ± arterial blood gas levels

ALT, alanine aminotransferase; AST, aspartate aminotransferase; LDH, lactate dehydrogenase; PT, prothrombin time; PTT, partial thromboplastin time.

necessity to evaluate for hypoxemia by measurement of arterial blood gases or pulse oximetry.

The patient who has undergone **liver transplantation** who now presents for anesthesia deserves special evaluation. Indices of hepatic function should be tested, including AST, ALT, alkaline phosphatase, LDH, and albumin levels, and PT and PTT. Immunosuppressant drugs have a myriad of side effects that should be recognized. Because cyclosporine and tacrolimus have serious potential for renal toxicity, BUN and creatinine should be evaluated. If renal function is abnormal, cyclosporin or tacrolimus levels need to be determined. Azathioprine is a myelosuppressant, so that a complete blood count is required for patients taking this drug. Corticosteroids are associated with sodium retention, edema, hypokalemia, alkalosis, and hyperglycemia, and their use requires evaluation of serum electrolytes and glucose levels.

RISK ASSESSMENT

Quantifying anesthetic risk in patients with hepatobiliary disease is difficult because of a paucity of data. Most studies of patients with hepatobiliary disease undergoing surgery are small, nonrandomized, retrospective reviews of patients with nonhomogeneous disease. Thus, the results may not be applicable to a different clinical setting. In addition, the anesthetic risk is often difficult to discriminate from the surgical risk. Clearly, intraabdominal surgical procedures, particularly those involving the hepatobiliary tree, carry a more serious risk than nonabdominal peripheral procedures. Events not necessarily attributable to anesthetic drug or technique, including bleeding, hypoxemia, hypercarbia, infection, and positive-pressure ventilation, may contribute to poor outcome in patients with underlying hepatobiliary dysfunction. Most anesthetic drugs and techniques, however, to some extent diminish perfusion and thus oxygenation to the hepatobiliary system. In the healthy patient or patient with mild hepatobiliary disease, a decrement in hepatic oxygenation usually produces no clinical effect. For the patient with more severe organ dysfunction, this decrement may have serious adverse consequences, including hepatic failure and death.

Another factor confounding risk assessment for patients with hepatobiliary disease is that much of the existing data are derived from patients who underwent procedures not commonly performed today. For example, many patients who underwent surgical exploration for diagnostic purposes could now be diagnosed by less invasive means. Similarly, high-mortality procedures such as establishment of portosystemic shunts are often unnecessary in the modern era of medical treatments and nonoperative modalities such as the use of transjugular intrahepatic portosystemic shunts. Although some recommendations can be made concerning operative risk in patients with hepatobiliary disease (see below), the anesthesiologist frequently must rely on a clinical assessment of the individual patient, results of the diagnostic evaluation, and knowledge of his or her own practice setting.

Acute viral hepatitis is an indication for postponement of elective surgery because many older studies suggest a very high morbidity (11%) and mortality (10%) in such cases. Most experts recommend delaying elective procedures until 4 weeks or more after blood tests have normalized. Unfortunately, data on surgery in the presence of acute or chronic **alcoholic hepatitis** are more scant, but available results suggest that postponing elective operations in this setting as well is prudent. The decision to proceed with urgent or emergent surgery in the patient with acute hepatitis is based on the risks and benefits as judged by the anesthesiologist, surgeon, and consultants involved. Routine screening of liver function in healthy patients presenting for surgery is not indicated, but if such a screen yields an abnormal result, prudence dictates postponing elective procedures until the cause of the findings is identified. Often the diagnosis is determined by history, examination, and serologic testing. If not, more expensive radiologic investigation with abdominal ultrasonography or computed tomography may be used. In some cases, a diagnosis may be established only by tissue biopsy (transvenous or transabdominal needle technique) or an open surgical approach.

Attention to history, physical examination, laboratory values, and results of prior diagnostic studies are important in patients with **chronic hepatitis**. Patients who are asymptomatic or have mild symptoms of disease usually undergo anesthesia safely. Patients with hyperbilirubinemia and cirrhosis may demonstrate perioperative increases in bilirubin level, but this is usually asymptomatic and self-limited. Similarly, those with ascites may have a temporary increase in ascitic fluid postoperatively.

The surgical risk of patients with **cirrhosis** has been investigated more thoroughly than that of patients with any other hepatobiliary disease. The Child-Turcotte classification (Table 9-4), originally designed for patients undergoing portacaval shunt procedures, is widely used and easily applied to estimate operative risk. Pugh later proposed a modification to the Child-Turcotte classification that eliminated nutritional status but incorporated degree of PT prolongation into a risk estimate for patients under-

Table 9-4. Operative risk of the patient with cirrhosis: Child-Turcotte classification

Class	A	B	C
Albumin	>3.5 g/dL	3.0–3.5 g/dL	<3.0 g/dL
Bilirubin	<2.0 mg/dL	2.0–3.0 mg/dL	>3.0 mg/dL
Ascites	None	Controlled	Refractory
Encephalopathy	None	Mild	Advanced
Nutritional status	Excellent	Good	Poor
Operative mortality for major surgery	0–10%	4–31%	19–76%
Pugh's modification*: Prothrombin time (PT) prolongation	<4.0 sec	4.0–6.0 sec	>6.0 sec

*Pugh substituted *PT prolongation* for *nutritional status*. He assigned 1 point for each item in Child-Turcotte class A, 2 points for each item in class B, and 3 points for each item in class C. In Pugh's modification, a total of 5 to 15 points is possible, with the following risk stratification: ≤6, good; 7–9, moderate; ≥10, poor.

going esophageal transection for bleeding varices (see Table 9-4). Pugh's classification also differed from the Child-Turcotte classification in that points were assigned to each component assessed (PT, bilirubin, etc.), depending on the severity of perturbation, and operative risk was determined by the total points. Despite problems with the Child-Turcotte classification (e.g., lack of quantification of ascites, encephalopathy, and nutritional status), no other system of perioperative risk stratification has achieved clinical superiority, either in its risk prediction or in its utility for evaluation of cirrhotic patients undergoing shunt or nonshunt procedures. Preoperative Child-Turcotte classification has been shown to predict not only operative mortality but also morbidity, including hepatic failure, bleeding, infection, and multiorgan failure. Risk factors not included in this classification system but also demonstrated to increase operative risk are emergent nature of the procedure, PT prolongation greater than 3 seconds *and* refractory to correction with vitamin K, and the presence of infection. Thus, the anesthesiologist preparing a Child-Turcotte class C patient for abdominal surgery must be particularly attentive to preoperative interventions designed to maximize the patient's condition (e.g., instituting nutritional support, see Chapter 16), intraoperative measures taken to adequately monitor and treat potential problems, and delivery of postoperative care in an appropriate setting where interventions can be made if complications arise.

As discussed previously, the initial management of acute **cholecystitis** is usually nonoperative medical therapy consisting of bowel rest, hydration, and administration of antibiotics. Patients who require emergent cholecystectomy are those with complicated cholecystitis who may have a higher anesthetic risk because of a more severe illness.

As with patients with acute cholecystitis, patients with acute **pancreatitis** who require operative intervention are at higher risk for perioperative complications because of more severe disease. Usually, acute pancreatitis is managed nonoperatively, with fluid resuscitation, bowel rest, antibiotic administration, nutritional changes, and other supportive therapies. Radiologic drainage of infected intraabdominal fluid collections may be required. The patient for whom surgical intervention is deemed necessary is the rarity in whom other methods of treatment have failed, predicting a more complicated case with higher risk for morbidity and mortality. Although no specific predictors of perioperative risk have been identified for the patient with acute pancreatitis, the traditional Ranson's criteria (Table 9-5) have been used extensively in evaluating medical patients to describe mortality from the disease. Patients meeting fewer than three of Ranson's criteria after 48 hours have a more benign disease course, whereas those with three or more risk factors have a significantly increased mortality, on the order of 20% to 30%.

The perioperative risk of patients with **chronic pancreatitis** is unknown, but with a standard, careful preoperative evaluation and appropriate anesthetic technique, many patients have undergone successful surgical procedures without negative outcome.

After **orthotopic liver transplantation,** patients may present to the operating room for a myriad of interventions with a variety of attendant risks. The perioperative risk of the patient is generally related to the surgical disease itself plus the underlying function of

Table 9-5. Ranson's criteria for severity of acute pancreatitis

On admission
  Age >55 yr
  Serum glucose >200 mg/dL
  WBC >16,000/mm^3
  LDH >350 IU/L
  AST >250 IU/L
Within 48 hours
  Serum calcium <8 mg/dL
  PaO$_2$ <60 mm Hg
  Base deficit >4 mEq/L
  BUN increase >5 mg/dL
  Hematocrit fall >10%
  Fluid sequestration >6 L

AST, aspartate aminotransferase; BUN, blood urea nitrogen; LDH, lactate dehydrogenase; PaO$_2$, arterial partial pressure of oxygen; WBC, white blood cell count.

the transplanted liver. Complications of immunosuppressive therapy, as detailed in Table 9-1, may increase the perioperative risk of the patient who has undergone liver transplantation.

MEDICATIONS

In general, patients with hepatobiliary disease presenting for surgery should be maintained on their usual medical regimen. Individual assessment of each patient and the nature of the procedure, however, may result in minor alterations in the patient's medications.

Injected interferon-α is used in the treatment of chronic hepatitis B and hepatitis C. Therapy should be continued in the perioperative period, but the anesthesiologist should be familiar with the drug's side effects, including flulike symptoms, fatigue, myalgias, nausea, and bone marrow suppression resulting in leukopenia and thrombocytopenia. Rarely, interferon use may cause hypothyroidism. If symptoms or signs of hypothyroidism are present, thyroid-stimulating hormone level should be measured (see Chapter 6). Patients with chronic hepatitis C may be taking combination therapy with interferon-α and ribavirin, a nucleoside analog that may cause hemolytic anemia, cough, pruritus, and rash.

Patients with cirrhosis frequently require many medications, including diuretics to treat ascites, laxatives to control encephalopathy, β-blockers to diminish risk of variceal bleeding, and vitamin K to normalize a prolonged PT. Most medications should be continued before and after surgery, although modifications may be made (e.g., diuretics may be held the day of surgery) for the patient undergoing major surgery with the potential for large volume shifts or intraoperative hemorrhage.

For the patient receiving immunosuppressant therapy after a hepatic transplant, continuing immunosuppression postoperatively is of paramount importance. Administration of medications via a nasogastric tube should be considered for the patient who is unable to swallow oral medications. Patients who are taking corticosteroids should be considered for "stress-dose" steroid coverage when undergoing any but minor surgery (see Chapter 15).

PERIOPERATIVE CARE

A rapid-sequence induction must be considered for most patients with hepatobiliary disease who are to undergo general anesthesia. This usually includes patients with acute cholecystitis or pancreatitis. Similarly, the patient with advanced cirrhotic liver disease may be at risk for aspiration due to ascites and diminished gastrointestinal motility. These patients should be premedicated with agents to reduce gastric volume and acidity. Typically, a histamine$_2$ antagonist, sodium bicitrate, and a promotility agent (metoclopramide or cisapride) in the unobstructed patient should be prescribed preoperatively.

Hematologic and nutritional issues should be carefully evaluated preoperatively in the patient with hepatobiliary disease. Because many of these patients are coagulopathic and anemic, correction of aberrant hematologic values should be attempted, especially if the planned procedure carries a significant risk of bleeding. PT prolongation may be the result of impaired hepatic synthesis of clotting factors or insufficiency of vitamin K because of poor dietary intake, impaired intestinal absorption, or antibiotic treatment. Because patients with hepatobiliary disease may have vitamin K deficiency, a preoperative trial of vitamin K therapy is worthwhile. The prolonged PT, if caused by vitamin K insufficiency, should correct within 24 to 48 hours after parenteral injections of vitamin K (10 mg subcutaneously once a day). Poor nutritional status contributes to altered protein binding of anesthetic agents, transudation of fluids to extravascular spaces due to low oncotic pressure, poor wound healing, and overall increased morbidity. Thus, nutritional supplementation should be considered (see Chapter 16).

Central venous access may be required for large-bore intravenous cannulation, measurement of central venous pressures, or administration of vasoactive drugs. Arterial line placement must be considered in the patient with hepatic dysfunction for purposes of blood sampling and blood pressure monitoring. Finally, pulmonary artery catheter (PAC) monitoring may be appropriate in the patient with severe hepatic dysfunction because the pathophysiology often mimics a septic state, with a hyperdynamic cardiac output and systemic hypotension due to low vascular tone. A PAC may be useful to determine the cause of hypotension and guide appropriate volume replacement and inotropic or vasopressor support. In addition, a PAC may be useful in managing the severely ill patient with acute cholecystitis or acute pancreatitis, who may be septic and at risk for respiratory or renal failure. Transesophageal echocardiography might be an alternative monitoring modality in patients with severe hepatobiliary disease, but its use is usually contraindicated in the presence of a coagulopathy or esophageal varices. Any patient with hepatobiliary disease who merits intraoperative invasive monitoring deserves consideration for postoperative care in an intensive care unit

(ICU). In an ICU, the patient can be closely monitored and treated for hypovolemia due to perioperative volume shifts, bleeding, coagulopathy, respiratory failure, and renal failure due to sepsis or the hepatorenal syndrome.

Nasogastric or orogastric tube placement must be approached cautiously in cirrhotic patients who are at risk for bleeding from esophageal varices. If tube placement is necessary for gastric decompression or administration of medications, however, the tube should be used because clinical studies of anesthetized patients at risk for variceal bleeding have not shown an increased incidence of this complication after tube placement.

Regional anesthesia may be contraindicated in many patients with hepatobiliary disease due to coagulopathies with an increased risk of bleeding or hematoma formation. However, patients whose condition has been well compensated (e.g., some patients with chronic hepatitis) may be appropriate candidates for a regional anesthetic technique if laboratory values are in an acceptable range.

The primary physiologic goal is to maintain appropriate intraoperative hepatic perfusion via support of cardiac output, blood volume, blood pressure, oxygenation, and ventilation. Avoidance of hypotension, hypoxia, and hypocarbia, all of which may produce an ischemic insult to the liver, is important.

Specific anesthetic agents are chosen based on the goals outlined above and on the pharmacokinetic and pharmacodynamic properties of the drugs. Benzodiazepines may be used for preoperative sedation, but should be used cautiously for two reasons: (a) many (e.g., midazolam hydrochloride) are highly protein bound and thus present in a higher free fraction in the hypoalbuminemic patient, and (b) circulating endogenous agonists to the γ-aminobutyric acid receptor are found in encephalopathic patients with cirrhotic liver disease, which makes these patients more sensitive to the effects of benzodiazepines. In addition, benzodiazepines that undergo oxidative metabolism (e.g., diazepam, midazolam hydrochloride) have prolonged action in patients with liver insufficiency. Opiates should be used cautiously in the patient with hepatic dysfunction due to possible prolonged effects. Fentanyl and sufentanil citrate do not demonstrate altered pharmacokinetics in cirrhotic patients when administered in single doses, but alfentanil hydrochloride, meperidine hydrochloride and, to a lesser extent, morphine clearances are reduced in these patients. Remifentanil hydrochloride has not been shown to accumulate in patients with severe hepatic failure, even after lengthy infusions. Opiates occasionally cause spasm of the sphincter of Oddi, which may be problematic in the patient with biliary obstruction. If spasm occurs, it may be reversed with naloxone hydrochloride or glucagon or, less successfully, with atropine sulfate or nitroglycerin. Titration to effect should be the guiding principle with use of benzodiazepines or opiates in patients with hepatic disease.

Of the volatile anesthetics, isoflurane and sevoflurane are probably most appropriate for the patient with hepatic dysfunction. These agents carry the lowest risk of impairing hepatic blood flow or resulting in abnormal perioperative liver function tests based on laboratory and clinical studies. Clearly, halothane should be avoided in patients with hepatic disease because of its deleterious effects on liver perfusion. In addition, as with any patient, the rare but real risk of halothane hepatitis should be considered. Nitrous oxide use is somewhat controversial because some animal studies have demonstrated modestly diminished portal and hepatic blood flow with this anesthetic. The potential for nitrous oxide–induced intestinal distention in long surgical procedures is cited as a reason to avoid its use in patients with severe hepatic dysfunction. Nitrous oxide has been widely and successfully used in patients with hepatic disease, however, without demonstrable ill effect.

Choice of muscle relaxants in patients with hepatobiliary disease should be based on mechanisms of metabolism and clearance. Those drugs dependent on hepatic metabolism or clearance (e.g., vecuronium bromide, rocuronium bromide) are best avoided because of the possibility of prolonged effects. Atracurium besylate and cisatracurium besylate, which are degraded independent of the liver, are safe choices.

Intraoperative laboratory monitoring should be carefully considered, particularly during procedures that are lengthy or complicated by blood loss. Values that should be checked include glucose, calcium, hematocrit, PT, PTT, platelet count, fibrinogen, and D-dimer if disseminated intravascular coagulation is suspected.

Temperature monitoring and active warming measures (e.g., use of heated intravenous fluids, forced warmed air blankets) are extremely important in the patient with hepatic disease because hypothermia impairs coagulation.

This chapter has reviewed the importance of hepatobiliary disease to perioperative management, including the implications of hepatitis, cirrhosis, cholelithiasis, pancreatitis, and prior hepatic transplantation. History and physical examination are the most important elements for diagnosing the presence of hepatobiliary disease. These, in concert with the appropriate diagnostic tests, can usually guide the clinician to an accurate estimation of operative risk and to a plan for a safe, effective anesthetic. The anesthesiologist must appreciate the vast implications of hepatobiliary disease, including common alterations to the hematologic, neurologic, cardiovascular, pulmonary, and renal systems.

CASE STUDY

A 35-year-old man presents for anesthetic evaluation for an elective inguinal herniorrhaphy. The patient states that during the past 2 weeks he has felt very tired and had a slight fever, sore throat, cough, nausea, and dark urine. The patient is still fatigued but is feeling better. Further questioning reveals that the patient returned from a vacation 6 weeks earlier. During his trip, he ate shellfish and was exposed to poor sanitation. He complains of anorexia and has lost 3 pounds. His fluid intake has increased, and the urine color became normal over the last 24 hours. He has had some discomfort in his epigastric area, which he attributes to changes in his eating habits. The review of the cardiovascular system is negative. The patient does not smoke and occasionally drinks alcohol. Current medications are a multivitamin and acetaminophen for his fever. He denies allergies or family history of problems with anesthetics.

Physical examination reveals a man who appears acutely ill. His blood pressure is 105/60 mm Hg, heart rate is 108 beats per minute, and temperature is 37.8°C. He is pale and icteric, and has dry oral mucosa and ecchymoses on his lower extremities. His liver is palpable 5 cm below the right costal margin, is tender, and spans 16 cm. A large and reducible right inguinal hernia is present. Cardiac, pulmonary, and neurologic examinations are normal.

The patient has signs and symptoms of an acute viral illness, which is most likely hepatitis A. The history is quite typical. The patient vacationed in places with poor sanitation and ingested shellfish. After a 20- to 35-day incubation period, the patient developed prodromal symptoms (fatigue, fever, sore throat, nausea) of acute viral hepatitis and recently became clinically jaundiced. Although the history in this case is very suggestive of hepatitis A, confirming the cause of the patient's illness is important. A hepatitis screen (HB$_s$Ag, anti-HBs, anti-HCV) and measurement of IgM anti-HAV are indicated. However, hepatitis C antibody may not become measurable for 4 to 6 months. Levels of electrolytes, BUN, creatinine, AST, ALT, alkaline phosphatase, and bilirubin need to be checked and a complete blood cell count and PT measured.

Anesthesia and surgery in the setting of acute viral hepatitis are associated with significant morbidity and mortality. Therefore, any elective surgery should be postponed until at least 4 weeks after complete clinical recovery and normalization of ALT, AST, and bilirubin levels. In the case of emergent and urgent surgery, the benefits of the procedure must be weighed against the risks associated with the potential complications of anesthesia and surgery in the setting of acute viral hepatitis. In such cases, discussions among the patient and surgical and anesthesia teams are of utmost importance in planning care to optimize outcome and avoid hepatic decompensation.

In the present case, the patient was informed of the clinical diagnosis of hepatitis and told to follow up with his primary care physician. He was instructed to have his surgery rescheduled for no earlier than 12 weeks later. At that time, all signs and symptoms described above had resolved, and transaminase levels, bilirubin level, and PT were within normal limits. Given the complete clinical and laboratory resolution of his acute disease, the options of local, regional, and general anesthesia were discussed, and the patient opted to have an inguinal nerve block. The risks of transmission of hepatitis A to health care providers in this case is practically nil given that a hepatitis A carrier state and progression to chronic disease do not occur.

BIBLIOGRAPHY

Aranha GV, Greenlee HB. Intra-abdominal surgery in patients with advanced cirrhosis. *Arch Surg* 1986;121:275–277.

Bito H, Ikeda K. Renal and hepatic function in surgical patients after low-flow sevoflurane or isoflurane anesthesia. *Anesth Analg* 1996; 82:173–176.

Child CG. Surgery and portal hypertension. In: Child CG, ed. *The liver and portal hypertension*. Philadelphia: WB Saunders, 1964:1–85.

Dershwitz M, Hoke JF, Rosow CE, et al. Pharmacokinetics and pharmacodynamics of remifentanil in volunteer subjects with severe liver disease. *Anesthesiology* 1996;84:812–820.

Fried MW. Therapy of chronic viral hepatitis. *Med Clin North Am* 1996;80:957–971.

Friedman LS, Maddrey WC. Surgery in the patient with liver disease. *Med Clin North Am* 1987;71:453–476.

Gelman S. General anesthesia and hepatic circulation. *Can J Physiol Pharmacol* 1987;65:1762–1779.

Gholson CF, Provenza JM, Bacon BR. Hepatologic considerations in patients with parenchymal liver disease undergoing surgery. *Am J Gastroenterol* 1990;85:487–496.

Isselbacher KJ, Podolsky DK, Dienstag JL, et al. Approach to the patient with liver disease: liver and biliary tract disease. In: Fauci AS, Braunwald E, Isselbacher KS, et al., eds. *Harrison's principles of internal medicine*, vol 2, 14th ed. New York: McGraw-Hill, 1998:1660–1751.

Mammen EF. Coagulation abnormalities in liver disease. *Hematol Oncol Clin North Am* 1992;6:1247–1257.

Moseley RH. Evaluation of abnormal liver function tests. *Med Clin North Am* 1996;80:887–907.

Runyon BA. Surgical procedures are well tolerated by patients with asymptomatic chronic hepatitis. *J Clin Gastroenterol* 1986;8:542–544.

Sjögren MH. Serologic diagnosis of viral hepatitis. *Med Clin North Am* 1996;80:929–955.

Musculoskeletal and Autoimmune Diseases

Jane Ballantyne

This chapter reviews a group of common musculoskeletal diseases that are autoimmune in origin and whose most obvious features are their joint and skin involvement. This group comprises **rheumatoid arthritis, ankylosing spondylitis, systemic lupus erythematosus**, and **scleroderma**. Other less common autoimmune connective tissue diseases (including **polyarteritis nodosa, dermatomyositis, polymyositis, polymyalgia rheumatica,** and **mixed connective tissue diseases**) are not reviewed here, but the principles of this chapter apply to all connective tissue diseases. **Osteoarthritis**, although not an autoimmune disorder, is the most common and ubiquitous of the musculoskeletal diseases and is included here for comparison. **Kyphoscoliosis**, a possible manifestation of the musculoskeletal diseases, has important anesthetic implications and is considered as a separate entity.

The autoimmune group of diseases are non–organ specific, connective tissue disorders with lesions affecting joints, skin, glomeruli, serous membranes, and blood vessels. They are systemic diseases with a wide range of clinical manifestations. Osteoarthritis, on the other hand, is a degenerative disease affecting only the joints and is not a systemic disease. Treatment of the musculoskeletal and autoimmune diseases is largely palliative and aimed at suppressing the inflammatory or immunologic process to improve symptoms and prevent progressive damage. In osteoarthritis, nonsteroidal antiinflammatory drugs (NSAIDs) are the mainstay of drug treatment. In the autoimmune group, specific immunosuppressant and antirheumatic drugs often are added (Table 10-1). Significant toxicity is associated with all the drugs used in the treatment of these musculoskeletal diseases, and drug toxicity is an important consideration when evaluating patients with these diseases (Table 10-2).

The following is a description of the clinical characteristics of the musculoskeletal diseases that occur commonly and are of particular significance to anesthesiologists. Although each of the diseases in the autoimmune group tends to display certain characteristics, the individual patient may exhibit any of the features of connective tissue disorders. Thus, the clinical features of these diseases may overlap. Tables 10-3 and 10-4 summarize the disease characteristics.

Table 10-1. Common treatment modes for musculoskeletal and autoimmune diseases

Treatment	Rheumatoid arthritis	Osteoarthritis	Ankylosing spondylitis	Systemic lupus erythematosus	Scleroderma
Physical therapy	X	X	X	X	X
NSAIDs	X	X	X		X
Immunosuppressants (commonly methotrexate sodium)	X				
DMARDs [commonly hydroxychloroquine sulfate (Plaquenil)]	X			X	
Steroids	X			X	
Surgery	X	X	X		

DMARDs, disease-modifying antirheumatoid drugs; NSAIDs, nonsteroidal antiinflammatory drugs.

Table 10-2. Side effects of drugs used to treat musculoskeletal and autoimmune diseases

Drug category	Drug	Side effects
Antiinflammatory drugs	Aspirin/NSAIDs	Gastric erosion
		Gastrointestinal hemorrhage
		Platelet dysfunction
		Renal dysfunction
Immunosuppressants	Methotrexate sodium/ azathioprine	Myelosuppression
		Mucositis
		Hepatotoxicity
		Pneumonitis (rare, only with methotrexate)
DMARDs	Gold	Proteinuria and nephrotic syndrome
		Myelosuppression
		Skin rashes
	Phenacetin/ penicillamine	Nephropathy
	Chloroquine/ hydroxychloroquine sulfate (Plaquenil)	Cataracts
		Retinopathy
		Photosensitivity
Steroids	Prednisone	Depression of stress response
		Depression of response to infection
		Glucose intolerance
		Gastrointestinal hemorrhage
		Hypertension
		Hypokalemic alkalosis
		Proximal myopathy
		Cataracts

DMARDs, disease-modifying antirheumatoid drugs; NSAIDs, nonsteroidal antiinflammatory drugs.

Table 10-3. Summary of characteristics of musculoskeletal and autoimmune diseases

	Rheumatoid arthritis	Osteoarthritis	Ankylosing spondylitis	Systemic lupus erythematosus	Scleroderma
Disease description	Chronic inflammatory disease of unknown etiology characterized by symmetric polyarthropathy and significant systemic involvement	Degenerative process affecting articular cartilage; minimal inflammatory reaction	Back pain characterized by morning stiffness that improves with exercise	Multisystem chronic inflammatory disease characterized by antinuclear antibody production	Disease characterized by inflammation, vascular sclerosis, and fibrosis of the skin and viscera
Pain	Morning stiffness, resolves slowly	Pain on movement, improves with rest	Morning stiffness, relieved by exercise	Not characteristic	Not characteristic
Markers	Proximal phalangeal involvement and swelling; ulnar deviation	Heberden's nodes on distal interphalangeal joints	Radiographic evidence of sacroiliitis, kyphosis	Malar (butterfly) rash	Contractures (especially of the fingers), mask-like face
Family history	Rare		Common		
Gender/age	Women, 30–50 yr	Men and women, elderly	Men, 20–30 yr	Women, 20–40 yr	Women, 30–50 yr
Joint involvement	Symmetric polyarthropathy	Monoarthropathy or asymmetric polyarthropathy	Asymmetric oligoarthropathy	Symmetric polyarthropathy (hands, wrists, elbows, knees, ankles) (90%); avascular necrosis (rare)	Mild inflammatory arthritis possible
Rheumatoid factor	Positive/negative	Negative	Negative	Positive/negative	Positive/negative
Antinuclear factor	Positive/negative	Negative	Negative	Positive	Positive
HLA-B27	Negative	Negative	Positive	Negative	Negative

Table 10-4. Summary of characteristic systemic involvement in musculoskeletal and autoimmune diseases

	Rheumatoid arthritis	Osteoarthritis	Ankylosing spondylitis	Systemic lupus erythematosus	Scleroderma
Cardiovascular	Pericardial effusion, aortic regurgitation, conduction abnormalities, valvular fibrosis; coronary arteritis, Raynaud's phenomenon in some	None associated	Cardiomegaly, aortic regurgitation, conduction abnormalities	Pericarditis, myocarditis, conduction abnormalities, tachycardia and CHF may develop; Libman-Sacks endocarditis (involving aortic and mitral valves), Raynaud's phenomenon in some	HTN due to intimal fibrosis of arterial walls; systemic and pulmonary HTN; pulmonary HTN due to pulmonary fibrosis; vessel wall changes; sclerosis of coronary arteries and conduction system; pericarditis and pericardial effusion; oral or nasal telangiectasia
Pulmonary	Pulmonary fibrosis, pleural effusion	None associated	Pulmonary fibrosis	Lupus pneumonia, pulmonary infiltrates, restrictive disease, pleural effusion, dry cough, dyspnea, hypoxia	Diffuse interstitial pulmonary fibrosis; reduced pulmonary compliance; decreased diffusion capacity (major cause of morbidity and mortality)
Renal	Rarely involved	None associated	None associated	Glomerulonephritis with proteinuria and resultant hypoalbuminemia; hematuria; frequent oliguric renal failure	Impaired renal perfusion and renal HTN

continued

Table 10-4. *Continued*

	Rheumatoid arthritis	Osteoarthritis	Ankylosing spondylitis	Systemic lupus erythematosus	Scleroderma
Liver	None associated	None associated	None associated	Abnormal LFTs common; lupoid hepatitis can develop (recurrent jaundice, hepatomegaly, hyperglobulinemia)	—
Neuro-muscular	Atlanto-occipital instability, peripheral neuropathy, mononeuritis multiplex, entrapment neuropathies	Entrapment neuropathies	None associated	Proximal myopathy; elevated creatine kinase	Proximal myopathy; elevated creatine kinase
Skin	None associated	None associated	None associated	Nasal malar erythematous rash (butterfly rash), alopecia	Initial thickening and edema; tightening as sclerosis progresses
Ocular	Keratoconjunctivitis (Sjögren's syndrome)	None associated	Conjunctivitis, uveitis	—	—
Other	Normochromic, normocytic anemia	—	Ulcerative colitis	Coagulopathy	Xerostomia, hypomotility, dysphagia, malabsorption (vitamin K deficiency, coagulopathy)

CHF, congestive heart failure; HTN, hypertension; LFTs, liver function tests; Libman-Sacks endocarditis, nonbacterial endocarditis associated with systemic lupus erythematosus.

CLINICAL CHARACTERISTICS

Rheumatoid Arthritis

Rheumatoid arthritis (RA) is a chronic inflammatory disease of unknown etiology characterized by symmetric polyarthropathy, significant systemic involvement, and general ill health. It occurs predominantly in women (in a ratio of 3:1) during middle age (30 to 50 years). Normally the onset is insidious, but it may be acute or chronic relapsing. The small joints of the hands and feet are most commonly involved, but large synovial joints (hips, knees, elbows) are frequently affected. Ulnar deviation and proximal phalangeal involvement with fusiform swelling are markers of the disease. Morning stiffness that resolves slowly over the course of the day is characteristic of the active disease. The joint disease may be severe and extremely disabling.

Of particular importance to anesthesiologists is the prevalence of atlanto-occipital instability, which has the potential to cause acute or chronic cord compression and death. Radiologically demonstrable instability is present in as many as 25% of patients with RA, although few patients have symptoms (7%), and death during normal activity is almost unheard of. The instability is due to laxity of the atlantoaxial joint ligaments, usually with erosion of the odontoid peg. The presence of an intact odontoid peg increases risk of cord compression. Subluxation can occur with neck flexion during endotracheal intubation, even in asymptomatic patients, and can result in significant spinal cord or vertebral artery damage, or even death.[1,2] Endotracheal intubation is also difficult because of limited neck mobility, limited mouth opening (temporomandibular joint involvement), and fixation of the vocal cords (cricoarytenoid involvement). Although cricoarytenoid joint involvement is rare and usually associated only with severe disease, it may produce vocal cord fixation and limit the size of the laryngeal inlet.

Generalized manifestations of RA are fatigue, general malaise, occasional fever and chills, and chronic anemia. Clinically significant organ involvement is rare but can occur and should be sought. Pericardial effusion is the most common cardiac manifestation, but aortic insufficiency, conduction abnormalities, valvular fibrosis, or coronary arteritis may occur. As many as 50% of patients have abnormal pulmonary function (restrictive disease) due to the joint disease, but the restriction is rarely clinically significant, and lung involvement per se is extremely rare. Rheumatoid nodules, pulmonary fibrosis (diffuse fibronodular infiltration), and pleural effusions occur occasionally.[3] Secondary amyloidosis may affect the kidneys and liver, but otherwise renal or hepatic involvement is unlikely. The skin is not affected, but Sjögren's syndrome (a syndrome of reduced lachrymal and salivary secretions associated with RA and other non–organ specific autoimmune diseases) may cause dryness of the mucus membranes and keratoconjunctivitis.

Osteoarthritis

Osteoarthritis is a common degenerative disorder of the articular cartilage that is related to age, obesity, genetic predisposition, and previous joint injury. On radiograph, the disease is universal after the age of 55 years. Characteristically, the joint involvement is asymmetric and involves the hands, cervical and lumbar spine, knees, and hips. Fibrous nodules (Heberden's nodes) on the distal interphalangeal joints are markers of the disease. Joint pain worsens on movement and throughout the day, and improves with rest. Joint stiffness responds to gentle exercise over the course of 10 to 15 minutes. The inflammatory reaction and pain tend to fluctuate throughout the course of the disease.

Ankylosing Spondylitis

Ankylosing spondylitis is a disease mainly of young adult men (20 to 30 years) and has a 6% familial incidence. The sacroiliac joints are invariably affected, causing low back pain and morning stiffness that improves with exercise. The disease may also involve the spine, initially in the lumbosacral region, progressing to the thoracic and cervical spine. When the spine is involved, the ribs fuse to the vertebral bodies. Other joints may be involved, particularly the hips, knees, and ankles. The arthropathy differs from that of RA in that it is asymmetrical and affects large joints more than small joints. In severe cases, bony ankylosis develops and the intervertebral ligaments calcify and later ossify; the result is a rigid "bamboo" spine that lacks the normal lumbosacral curvature. Excessive manipulation of the ankylotic cervical spine during endotracheal intubation can result in spinal cord trauma. Many mild cases never present to a physician. In the majority (70% to 80%) of those cases that do present, patients maintain normal or near normal activity with minimal deformity, provided they receive appropriate treatment. In a small number of severe cases, rigidity of the spine and kyphosis develop rapidly, over 3 to 5 years. More commonly, the disease progresses slowly; it may remit at any stage or be relapsing and remitting.[4]

The disease may result in general ill health. Involvement of the eyes (uveitis and conjunctivitis) is common (25% to 40% of cases). Ulcerative colitis is more common in patients with ankylosing spondylitis than in the general population, and vice versa. Rarely, aortitis is present, with resultant aortic insufficiency. In severe disease, some degree of respiratory failure is inevitable because of the combined fixed rib cage and kyphosis; the severity depends on the amount of deformity and ankylosis. Pulmonary fibrosis (fibrosing alveolitis) may occur, and its presence worsens the respiratory failure.

Systemic Lupus Erythematosus

Systemic lupus erythematosus (SLE) is a multisystem chronic inflammatory disease characterized by antinuclear antibody production. The disease usually is manifested in young women 20 to 40 years of age (90% of cases). The most common presentation consists of fever, arthralgia, general malaise, and weight loss. The onset of the disease may be induced by drugs (hydralazine hydrochloride, procainamide hydrochloride, isoniazid, penicillamine, methyldopa, anticonvulsants). The characteristic facial rash—the "butterfly" rash across the nose and upper cheeks—is a marker of the disease but is not always present. Joint and skin involvement occurs in most patients (80% to 90%), but involvement of other systems (kidneys, lungs, cardiovascular system) is also common. Typically, episodic relapses and remissions occur that last months to years, but life expectancy is normal or near normal. Significant renal or cerebral involvement decreases survival. Pregnancy, surgery, infection, and other stressors may exacerbate the disease.

The arthralgia is a migratory, usually symmetrical polyarthralgia, not unlike that in RA, but is very rarely deforming. The small joints of the hands are affected, as well as elbows, shoulders, knees, and ankles. The most common skin features are nonspecific erythema, photosensitivity, alopecia, and malar (butterfly) rash. Other features include blocked follicles, telangiectasia, nail fold infarcts, oral and nasal mucosal ulceration, and Raynaud's phenomenon (intermittent, cold-precipitated attacks of vasospasm, pallor, or cyanosis of the digits, without evidence of arterial occlusive disease). Some form of laryngeal involvement (mucosal ulceration, cricoarytenoid arthritis, laryngeal nerve palsy) is relatively common (30%).

Renal involvement is common (60%) and associated with a poor prognosis. The glomeruli are damaged by antigen-antibody complexes, which results in glomerulonephritis. The presentation is usually of nephrotic syndrome (see Chapter 8), although less commonly asymptomatic proteinuria, oliguric renal failure with hypertension, or an acute nephritic syndrome is seen. Hematuria may be present. Circulating anticoagulants may increase prothrombin time (PT) and partial thromboplastin time (PTT) (see Chapter 7). Lung involvement (occurring in approximately 50% of cases) can result in pleurisy with effusions, intrapulmonary disease due to patchy consolidation and collapse, pulmonary infiltrates, or lupus pneumonitis. Dry cough, dyspnea, and hypoxia are common. Cardiac involvement occurs in approximately 40% of patients. Pericarditis is the most common cardiac manifestation, and sometimes the first indication of SLE. Myocarditis with conduction abnormalities, a persistent tachycardia, and gradual development of congestive cardiac failure may occur. Libman-Sacks endocarditis (a nonbacterial endocarditis associated with SLE) involves the aortic and mitral valves. The nervous system is damaged by arteritis and ischemia. This may result in cranial or peripheral nerve lesions. A peripheral sensory neuropathy is the most common neurologic complication. Central nervous system involvement—resulting in phobias, confusion, depression and, rarely, epilepsy—is associated with a poor prognosis. Generalized lymphadenopathy, with or without hepatosplenomegaly, may be noted. Anemia and leukopenia may occur. Thrombocytopenia with purpura is relatively common (30%).

Scleroderma

Scleroderma is a disease affecting primarily middle-aged women, characterized by inflammation, vascular sclerosis, and fibrosis of the skin and viscera. The disease presents with lassitude, fever, and weight loss. Although initially edematous, the skin becomes smooth, waxy, and tight, especially over the hands, ankles, and face, so that the patient with advanced disease has a characteristic masklike face with contracted, immobile fingers. The sclerosis of the skin of the face and neck may limit mouth opening and neck extension. Raynaud's phenomenon and telangiectasia are common. The sicca syndrome (reduced lachrymal and salivary secretions) develops in 5%. Involvement of the viscera most frequently affects the gastrointestinal tract, especially the esophagus. Dysphagia is common (65%). Rarely, hypomotility of the entire gastrointestinal tract occurs, with dilatation, malabsorption, and steatorrhea. Relaxation of the lower esophageal sphincter may cause reflux. The disease is slowly progressive, with death usually the result of renal, heart, or lung complications.

Involvement of other systems is less common, tends to occur late in the disease, and is often the harbinger of death. Progressive renal failure, with or without hypertension, results from impaired renal perfusion, usually occurs late in the disease, and is often fatal. Pericardial effusion, cardiomyopathy, and heart failure are rare but usually fatal. Diffuse interstitial pulmonary fibrosis progresses to respiratory failure and is a major cause of morbidity and mortality.

Kyphoscoliosis

Kyphoscoliosis is a deformity of the vertebral column with anterior flexion (kyphosis) and lateral curvature (scoliosis) of the spine. The ribs are deformed secondarily. Eighty percent of cases are idiopathic, commencing late in childhood with rapid progression during periods of rapid skeletal growth. Treatment is aimed at early surgical correction. Diseases of the neuromuscular system, including muscular dystrophy, cerebral palsy, ankylosing spondylitis, and poliomyelitis, may cause kyphoscoliosis. A curvature of 40% or greater is considered severe. A severe kyphosis may make airway management and endotracheal intubation extremely difficult.

Morbidity is associated with the inevitable pulmonary and subsequent cardiac dysfunction.[5] As the curvature worsens, the lungs become compressed, which results in restrictive incapacity. The abnormal mechanical function of the rib cage further increases the work of breathing, which hastens the development of respiratory failure. A poor cough results in frequent pulmonary infections. Later, pulmonary hypertension develops because of the compression and hypoxia, and progresses to right heart failure and death.

HISTORY

Although the most obvious features of this group of diseases are their joint and skin manifestations, the diseases (except osteoarthritis) are systemic and thus necessitate a thorough evaluation of each system. Guidelines for the assessment of the major organ systems are found in the appropriate chapters of this book. This chapter concentrates on the clinical features of the named diseases that are specific to these diseases. Key factors in the histories of these patients in general are lifestyle, the degree of disability, and exercise tolerance. Drug history is vitally important because all of the drugs used to treat these diseases have potentially serious side effects (see Tables 10-1 and 10-2), which may exacerbate or be the sole cause of some of the systemic manifestations of the diseases.[6] A history of how anesthesia and surgery were tolerated in the past is useful, particularly if intubation may be difficult.

Rheumatoid Arthritis

Every system must be carefully assessed. As a rule, the extraarticular manifestations of RA occur in individuals with high titers of rheumatoid factor, so that a finding of high titers may be a useful marker of systemic involvement. The joint disease, if it has resulted in severe deformity, has obvious implications for anesthesia, particularly in terms of neck mobility and airway management and positioning. Symptoms of nerve compression should be sought. If neck movements induce neurologic symptoms, this should be noted so that the positions that trigger symptoms can be avoided during anesthesia. Symptoms of atlanto-occipital instability (syncope, visual changes, neurologic deficits) should be sought. Symptoms of airway obstruction (dyspnea, stridor, hoarseness) should also be sought. Hoarseness may indicate either an acute cricoarytenoiditis or rigidity of the vocal cords due to chronic involvement of the cricoarytenoid joints. The degree of disability and functional impairment should be established because severe functional impairment may mask cardiac and other symptoms.

Osteoarthritis

No systemic involvement occurs in osteoarthritis, and a routine anesthesia preoperative history suffices. As with all disabling diseases, the degree of disability and functional impairment should be established because severe functional impairment may mask cardiac and other symptoms.

Ankylosing Spondylitis

Although the majority of cases (80% to 90%) are mild and result in minimal functional impairment, severe disease presents enormous problems to the anesthesiologist, chiefly related to the airway and lung function. Ankylosing spondylitis is a systemic disease, and a detailed assessment of the systems is mandatory. With reference to the airway, symptoms of airway obstruction (dyspnea, stridor) should be sought. Because the lung function of these patients is frequently impaired, the history taking should focus on determining the severity of any impairment and the possibilities for improving the present pulmonary status. Evidence of pulmonary infection (malaise, fever, chills, cough, pleuritic pain, dyspnea) should be actively sought.

Systemic Lupus Erythematosus

Surprisingly, although the clinical picture of SLE is one of multisystem organ failure, few anesthetic issues specific to SLE exist.

Although the arthropathy mimics that of RA, serious deformity is rare, so that the airway is not affected, and positioning is not particularly a problem. As with all diseases in this class, the history taking should be aimed at thoroughly assessing each system, with emphasis on functional status. The disease shows a range of severity, with patients at one end of the spectrum requiring little or no special attention and patients with severe disease presenting with a host of risk factors. The history should focus on the pulmonary status; the presence or absence of pulmonary infection; renal, hepatic, and cardiac function; and the coagulation status.

Scleroderma

Scleroderma affects primarily the skin and viscera. The skin changes of the face and neck may make endotracheal intubation difficult. Late and severe disease presents significant systemic problems—in particular, renal, cardiac, and respiratory failure. The history should assess each system carefully because they all can be involved. The patient should be asked whether difficulty is experienced in mouth opening and neck mobility, whether dysphagia is present and severe, and whether there is a history of regurgitation, with or without aspiration. A history of nose bleeds should be sought. Evidence of malabsorption (diarrhea, steatorrhea) or nutritional deficiency (weight loss) (see Chapter 16), and symptoms of Raynaud's phenomenon (intermittent cyanotic, cool digits) should be sought.

Kyphoscoliosis

The history should focus on establishing the degree of cardiopulmonary dysfunction. Dyspnea, tachypnea, bronchospasm, cough, fatigue, general malaise, and epigastric pain are common symptoms of worsening cardiopulmonary function. Evidence of pulmonary infection (dry or productive cough, fever, chills, pleuritic pain) should be actively sought.

PHYSICAL FINDINGS

Every patient should receive a systematic physical examination that looks for the markers of serious disease—weight loss; dry skin, eyes, and mucus membranes; skin changes; edema; and signs of pulmonary or cardiac failure. Many of these patients have some degree of pulmonary dysfunction, so that the respiratory system should be examined thoroughly, and signs of chest infection should be identified or excluded. An area of specific concern for these patients is their mobility, especially their neck mobility. If a patient is severely disabled, extra time is needed to test for mobility. The patient should be put through his or her full range of active movements. Note should be taken of whether movements are limited and whether any particular position induces pain or other neurologic symptoms so that the position can be avoided during anesthesia. The feasibility of regional anesthesia should be assessed in terms of whether the patient can be comfortably positioned for placement of the block. In cases of severe deformity, venous access may be limited; in such cases, the need for central access should be assessed. Skin changes, notably those in SLE and scleroderma, may preclude regional anesthesia and increase the difficulty of gaining venous access. When skin involvement is extensive, the skin over potential sites for regional anesthesia and venous access should be examined.

A thorough airway evaluation is warranted in all patients in this diagnostic group. These patients may have limited neck mobility, kyphoscoliosis, atlanto-occipital instability, a small laryngeal inlet, or limited mouth opening. The patient should be put through his or her full range of active neck movements, with note taken of whether any pain or limitation of movement occurs and whether any position induces neurologic symptoms. The presence of any hoarseness should be noted. The extent of mouth opening should be established, and the airway should be categorized according to the Mallampati classification (see Chapter 14). The presence or absence of telangiectasia should be noted in patients with SLE and scleroderma. The thyromental distance should be measured (a distance of less than 6 cm may contribute to difficulty of intubation).[7] Overall, an assessment should be made as to whether endotracheal intubation is likely to be safely accomplished using standard direct laryngoscopy, or whether a fiberoptic scope is needed.

DIAGNOSTIC TESTING

The reader is referred to Chapter 2 for age-specific and disease-specific guidelines for routine preoperative testing in healthy patients. Patients with musculoskeletal disease present with a wide range of systemic involvement, and the need for additional tests is a matter of clinical judgment based on consideration of the individual patient. Most patients with connective tissue disease (with the exception of those with mild disease and minimal systemic involvement), need a chest radiograph (CXR). Patients with RA should receive lateral radiographs of the neck in flexion and extension to identify or exclude atlanto-occipital instability. The separation of the odontoid process from the posterior margin of the anterior arch of the atlas should be less than 3 mm with the neck in flexion. PT and PTT should be measured in patients with SLE.

All patients with cardiac involvement by history or physical examination should have at least an electrocardiogram (ECG), CXR, complete blood cell count (CBC), and assessment of blood urea nitrogen (BUN) and creatinine, with a possibility of further tests (exercise or stress ECG, radionucleotide scan, or echocardiogram) as needed. Patients with severe disability may be unable to stress themselves to the point of angina or functional impairment and may have significant cardiac disease without symptoms. In these patients, the use of electrocardiography and cardiac imaging techniques in conjunction with pharmacologic stressors [e.g., dipyridamole (Persantine), dobutamine hydrochloride] may be the only way of detecting cardiac involvement or of obtaining a measure of its severity (see Chapter 3).

All patients with pulmonary involvement should have an ECG and CXR. Pulmonary function tests can be helpful when assessing the risks and advisability of positive-pressure ventilation in patients with serious pulmonary disease.[8] Measurement of blood gas levels on room air identifies patients with severe hypoxia and chronic, compensated hypercarbia and serves not only as an indication of the severity and chronicity of the disease but also as a guide to the ventilation parameters that should be chosen (see Chapter 5). The 1-second forced expiratory volume (FEV_1) and the peak flow provide a measure of the obstructive component of the disease and can be used to determine whether bronchodilator therapy improves the obstructive component. A measure of vital capacity is a useful guide to the severity of the restrictive component of the disease and to the feasibility of an early wean from ventilation. Extubation and weaning are usually delayed in patients whose vital capacity is 1 L or less, because these patients usually cannot sustain an adequate ventilatory effort during the immediate post-surgical recovery period. More sophisticated pulmonary function tests probably do not contribute to the anesthetic management of patients for nonpulmonary surgery[9] (see Chapter 5).

For all patients at risk of renal disease (notably patients with SLE and scleroderma, and patients taking steroids, gold, phenacetin, or penicillamine), levels of electrolytes, BUN, and creatinine should be measured. For all patients with general debilitation, malnutrition, or malabsorption (the latter being relatively common in patients with scleroderma), CBC, PT, PTT, and albumin level should be determined (see Chapter 16). Levels of electrolytes, BUN, creatinine, and glucose should be measured for patients on steroids, whereas levels of electrolytes, BUN, and creatinine, and CBC should be measured for patients on gold therapy. Patients undergoing prosthetic surgery need urinalysis to exclude urinary tract infection. Table 10-5 summarizes the recommended disease-specific tests.

Table 10-5. Preoperative testing guidelines: tests recommended in addition to routine age-specific and surgery-specific testing

Category	Recommended tests
Rheumatoid arthritis	CXR, lateral radiographs of the neck in flexion and extension
Osteoarthritis	None
Ankylosing spondylitis	CXR
Systemic lupus	CXR, PT, PTT
Scleroderma	CXR
Kyphoscoliosis	CXR
Cardiac involvement	ECG, CXR, CBC, BUN, creatinine
Pulmonary involvement	ECG, CXR, ABGs, vital capacity
Renal involvement	Electrolytes, BUN, creatinine
Debilitation, weight loss	CBC, PT, PTT, electrolytes
Steroid therapy	Electrolytes, BUN, creatinine, glucose
Gold therapy	Electrolytes, BUN, creatinine, CBC
Preprosthetic surgery	Urinalysis

ABGs, arterial blood gases; BUN, blood urea nitrogen; CBC, complete blood cell count; CXR, chest radiograph; ECG, electrocardiogram; PT, prothrombin time; PTT, partial thromboplastin time.

IMPLICATIONS OF DISEASE ON RISK AND RISK MODIFICATION

The impact of these diseases on perioperative risks and complications are related to the diseases, the drugs used to treat the diseases, and the surgery. A checklist of measures to modify risk is presented in Table 10-6.

Disease-Related Implications

As a group, these patients tolerate surgery better if their disease and the systemic components of their disease are optimally controlled preoperatively. For severely affected and incapacitated patients, factors such as maintenance of mobility, nutritional status, metabolic stability, prevention and treatment of infection, skin care, and optimization of drug therapy can all contribute to improved outcome after surgery. For patients with significant pulmonary involvement, the risk of postoperative pulmonary complications can be decreased by measures taken over several weeks preoperatively, including cessation of smoking for 8 weeks, bronchodilator therapy, measures to mobilize secretions, and treatment of sources of infection[10,11] (see Chapter 5).

Drug Considerations

The drugs used to treat the musculoskeletal diseases and their side effects are summarized in Tables 10-1 and 10-2. NSAIDs are used to treat pain and inflammation in these conditions, but despite their widespread use, they are not benign drugs. Of particular relevance during the perioperative period is their propensity to depress platelet function, which can result in postsurgical bleeding or hematoma formation. In the case of aspirin, this effect lasts for the lifespan of the platelets (7 to 10 days), and aspirin therapy is usually withheld for 7 to 10 days before surgery. In the case of other NSAIDs, the effect is reversed on discontinuation of the drug, and its duration therefore depends on the half-life of the drug. Whether nonsalicylate NSAIDs actually need to be withheld before surgery is unclear,[12] but most surgeons advise their patients to discontinue these drugs for at least 24 hours before surgery. Acetaminophen can be safely substituted but is less effective for pain management than the NSAIDs. Gastrointestinal hemorrhage and renal dysfunction are other relevant side effects of NSAIDs. The elderly are at particular risk of NSAID side effects.

The corticosteroids have a wide range of adverse effects that can influence surgical outcome. Patients on chronic steroid therapy need an increase in steroid dosage to cover the surgical period ("stress-dose" steroid therapy) (see Chapter 15). The additional steroids further increase the risk of steroid-related complications. Steroid-treated patients are likely to develop glucose intolerance, various metabolic derangements, hypertension, and gastrointestinal hemorrhage, factors that may be induced, or made worse, by the surgery itself. Steroid therapy can retard wound healing and increase infection risks. Patients with SLE are heavily dependent on steroids. The increasing popularity and success of more specific

Table 10-6. Preoperative preparation for patients with musculoskeletal and autoimmune diseases

Risk modification

General debilitation

Improve nutritional status

Achieve metabolic stability

Provide skin care

Treat infection

Maintain mobility

Optimize drug therapy

Aspirin and other NSAIDs

Stop aspirin 7–10 d and other NSAIDs 24–48 h before surgery

Steroids

Minimize use if possible

Anemia

Improve nutritional status

Give iron for iron deficiency

Give erythropoietin in renal failure

Blood transfusion

Have patient donate blood for autologous transfusion, 1 unit weekly until 7 d preoperatively, guided by hematocrit

Pulmonary involvement

Provide physical therapy

Treat infection

Use bronchodilators

Cardiac and other systems involvement

Optimize

Urinary tract infection

Identify and treat infection

Anesthesia preoperative visit

Ensure medical condition is optimal

Discuss following points:

Choice of anesthetic

Pain management options

Need for blood transfusion

Need for awake intubation

Need for postoperative ventilation and intensive care

Need for wake-up test

Provide medication, as needed

Regular medications

Anxiety-reducing drugs

Antacids

Bronchodilators

"Stress-dose" steroids

Psychological preparation

NSAIDs, nonsteroidal antiinflammatory drugs.

immunosuppressant therapy (notably methotrexate sodium) have resulted in less reliance on steroids, especially for patients with RA. Although these immunosuppressants are associated with toxicity in some patients (see Table 10-2), many patients are unaffected, and the reduction or obviation of steroid use has markedly improved patients' overall condition and perioperative risks, although their long-term outcome is not improved.[13-16] The risk of developing perioperative renal failure is increased by the use of NSAIDs, gold, phenacetin, and penicillamine.

Surgical Considerations

Patients with musculoskeletal disease present for the same surgeries as the general population. However, they present most frequently for joint and spine surgery. Because these surgeries are almost unique to this population, their risks are closely linked to the diseases themselves, and considering them here is appropriate. Prosthetic joint surgery is usually successful and results in a marked improvement in quality of life. Two issues, however, plague the long-term success of joint replacement therapy: infection and failure to mobilize. In general terms, optimizing the patient's physical and medical condition preoperatively improves recovery after joint surgery. More specifically, any infection should be actively treated before surgery, and surgery should be postponed if it is not under control. Patients should understand the importance of aggressive and often painful postoperative mobilization and be prepared for it mentally. Blood transfusion may be needed, especially during repeated procedures, which may be associated with large blood losses. The use of donated blood can be minimized by achieving reasonable preoperative hemoglobin levels (with iron in iron deficiency, erythropoietin in renal failure, and nutrition in general debilitation), by using preoperative blood donation and autologous transfusion[17] and by performing blood-salvaging procedures. Patients can donate autologous blood, usually at the rate of 1 unit every 7 days until 7 days before surgery, as guided by hemoglobin levels.

Corrective spine surgery (e.g., kyphoscoliosis correction) carries a high risk. A significant risk exists of spinal cord ischemia due to direct surgical trauma, stretching, impaired blood supply, and massive blood loss. Prolonged postoperative intensive care is likely to be needed because of the extensive nature of the surgery in patients who tend to be in poor condition preoperatively. As with prosthetic joint surgery, measures to increase preoperative hemoglobin levels and reduce the need for donated blood are helpful. Measures to improve general status and pulmonary function in particular (see Table 10-6) are also contributory.

PREOPERATIVE PREPARATION

Measures for reducing perioperative risk are discussed in the section Implications of Disease on Risk and Risk Modification (above) and tabulated in Table 10-6. The primary role of the anesthesiologist at the preoperative visit is to ensure that the patient is optimally prepared for surgery. Patients with mild disease and minimal deformity present few issues other than those related to their drug therapy, their surgery, their need for blood transfusion, their choice of anesthetic, and their pain-management options. On the other hand, patients with severe disease present with multiple issues, not only because of the systemic nature of their disease but also because the joint disease can involve the cervical or thoracic spine, the atlanto-occipital axis, or the larynx, so that the establishment of an artificial airway is potentially hazardous. Many patients with kyphoscoliosis and with the rheumatic diseases have poor ventilatory function, which not only increases the risk of hypoxia during protracted endotracheal intubation but may necessitate postoperative ventilation and intensive care. Some of these patients will need an awake intubation. Some will need to be awake after intubation so their positioning can be optimized before surgery or neurologic function can be tested during surgery (a wake-up test). Some will need to remain intubated postoperatively. The plan for airway management, intubation, and postoperative care should be discussed in detail with the patient. Patient cooperation is integral to safe airway management, and patients need explanations so that they understand what is likely to happen to them, how it can be made as comfortable as possible, and why their cooperation is important. Premedication should be prescribed as needed (see Table 10-6).

SPECIAL ANESTHETIC CONSIDERATIONS

Choice of Anesthetic

The choice of anesthetic is determined by patient preference, suitability of anesthetic choice for surgery, and feasibility. Particular issues for the severely affected of this group of patients are the hazards of endotracheal intubation and the deleterious effects of prolonged artificial ventilation in those with severe pulmonary disease. A good rule of thumb with regard to very sick patients is to choose the simplest reasonable anesthetic option. If surgery can be accomplished under a peripheral nerve block, this is often the best choice and avoids the need for intubation and ventilation, and the hazards of central neuraxial blockade anesthesia (vasodilation, fluid shifts, high block, emergent intubation). When peripheral nerve blockade is not an option, anesthetic delivered via a simple mask (or laryngeal mask airway) with a spontaneously breathing patient may be the best option, especially for a short procedure. Provided it is feasible in terms of positioning and the patient's general condition, regional anesthesia may be a good choice, especially for lower extremity procedures. Whether or not regional anesthesia should be used specifically to avoid intubation in cases in which a difficult intubation is likely remains controversial. Some anesthesiologists insist on establishing a secure artificial airway under controlled conditions in all these patients before surgery begins, so that no possibility exists of having to intubate under emergent conditions (e.g., high spinal, local anesthetic overdose or cardiac event). Others argue that, when the benefit of avoiding intubation and ventilation outweighs the risk of possibly having to establish an airway under uncontrolled conditions, regional anesthesia is the safest option and should be used provided the patient has an accessible and straightforward mask airway. Whether or not the benefit does exceed the risk obviously depends on the individual patient and is a matter of clinical judgment. The patient with very severe pulmonary dysfunction and respiratory failure is unlikely to cope with breathing spontaneously while immobilized and stressed by surgery. In this case, intubation with ventilation is probably the best option. Combined general and regional anesthesia may be helpful for minimizing general anesthetic requirements and providing intraoperative and postoperative analgesia. The literature contains very little convincing evidence that choice of anesthetic per se affects long-term postsurgical outcome, although evidence exists that extension of epidural anesthesia and analgesia (with local anesthetics) into the postoperative period may reduce the incidence of deep venous thrombosis and postoperative pulmonary embolus.[18] Another conflict with the use of regional anesthesia in orthopedic patients is the practice of using deep venous thrombosis prophylaxis in those undergoing lower extremity procedures, particularly joint replacements. In these patients, the risk of deep venous thrombosis and subsequent pulmonary embolus is high because of a combination of prolonged immobility during and after surgery, surgical manipulation of the femoral vein, and decreased venous blood flow. Therefore, deep venous thrombosis prophylaxis is used routinely. Epidural catheters may have to be removed early in patients who are started on prophylactic anticoagulation (within 48 hours of the first dose of warfarin sodium).[19,20] Spinal and epidural anesthesia should be completely avoided in patients who are taking (or are due to take) low-molecular-weight heparin with twice daily dosing (the routine dosing regime in the United States)[21,22] (see Chapter 7).

Intravenous Access

In the case of gross disability or extensive skin involvement, obtaining venous access may be difficult. Some procedures (including second hip replacement and corrective spinal surgery) are associated with massive blood loss, so that at least one large intravenous line will be needed. A central line or (rarely) a peripheral vein cutdown may be needed.

Steroid Coverage

Perioperative management and anesthetic considerations for patients taking corticosteroid therapy are discussed in Chapter 15.

Monitoring

Standard monitors (ECG, pulse oximeter, instruments for intermittent noninvasive measurement of blood pressure, capnograph, temperature probe, esophageal stethoscope, nerve stimulator) are used. Direct arterial pressure monitoring (via an arterial line) is useful when rapid blood pressure control is needed (e.g., for sick cardiac patients) and when massive blood loss is anticipated. Arterial lines are best avoided in patients with Raynaud's disease because of the theoretical risk of inducing vasospasm. The need for right or left heart monitoring is dictated by the nature of the surgery and the patient's cardiac status. Motor or somatosensory evoked potentials or motor nerve stimulation may be used as a measure of spinal cord and nerve root integrity during spinal surgery.

Intubation

If a difficult intubation is predicted, preparation of airway equipment is important. Appropriate help should be available (e.g., a surgeon and a second anesthesiologist). Sometimes, as in the case of extreme kyphosis, an elective tracheostomy must be performed.

Positioning

Because extreme deformity may preclude positioning in a standard position, and because in some patients the skin is susceptible to breakdown and ischemia, extra time is required for careful positioning and padding. Special care should be given to the eyes because of the likelihood of Sjögren's syndrome and keratoconjunctivitis.

Patient Warming

Maintenance of normal body temperature is particularly important in thin, debilitated patients, who lose heat rapidly. Patients with massive blood loss also cool rapidly. Peripheral warming reduces the incidence of vasospasm in patients with Raynaud's disease. The use of hot-air blankets is probably the most efficient way of providing heat.[23] Intravenous fluids, particularly blood, should be warmed.

CASE STUDY

A 45-year-old man with ankylosing spondylitis, diagnosed at age 20 and showing rapid progression in the last 15 years, has severe ankylosis of the cervical and thoracic spine, with a kyphosis to 45 degrees. He has a limited range of movement and pain in the right hip. He can walk unaided but only with difficulty, and he generally uses a motorized wheelchair. The surgeons plan corrective spine surgery, with the aim of reducing the kyphosis by 5 to 10 degrees and easing the difficulties associated with his activities of daily living. Harrington rods will be placed from C6 through T10.

In the review of systems, no chest pain, hypertension, orthopnea, or paroxysmal nocturnal dyspnea are found to be present. The patient develops ankle edema at the end of the day, which improves with bed rest, and has improved markedly since starting diuretic therapy. The patient has no history of syncope or palpitations. He complains of dyspnea that is markedly worse on exertion. No stridor, wheezing, or history of chest infection is found. The patient has never been a smoker. He has a good appetite and no history of abdominal pain, heartburn, reflux, or diarrhea.

The patient had a tonsillectomy at age 5, without complications. There is no family history of anesthetic problems, but the patient's father also had ankylosing spondylitis and died of respiratory failure at age 35.

The patient has no allergies. He takes naproxen sodium 500 mg twice daily, furosemide 40 mg per day, and potassium 10 mEq per day.

On physical examination, an obvious thoracic and cervical kyphosis to approximately 45 degrees is seen, with mild scoliosis to the left. The patient is thin but appears well nourished. He weighs 130 lb. His skin is in good condition, with no pressure sores or ulcers. He has normal vital signs. An early, blowing diastolic heart murmur is present, maximal in the second left intercostal space, and a split second heart sound with pulmonary accentuation is heard. The maximum cardiac impulse can be felt in the fifth intercostal space, midaxillary line. The jugular venous pressure is not raised, and no hepatomegaly or peripheral edema are noted. The respiratory rate is 18 per minute. Chest expansion is poor and is worse on the left than on the right. The chest wall is rigid, and the breathing is predominantly diaphragmatic. No adventitious lung sounds are heard. No cyanosis or clubbing is noted. Specific examination of the airway reveals complete ankylosis of the thoracic and cervical spinal column. There is no flexion or extension of the neck and minimal neck rotation. Mouth opening is limited to 2 cm. Surgical access to the trachea is limited because of the fixed neck flexion.

Diagnostic testing reveals normal levels of electrolytes, BUN, and creatinine. The hematocrit is 35 mg per dL, with a normocytic, normochromic picture. The white cell count is normal. The ECG reveals a right-axis deviation and normal sinus rhythm. The CXR shows severe kyphoscoliosis, with right mediastinal shift. The heart appears normal in size. The lung fields are reduced, but no focal opacities are seen. Cardiac catheter results show pulmonary artery pressure of 60/30 mm Hg, pulmonary arterial occlusion pressure of 12 mm Hg, normal left ventricular function, ejection fraction of 55%, and normal coronary vasculature. Echocardiography confirms grade 2 (mild to moderately severe) aortic insufficiency with a normal left ventricular ejection fraction of 60%. Pulmonary function tests show arterial partial pressure of oxygen of 75 mm Hg, arterial partial pressure of carbon dioxide of 40 mm Hg, pH of 7.4, FEV_1/forced vital capacity of 90%, and vital capacity of 950 mL; results are reported as pure restrictive disease with no obstructive component and no response to bronchodilators.

Overall Impression

This patient with severe kyphosis and cervical and thoracic ankylosis has severe restrictive pulmonary disease, with secondary pulmonary hypertension and mild right heart failure, which is well controlled by diuretic treatment. He has mild aortic insufficiency with no hemodynamic consequence. His medical condition is optimal. Important anesthetic considerations are (a) a difficult intubation and possible difficulty in establishing a mask airway; (b) the need for prolonged ventilation and intensive care management; (c) the potential for worsening pulmonary hypertension and right heart failure due to anesthetic drugs, prolonged immobility, and fluid shifts; and (d) the potential for spinal cord ischemia resulting in permanent neurologic damage, worsened by hypovolemia and hypotension.

Risk Modification

No evidence is found of pulmonary infection, and the patient's general condition and nutritional status are good. Because he has a chronically borderline-low hemoglobin level, he will not donate his blood for autotransfusion. The risks of homologous transfusion should be explained. A preoperative course of erythropoietin therapy could be considered (see Chapter 7).

Preoperative Preparation

This surgery must be performed under general endotracheal anesthesia. Regional anesthesia is not an option and need not be discussed. Although no aspiration risk is obvious in this patient, because of the combination of difficult intubation, possible difficult mask airway establishment, and poor surgical access to the trachea, an awake intubation (preferably with a fiberoptic scope) is probably the safest option for intubation. The rationale for the awake intubation and the process for achieving it should be discussed with the patient. If he is unable or unwilling to cooperate with an awake intubation, it would be reasonable to offer an inhalation induction, with intubation under deep inhalational anesthesia, as an alternative. Because the patient has severe restrictive lung disease with a vital capacity of only 950 mL, he will be electively ventilated postoperatively, and therefore must stay in the intensive care unit. This should be explained and discussed with the patient. Invasive monitoring (via arterial and pulmonary artery catheter) is likely to be used and should be explained. Some method of determining spinal cord and nerve root integrity during surgery will be used. In many centers, the wake-up test has been superseded by advanced electrophysiologic monitoring, but if the wake-up test is to be used, it should be explained to the patient. The mainstay of pain control will be systemic opioid treatment, which is best achieved during the early postoperative phase with an intravenous infusion and later with patient-controlled analgesia, which should be explained.

On the day of surgery, the patient should take his usual medications, except for naproxen sodium, which should be discontinued for at least 24 hours before surgery, preferably for 48 hours. The use of anxiety-reducing premedication in an unmonitored situation is not advisable because this patient has a fixed and severely restricted tidal volume and is dependent on his high respiratory rate for adequate oxygenation. Any drug with the potential to reduce his respiratory rate (including all sedatives) should be avoided. Although no clear risk factors exist for regurgitation, aspiration is always a concern during prolonged intubation, and because a prolonged intubation can be predicted, giving the patient a histamine$_2$ antagonist the night before and on the day of surgery is advisable. The dopamine antagonists should be avoided because of their sedating effects.

REFERENCES

1. Funk D, Raymon F. Rheumatoid arthritis of the cricoarytenoid joints: an airway hazard. *Anesth Analg* 1975;54:742–745.
2. Smith PH, Sharp J, Kellgren JH. Natural history of rheumatoid cervical subluxations. *Ann Rheum Dis* 1972;31:222–226.
3. Cervantes-Perez P, Toro-Perez AH, Rodreguez-Jurado P. Pulmonary involvement in rheumatoid arthritis. *JAMA* 1980;243:1715–1719.
4. Gran JT. An epidemiological survey of the signs and symptoms of ankylosing spondylitis. *Clin Rheumatol* 1985;4:161–169.
5. Kafer ER. Respiratory and cardiovascular functions in scoliosis and the principles of anesthetic management. *Anesthesiology* 1980;52:339–351.
6. Felson DT, Anderson JJ, Meenan RF. The comparative efficacy and toxicity of second-line drugs in rheumatoid arthritis. *Arthritis Rheum* 1990;33:1449–1461.
7. Benumof J. Management of the difficult adult airway. *Anesthesiology* 1991;75:1087–1110.
8. Tisi GM. Preoperative identification and evaluation of the patient with lung disease. *Med Clin North Am* 1987;71:399–412.
9. Zibrac JD, O'Donnell CR, Marton K. Indications for pulmonary function testing. *Ann Intern Med* 1990;112:763–771.
10. Mohr DN, Lavender RC. Preoperative pulmonary evaluation. *Postgrad Med* 1996;100:241–256.
11. Okeson GC. Pulmonary dysfunction and surgical risk. *Postgrad Med* 1983;74:75–83.
12. Souter AJ, Fredman B, White PF. Controversies in the perioperative use of nonsteroidal antiinflammatory drugs. *Anesth Analg* 1994;79:1178–1190.
13. Harris ED. Rheumatoid arthritis. Pathophysiology and implications for therapy. *N Engl J Med* 1990;322:1277–1288.
14. Kremer JM, Phelps CT. Long-term prospective study of the use of methotrexate in the treatment of rheumatoid arthritis. *Arthritis Rheum* 1992;35:138–145.
15. Weinblatt ME, Weissman BN, Holdsworth DE, et al. Efficacy of low-dose methotrexate in rheumatoid arthritis. *N Engl J Med* 1985;312:818–823.
16. Weinblatt ME, Weissman BN, Holdsworth DE, et al. Long-term prospective study of methotrexate in the treatment of rheumatoid arthritis: 84–month update. *Arthritis Rheum* 1992;35:129–137.
17. Toy PT, Strauss RG, Stehling LC, et al. Predeposited autologous blood for elective surgery: a national multicenter study. *N Engl J Med* 1987;316:517–520.
18. Liu S, Carpenter R, Neal JM. Epidural anesthesia and analgesia. Their role in postoperative outcome. *Anesthesiology* 1995;82:1474–1506.
19. Horlocker TT, Wedel DH, Schlichtine JL. Postoperative epidural analgesia and oral anticoagulant therapy. *Anesth Analg* 1994;79:89–93.
20. Rauck RL. The anticoagulated patient. *Reg Anesth* 1996;21:51–56.
21. Horlocker TT, Keit JA. Low molecular weight heparin: biochemistry, pharmacology, perioperative prophylaxis regimens and

guidelines for regional anesthetic management. *Anesth Analg* 1997;85:874–885.

22. Horlocker TT, Wedel DJ. Spinal and epidural blockade and perioperative low molecular weight heparin: smooth sailing on the *Titanic*. *Anesth Analg* 1998;86:1153–1156.

23. Hynson JM, Sessler DI. Intraoperative warming therapies: a comparison of three devices. *J Clin Anesth* 1992;4:194–199.

Neurologic Disease

11A Central Nervous System Disorders

Deborah J. Culley and Gregory Crosby

The purpose of this chapter is to aid in the preoperative evaluation of patients with neurologic disease. Because the scope of neurologic diseases and their anesthetic implications are quite broad, this chapter has been limited to the evaluation of patients with **cerebrovascular disease** and **stroke**, **pituitary adenomas**, **seizure disorders**, **myopathies**, **multiple sclerosis**, **Parkinson's disease**, **myasthenia gravis**, and **dementia**.

CEREBROVASCULAR DISEASE AND STROKE

Stroke[1-5] is a focal neurologic deficit of sudden onset due to cerebral embolism, thrombosis, or hemorrhage. Symptoms may resolve over days to weeks or may result in permanent disability and death. Transient ischemic attacks, in contrast, are focal neurologic deficits of sudden onset that resolve within 24 hours. In both cases, hypertension, cardiac disease, diabetes mellitus, smoking, hyperlipidemia, age older than 75 years, male gender, and a positive family history are risk factors.

Although many strokes are idiopathic, the history and diagnostic workup should be reviewed in preparation for elective surgery. The results of cerebral Doppler ultrasonography or angiography, brain imaging, cardiac studies, and hematologic and coagulation studies may reveal the cause of the stroke and provide information concerning the risk of cerebral reinfarction at the time of surgery. Patients with high-grade carotid stenosis (see Chapter 4), intracranial aneurysm (see Chapter 11B), or atrial fibrillation (see Chapter 4) may warrant further preoperative evaluation or treatment. In the event that previously unrecognized cerebrovascular disease is suspected, delay of elective surgery may be appropriate until an evaluation has been performed.

An asymptomatic carotid bruit is not associated with a higher risk of perioperative stroke in patients undergoing elective noncerebrovascular surgery. Therefore, surgery need not be delayed in this circumstance, but referral for evaluation is in order because long-term neurologic outcome is improved by carotid endarterectomy in some patients (see Chapter 4). At the other extreme are data indicating that the risk of perioperative stroke is as much as tenfold greater in patients with a recent stroke. The reason for or duration of this increased vulnerability is unknown, but it may be prudent to defer an elective surgical procedure for a week or two, even though there is no proven benefit of doing so. Data concerning the patient with transient ischemic attacks are ambiguous. If the cause is amenable to medical or surgical management (e.g., use of anticoagulants for intramural cardiac thrombus or carotid endarterectomy), undertaking these treatments before an elective surgical procedure seems appropriate (see Chapter 4); however, data are conflicting on this point.

Patients should be questioned about medications. Medical management of cerebrovascular disease often includes antiplatelet or anticoagulant drugs that predispose to perioperative bleeding or represent a relative contraindication to use of certain types of regional anesthesia (see Chapter 7). The decision to decrease, stop, or otherwise modify anticoagulation therapy warrants careful consideration, however, because doing so may increase the patient's risk of stroke. Aspirin and other antiplatelet drugs except nonsalicylate nonsteroidal antiinflammatory drugs produce a permanent platelet defect; coagulation returns to normal only after new platelets are formed, a process that takes approximately 7 days. Nonsalicylate nonsteroidal antiinflammatory drugs have a reversible effect on platelet function that lasts only for the duration of the drug effect (usually hours to 1 day). Warfarin sodium has a long half-life of approximately 40 hours. Therefore, one must anticipate the need to discontinue these drugs or adjust dosages. A common approach to management of the surgical patient on warfarin sodium is to discontinue the drug and provide anticoagulation with heparin sodium; this allows for short-duration changes in coagulation because of the relatively short half-life. The recommendation is usually to stop heparin sodium 6 to 8 hours before administering a regional anesthetic or beginning a surgical procedure. Prothrombin time and activated partial thromboplastin time are often measured in patients with the potential for such drug-induced coagulopathies before elective surgery or regional anesthesia (see Chapter 7).

Another important consideration is that cerebrovascular disease is often associated with hypertension and diabetes mellitus and is a marker of ischemic heart disease. Thus, the patient's history, physical examination, and laboratory studies should be reviewed for evidence of angina, congestive heart failure, and exercise intolerance (see Chapters 3 and 4). Because chronic hypertension shifts the cerebral autoregulation curve to the right, recording the patient's normal blood pressure range is important because it is used to guide intraoperative blood pressure management. Finally, because hyperglycemia worsens ischemic brain injury, blood glucose levels should be well controlled preoperatively in the diabetic patient, and medications should be prescribed or adjusted preoperatively to avoid intraoperative hyperglycemia (see Chapter 6).

Documentation of preoperative neurologic deficits is essential. First, muscles paralyzed or weakened by an upper motor neuron lesion are resistant to neuromuscular blockade and, because of this, train-of-four monitoring is misleading. In addition, proliferation of extrajunctional receptors can result in a hyperkalemic response to the administration of succinylcholine chloride. Second, cranial nerve involvement may impair patients' ability to swallow, cough, or protect their airway. In the event of cranial nerve involvement, a history of pulmonary aspiration should be sought and appropriate prophylaxis [histamine$_2$ (H$_2$) antagonists such as ranitidine hydrochloride, gastric motility agents such as metoclopramide and bicitrate] considered. Third, anesthetic agents can transiently unmask or exacerbate previous neurologic deficits, particularly if the deficit is recent. Thus, a patient awakening from general anesthesia may seem to have had a new stroke when a benign, drug-induced unmasking of an unrecognized preexisting deficit is actually the cause.

PITUITARY ADENOMA

The pituitary gland lies within the sella turcica in close proximity to the cavernous sinus, carotid arteries, optic chiasm, and cranial nerves III to VI. Numerous types of tumors occur in that region, but pituitary adenomas[6-9] or microadenomas are the most common. Symptoms relate to excess hormone secretion, compression of adjacent structures, or hypopituitarism. Tumors can be functional or nonfunctional. Only a minority of pituitary tumors are hormone secreting; such tumors usually overproduce prolactin, growth hormone, adrenal corticotropin hormone (ACTH), or thyroid-stimulating hormone (TSH). Pituitary adenomas may occur as part of a multiple endocrine neoplasia syndrome. These familial syndromes involve various combinations of pheochromocytoma, pancreatic islet cell tumors, parathyroid tumors, and thyroid carcinoma. Almost all cases are treated surgically by partial hypophysectomy using a transsphenoidal approach. Preoperative evaluation should include an assessment of visual changes and review of systems affected by abnormal pituitary function.

Growth hormone–secreting tumors result in the clinical syndrome of acromegaly. This manifests as an overgrowth of skeletal, connective, and soft tissues and has important implications for airway management and cardiovascular function. Characteristic features include hypertrophy of facial bones and soft tissue and thickening of the nose, tongue, lips, turbinates, soft palate, and epiglottis. Hoarseness due to laryngeal stenosis induced by soft tissue hypertrophy, fixation of the vocal cords, recurrent laryngeal nerve palsy, or anterior fixation and chondrocalcinosis of the larynx can occur. A goiter may also occur due to growth hormone stimulation. In severe cases, these changes make mask ventilation, laryngoscopy, and tracheal intubation quite difficult. Sedative premedication should be used cautiously, but a drying agent such as glycopyrrolate reduces secretions and may facilitate airway management.

The cardiopulmonary system may be affected. Left ventricular hypertrophy occurs in untreated acromegalic patients due to interstitial fibrosis, muscular enlargement, and cardiomyopathy. The severity of left ventricular hypertrophy worsens with the duration of the disease process. Acromegalic patients have a 30% incidence of diabetes mellitus, an increased incidence of hypertension, and an accelerated course of atherosclerotic disease. Thus, a thorough cardiovascular assessment guided by exercise tolerance is important, especially in patients with long-standing, severe disease. If abnormalities are noted in exercise tolerance, further workup, including electrocardiography (ECG) and cardiac echocardiography, is recommended (see Chapters 3 and 4). Pulmonary function can be impaired by chronic subglottic stenosis and sleep apnea. Octreotide acetate is a somatostatin analog that inhibits growth hormone secretion, decreases laryngeal changes, and improves cardiac function in patients with acromegaly.

An ACTH-secreting pituitary tumor produces hypersecretion of cortisol and results in Cushing's disease. The diagnosis is confirmed by elevation of the serum ACTH level, absence of diurnal variation of ACTH level, or lack of ACTH suppression by dexamethasone. Cushing's disease affects multiple organ systems (see Chapter 6). The incidence of hypertension, ischemic heart disease, and left ventricular hypertrophy is increased. Asymmetric septal hypertrophy is reported; the cause is unknown, but the problem often resolves when cortisol levels are normalized. Coexisting obesity, moon facies, and the "buffalo hump" body habitus characteristic of Cushing's disease can make mask ventilation and direct tracheal intubation difficult. Fluid and electrolyte disorders, including water and sodium retention, hypokalemia, metabolic alkalosis, and hyperglycemia, are common. With the exception of increased sensitivity to neuromuscular blocking agents because of muscle wasting, anesthetic drug responses are unaltered in patients with an ACTH-secreting pituitary tumor.

The preoperative evaluation should focus on the cardiovascular, metabolic, and endocrine systems. In the asymptomatic patient, the cardiovascular workup consists of the standard history, physical examination, and laboratory tests. Additional testing, including ECG and echocardiography, may be appropriate in the patient with symptoms of cardiovascular involvement (see Chapters 3 and 4). Because metabolic disturbances are common, serum electrolyte and glucose levels should be measured, and administration of "stress-dose" steroids should be considered if perioperative adrenal insufficiency is suspected (see Chapter 15).

TSH-secreting tumors represent fewer than 1% of all pituitary adenomas. Because they cause hyperthyroidism, TSH-secreting tumors can produce tachycardia, arrhythmias, and a risk of thyroid storm (hyperpyrexia, cardiac failure, delirium, coma). An elevated serum TSH level that does not increase further after administration of exogenous TSH confirms the diagnosis. Preoperative control of hyperthyroidism is important and should be confirmed by physical examination and, if necessary, thyroid function tests and ECG. Definitive treatment includes administration of antithyroid drugs such as propylthiouracil, but rapid control of symptoms is achieved with β-blockers and dexamethasone, which suppresses release of TSH. The use of β-blockers prevents the clinical end organ effects of thyroxine (T_4) and inhibits the peripheral deiodination of thyroxine to form triiodothyronine (T_3), the active compound. Antithyroid drugs can, on rare occasion, produce hepatitis, agranulocytosis, thrombocytopenia, and hypoglycemia. Thus, depending on the patient's history and clinical evaluation, liver function tests (see Chapter 9), complete blood cell count (CBC), and measurement of electrolyte and glucose levels may be appropriate.

Prolactinomas are common pituitary adenomas that lead to prolactin hypersecretion and cause symptoms that include galactorrhea, amenorrhea, and infertility. They are generally small and not associated with any relevant perioperative anesthetic-related complications.

Pituitary tumors that do not secrete hormones remain clinically silent for a longer period. Presenting symptoms may therefore relate to the enlarging mass lesion, obstruction of cerebrospinal fluid drainage, or hypopituitarism. Pituitary enlargement usually manifests as headaches or visual field changes (bitemporal hemianopia) and decreased visual acuity due to optic nerve compression. Hypothyroidism and hypoadrenalism are common manifestations of pituitary insufficiency. Occasionally, emergent treatment is required for pituitary apoplexy—acute hemorrhage or tumor infarction producing an acute mass effect that can lead to symptoms of increased intracranial pressure, sudden blindness, and cranial nerve palsies.

In cases of hypopituitarism, initial symptoms are due to hypoadrenalism because thyroxine has a half-life of 7 days. Adrenal insufficiency is manifested by orthostatic hypotension, intravascular volume depletion, electrolyte disturbances such as hyperkalemia, hyponatremia, and hypoglycemia, and lethargy secondary to hyponatremia-induced cerebral edema. Thus, the preoperative evaluation of patients with hypopituitarism should include determinations of blood pressure and heart rate in both the supine and standing positions and measurement of electrolyte and glucose levels. Treatment consists of corticosteroid replacement with hydrocortisone or another steroid, particularly in the event of unexplained hemodynamic instability. Hypothyroidism carries a significant risk of pericardial effusion, cardiac tamponade, congestive heart failure, and ischemic heart disease, and these conditions should be sought during the preoperative evaluation (see Chapters 3 and 4). A pericardial effusion is suggested by chest pain, a pericardial friction rub, and an enlarged cardiac silhouette on chest radiograph. The presence of cardiac tamponade is suggested by faint heart sounds and pulsus paradoxus (a drop of more than 10 mm Hg in systolic blood pressure during inspiration). Echocardiography is indicated if pericardial effusion or tamponade is suggested by history or physical examination. Other problems of hypothyroidism include muscle weakness, altered levels of consciousness, coma, increased sensitivity to sedatives and opiates, and a tendency toward hypothermia, hyponatremia, and hypoglycemia. Hypothyroidism should be corrected before elective surgery. For emergent surgery in cases of severe hypothyroidism, treatment should begin with levothyroxine sodium, using careful monitoring for myocardial ischemia.

SEIZURE DISORDERS

Seizures[5,10–12] may be idiopathic or may occur in association with neurologic injury, structural brain lesions, hypoxia, fever, or metabolic disturbances such as hypoglycemia and alcohol withdrawal. Epilepsy is a chronic disorder characterized by recurrent and unpredictable seizures in the absence of an obvious provoking factor. Three percent of the population have epilepsy; of these, 25% to 30% have seizures more than once per month. Often the diagnosis is made by history combined with electroencephalography and laboratory tests. Epileptic seizures vary from brief lapses of attention to abnormal motor activity followed by prolonged periods of loss of consciousness.

Seizures usually are classified as either *partial* or *generalized*. Partial seizures have a focal cortical onset and can be further subdivided into *simple seizures*, *complex seizures*, and *seizures of partial onset with generalization*. Simple partial seizures produce no detectable alteration in consciousness and have an electrically limited distribution in the brain. Complex partial seizures, also known as *temporal lobe* or *psychomotor seizures*, typically begin locally and subsequently spread into multiple areas of the brain. They often involve automatisms and alterations of consciousness, and the patient is amnesic for the event. Partial onset with generalization is the classification used for seizures that begin focally and subsequently spread to involve much of the brain and brainstem. These events often lead to tonic or clonic convulsive seizures, which make them indistinguishable from generalized seizures.

Generalized seizures involve both cerebral hemispheres and are divided into *inhibitory* and *excitatory* forms. Excitatory generalized seizures include myoclonic, clonic, and tonic convulsions, all of which are characterized by repetitive muscle contractions. Rather than causing movement, inhibitory seizures stop movement. They include absence (petit mal) seizures, which are characterized by lapse of consciousness without convulsion or muscle activity, and atonic seizures, during which the patient loses muscle tone and falls. Pseudoseizures can mimic the above seizure types and are thought to represent psychiatric conditions without electrical alterations in the brain.

Preoperative evaluation of a patient with a seizure disorder should include notations on seizure cause, patterns and frequency, therapeutic regimen and side effects, as well as changes that suggest medical noncompliance, drug interactions, or a new pathologic process. These patients should be on a stable therapeutic regimen without evidence of an increase in seizure frequency or serious drug-related side effects. Under these circumstances, routine determination of serum levels of antiseizure medications is unwarranted. Determining whether serum levels are in the therapeutic range is important, however, when the surgical procedure is a craniotomy, the character or frequency of the seizures is changing, or a new drug has been added to the regimen.

Phenytoin (Dilantin), phenobarbital, carbamazepine, valproic acid, and gabapentin are commonly used to treat epilepsy. Use of these drugs presents several issues in the perioperative period. First, because many are not available in parenteral form, the patient should receive the usual dose of anticonvulsant medication orally on the day of surgery. A plan for seizure control should be developed for the patient who is unable to consume oral medications postoperatively. Often, this involves the use of intravenous phenytoin; however, care must be exercised because phenytoin has significant cardiovascular toxicity and can produce hypotension and conduction abnormalities. Second, most anticonvulsants have sedating properties. Dosages of premedicants and anesthetics may need to be adjusted accordingly. Third, a number of these agents are associated with electrolyte and liver function abnormalities. Accordingly, measurement of serum electrolyte levels and liver function tests should be considered, but preoperative measurement may not be necessary in the stable patient on chronic therapy. Finally, anticonvulsants cause induction of liver enzymes, which leads to more rapid metabolism of some nondepolarizing muscle relaxants and certain hypnotics and analgesics.

Medications known to lower seizure threshold should be avoided or used judiciously. These include penicillin, imipenem, meperidine hydrochloride, phenothiazines, and amitriptyline hydrochloride. Most anesthetic agents have both proconvulsant and anticonvulsant activity. Among the inhalational anesthetics, enflurane produces electroencephalographic epileptiform activity in both normal and epileptic patients with profound hypocarbia. Case reports suggest that halothane, isoflurane, sevoflurane, and nitrous oxide can provoke seizure-like activity, but such reports have not appeared for desflurane. Intravenous anesthetics have been implicated in the genesis of epileptiform activity. Methohexital sodium is epileptogenic in patients with psychomotor epilepsy but not in those with generalized convulsive disorders. Etomidate and ketamine hydrochloride also activate epileptogenic foci. Propofol can produce seizures in patients with central nervous system (CNS) pathology, but this effect seems to be dose dependent; sedative doses increase spike activity, whereas depression occurs at high dosages. The opioid fentanyl and some of its derivatives can induce electrocorticographic seizures in patients with preexisting epilepsy. These data notwithstanding, whether or not these electrophysiologic effects of anesthetics are neurologically meaningful is uncertain. In fact, most anesthetics possess anticonvulsant properties, and many have been used successfully to treat status epilepticus.

MYOPATHIES

Myopathies[13-16] are primary muscular disorders that cause acute or chronic muscle weakness. For simplification, they can be divided into four groups: *inherited*, *metabolic/endocrine*, *inflammatory*, and *toxic* myopathies. This discussion focuses on the common inherited myopathies, but much is generalizable to other myopathies.

The muscular dystrophies are inherited myopathies in which muscle fibers are destroyed and replaced by fibrous and fatty tissue, which leads to muscle weakness. Duchenne's and Becker's muscular dystrophies are X-linked recessive hereditary disorders characterized by painless degeneration and atrophy of skeletal muscles, without denervation. Lack of dystrophin protein, or presence of an abnormal form, causes muscle cell necrosis. The incidence of Duchenne's or pseudohypertrophic muscular dystrophy is 3 per 10,000 male births, whereas Becker's muscular dystrophy, which is thought to be a more benign form of Duchenne's disease, occurs in 3 of 100,000 male newborns.

Symptoms of Duchenne's muscular dystrophy become apparent in affected boys between the ages of 2 and 5 years. Proximal muscles are affected first, leading to characteristic symptoms such as a waddling gait, lumbar lordosis, frequent falling, and difficulty climbing stairs. Although proximal muscle wasting is apparent, more distal muscles become pseudohypertrophic from fatty infiltration. Because of progressive skeletal muscle wasting, joint contractures, and scoliosis, most patients require braces by age 10 and are confined to a wheelchair by age 12. Intellectual impairments are common but nonprogressive. Death frequently occurs by age 20, usually from pulmonary causes. The more benign form of the disease, Becker's muscular dystrophy, manifests with weakness between the ages of 5 and 15 years. These patients ambulate beyond age 15 and have a life expectancy of 40 to 50 years but ultimately develop the same problems as patients with Duchenne's disease. The diagnosis of Duchenne's or Becker's muscular dystrophy is suggested by a positive family history and characteristic physical findings. An elevated serum creatine phosphokinase level (often 20 to 100 times normal) and a myopathic pattern on electromyography (EMG) are nonspecific but suggest the diagnosis. Definitive diagnosis requires demonstration of abnormal or deficient dystrophin in biopsied muscle, or mutation and linkage analysis of peripheral blood leukocytes. No definitive treatment exists for these disorders, but prednisone slows progression. Because these patients develop contractures and kyphoscoliosis, orthopedic and spine procedures are particularly common.

With respect to preoperative evaluation, attention should be directed toward the pulmonary, cardiac, neuromuscular, and gastrointestinal systems. Respiratory and cardiac involvement are invariably present. Respiratory impairment results from weakness of the muscles of respiration. In Duchenne's disease, such weakness is usually present by age 10 and is compounded by the effects of contractures and progressive scoliosis. In fact, one of the primary indications for correction of scoliosis is that surgery decreases annual deterioration in vital capacity from 20% per year to just 5% per year. Muscle weakness also results in decreased ability to cough, accumulation of secretions, and a predisposition to pneumonia. Therefore, except in very mild cases, preoperative pulmonary function tests and a chest radiograph are advised. The incidence of sleep apnea and pulmonary hypertension is increased in patients with muscular dystrophy. Thus, patients should be questioned about snoring, sleep disturbances, and daytime somnolence (see Chapters 5 and 15), and premedication should be prescribed judiciously.

The risk of scoliosis surgery varies with vital capacity. If the vital capacity exceeds 45% of predicted, postoperative ventilation is unlikely to be necessary. When vital capacity is less than 30% of predicted, however, serious postoperative complications frequently occur. In such cases, patients should be made aware of the possibility that postoperative mechanical ventilation may be necessary.

Muscular dystrophy patients often have a cardiomyopathy, but the extent of cardiac involvement is difficult to determine by history because exercise tolerance can rarely be assessed. Therefore, formal cardiac evaluation, usually by noninvasive means such as ECG and echocardiography, is advised (see Chapters 3 and 4). Tall R waves in V_1 and deep, narrow Q waves in the precordial leads may be seen on the ECG due to scarring of the posterobasal portion of the left ventricle. In addition, a short PR interval and sinus arrhythmias are common, but sudden cardiac death is rare.

Because of the muscle abnormalities, muscular dystrophy patients have altered responses to neuromuscular blocking agents and susceptibility to malignant hyperthermia. Muscular dystrophy is associated with hyperkalemia, rhabdomyolysis, and life-threatening cardiac dysrhythmias after administration of succinylcholine chloride. Nondepolarizing muscle relaxants have been used successfully, but the possibility of a prolonged response must be considered. Because of the increased risk of malignant hyperthermia, succinylcholine chloride and other known triggering agents should be avoided. Although prophylactic administration of dantrolene sodium is not necessary, a high index of suspicion and careful intraoperative and postoperative monitoring for malignant hyperthermia, possibly for an extended period, are needed (see Chapter 14).

Other issues include adrenal suppression secondary to chronic steroid use and an increased risk of pulmonary aspiration. For the former, supplemental steroids are indicated in the perioperative period (see Chapter 15). Because decreased gastric emptying and weak laryngeal and pharyngeal musculature are found in muscular dystrophy patients, full-stomach precautions, including the administration of antacids and H_2 blockers, are recommended preoperatively, and a nasogastric tube should be considered for postoperative management.

Other inherited muscular dystrophies include limb-girdle, facioscapulohumeral, oculopharyngeal, and nemaline rod muscular dystrophy. Respiratory, laryngeal, and pharyngeal weakness and myocardial involvement occur to a variable extent in these patients. Patients with oculopharyngeal dystrophy, like patients with myasthenia, have greatly increased sensitivity to nondepolarizing muscle relaxants; complete paralysis can occur with 10% of the normal dose. Nemaline rod muscular dystrophy is associated with micrognathia and dental malocclusion, which may make tracheal intubation difficult; alternative approaches to intubation other than direct laryngoscopy should be considered.

MYOTONIC DYSTROPHIES

The myotonic dystrophies are a group of hereditary disorders characterized by persistent skeletal muscle contractions after stimulation. The cause is thought to be related to abnormal calcium metabolism, in which intracellular calcium released on muscle contraction fails to return to the sarcoplasmic reticulum. Neither general nor regional anesthesia nor muscle relaxants relieve these contractures, but infiltration of the muscle with local anesthetics may induce relaxation. Phenytoin, presumably due to its membrane-stabilizing properties, is the treatment of choice for patients requiring prolonged therapy.

Myotonia dystrophica is the most severe form of myotonic dystrophy. It is an autosomal dominant disorder with an incidence of 5 in 100,000. Symptoms appear in the second to third decade of life and include facial and sternocleidomastoid weakness, dysarthric speech, ptosis, and inability to relax from voluntary contractions. The triad of mental retardation, frontal baldness, and cataract formation is characteristic. Levels of creatine phosphokinase are elevated at all stages, and EMG shows high-frequency repetitive discharges.

Preoperative evaluation of patients with myotonic dystrophy must consider cardiac and respiratory abnormalities, pulmonary aspiration risk, associated disorders, and abnormal responses to drugs used for anesthesia.

Cardiac involvement is multifactorial. Cardiac dysrhythmias and conduction abnormalities are quite common and may precede other symptoms of the disease. A baseline ECG should be obtained and often reveals bradycardia and intraventricular conduction delays. However, these changes do not correlate with the severity of skeletal muscle involvement. Deaths from arrhythmias are common, but treatment of the arrhythmia may worsen cardiac conduction. Thus, antiarrhythmics must be used with caution, but the need to control cardiac rhythm should be anticipated because anesthesia and surgery may aggravate preexisting conduction blockade. All patients with myotonia dystrophica are assumed to have some degree of cardiomyopathy and may require formal evaluation, such as an ECG, if exercise tolerance cannot be assessed. Myocardial depression associated with anesthetic agents may be exaggerated. Finally, 20% of patients with myotonia have mitral valve prolapse or other valvular lesions that may require endocarditis prophylaxis (see Chapters 4 and 16).

Preexisting respiratory muscle weakness is a problem and contributes to the same difficulties discussed under the muscular dystrophies. In addition, sleep apnea with carbon dioxide retention and a depressed carbon dioxide response curve is well documented. This contributes to heightened sensitivity to respiratory depressants and increases the possibility of postoperative respiratory insufficiency.

Gastrointestinal hypomotility, combined with weakness of pharyngeal, laryngeal, and thoracic muscles, makes these patients vulnerable to pulmonary aspiration of gastric contents. The patient should be questioned about pulmonary aspiration, and prophylaxis should be considered.

These patients have increased risk of endocrine abnormalities, which may affect the course of anesthesia. The preoperative evaluation should specifically seek information regarding the presence of diabetes mellitus, hypothyroidism, and adrenal insufficiency. Thyroid function tests, glucose level, and electrolyte levels should be obtained as appropriate (see Chapter 6).

The muscular system requires special attention. Succinylcholine chloride must be avoided because it produces prolonged muscle contractions that can make ventilation of the lungs and intubation of the trachea difficult. The response to nondepolarizing muscle relaxants is normal, however. Although reversal of neuromuscular blockade can theoretically precipitate muscle contraction; it does not seem to occur when neostigmine is used for reversal. To eliminate the need for reversal, careful titration of short- or intermediate-acting muscle relaxants should be considered. Finally, aggressive measures should be used to maintain the patient's temperature in the normal range during surgery, because shivering precipitates myotonia.

MULTIPLE SCLEROSIS

Multiple sclerosis (MS)[5,17–19] is an acquired disease of the CNS characterized by demyelination of plaques within the brain and spinal cord. The precise etiology remains unknown, but autoimmune and viral causes in combination with genetic susceptibility have been implicated. The incidence of MS varies by geographic latitude; the incidence is lowest near the equator (1 in 100,000) and increases with distance from it. In North America, the incidence is 6 to 80 per 100,000, with urban dwellers and members of higher socioeconomic groups at greatest risk.

Symptoms usually develop between the ages of 20 and 40 years, and clinical manifestations reflect the site of CNS demyelination. Predilection for periventricular white matter, the optic nerves, pons, medulla, and spinal cord leads to the common clinical manifestations of optic neuritis, decreased visual acuity, diplopia, nystagmus, weakness, impotence, paresthesias, spasticity, ataxia, bladder dysfunction, and autonomic insufficiency. The disease is marked by periods of unpredictable exacerbations and remissions. Typically, symptoms develop over a few days, remain stable for a few weeks, and then improve. Improvement is most likely due to correction of nerve conduction and not remyelination. Hence, symptoms ultimately persist, and severe disability results. No specific diagnostic tests exist for MS. Evidence for the diagnosis includes neurologic abnormalities separated in both time and place; the presence of plaques on magnetic resonance images or computed tomographic scans of the head and spinal cord; delayed conduction on visual, somatosensory, and auditory evoked potentials; and elevated levels of cerebrospinal fluid immunoglobulin G and myelin basic protein.

Preoperative evaluation should focus on disease severity and progression, presence of associated disorders, drug therapy, and complications of therapeutic regimens. Documentation of the presence of symptoms and location of neurologic deficits is important because perioperative exacerbation is common. Autonomic insufficiency is of particular importance because of the possibility of perioperative hemodynamic instability. This condition is suggested by a history of impotence, bladder and bowel dysfunction, dizziness, or syncope. Physical evaluation therefore should include blood pressure and heart rate determinations in the supine and sitting positions. As the disease progresses, spasticity, contractures, and limitation of movement can occur. This can make surgical positioning difficult and occasionally complicate airway management. Cranial nerve involvement is common in MS. In particular, patients should be questioned about a history of upper airway incompetence, inability to clear secretions, and aspiration. Finally, 5% of patients with MS have a seizure disorder.

No definitive therapy exists for MS. Therapeutic modalities are directed toward amelioration of acute exacerbations, the prevention of relapses, and relief of symptoms. Immunosuppression with ACTH, corticosteroids, and immunosuppressive agents such as azathioprine and cyclophosphamide enhance recovery from acute episodes and reduce the number of relapses in some patients but do not alter the ultimate course of the disease. Patients treated over the long term with steroids or ACTH require supplemental steroids during the perioperative period (see Chapter 15). A CBC and liver function tests should be obtained in the patient taking azathioprine because it suppresses the bone marrow and impairs liver function. Measurement of serum electrolyte levels is indicated in the patient taking cyclophosphamide because it can produce the syndrome of inappropriate secretion of antidiuretic hormone and lead to perioperative water intoxication and hyponatremia. Bladder dysfunction and muscle spasticity are often treated with diazepam, dantrolene sodium, or baclofen. Dantrolene sodium produces liver function abnormalities, so liver function tests are indicated. Baclofen is known to prolong the action of sedatives and hypnotics.

MS patients are exquisitely sensitive to hyperthermia, so careful temperature management is critical. As little as a 0.5°C increase in body temperature can make subclinical lesions clinically apparent. Thus, the ability to prevent and treat even a mild hyperthermic response is critical, and one should avoid warming the patient.

Surgery and anesthesia have been alleged to exacerbate MS, but the evidence is entirely anecdotal; preoperative documentation of deficits avoids such confusion. The response to muscle relaxants may be abnormal. MS patients with severe neurologic disability and associated muscle atrophy are at risk for succinylcholine chloride–induced hyperkalemia, but succinylcholine chloride has been used safely in patients in remission and those with mild neurologic symptoms. Resistance to nondepolarizing muscle relaxants has been reported in MS, perhaps because upper motor neuron lesions cause proliferation of extrajunctional cholinergic receptors.

Controversy exists concerning the use of regional anesthesia in patients with MS. Based on the hypothesis that the blood-brain barrier is more permeable to local anesthetics or that demyelination predisposes the spinal cord to local anesthetic toxicity, some authorities suggest that epidural anesthesia is more appropriate than spinal anesthesia because cerebrospinal fluid concentrations of local anesthetic are lower. No large, well-controlled studies exist to resolve the issue, however, and case reports can be found of both acute exacerbations of MS after spinal anesthesia and of uncomplicated use of spinal and epidural anesthesia. In fact, acute exacerbations of MS have not been shown to occur more commonly after anesthesia (regional or general) than in normal daily life.

PARKINSON'S DISEASE (PARALYSIS AGITANS)

Parkinson's disease[5,19–21] (Table 11A-1) is a neurodegenerative disorder characterized by neuronal loss and reactive gliosis of the nigrostriatal dopaminergic system of the basal ganglia. Parkinson's disease is typically idiopathic, but other neurodegenerative diseases, stroke, and dopaminergic receptor antagonists such as haloperidol, chlorpromazine (Thorazine), droperidol, prochlorperazine maleate, and metoclopramide may exacerbate the condition. Emotional stress, which is unavoidable in the perioperative period, can exacerbate the disease. Clinical manifestations of Parkinson's disease result from decreased dopaminergic transmission within the basal ganglia and include resting rhythmic tremor (4 to 8 per second), muscular rigidity, bradykinesia, and gait disturbances. Paucity of spontaneous movement, fixed facial expressions (masked facies), monotonous voice, and a shuffling gait are characteristic. Autonomic nervous system dysfunction can occur, impairing the response to hypovolemia, and 25% of affected patients and 50% of advanced cases have an associated dementia. Parkinson's patients have essentially no sensory changes, however, and deep tendon and plantar reflexes remain normal. Eventually, the disease produces incapacitating tremor and rigidity.

Table 11A-1. Classification and grading scale for Parkinson's disease

Stage	Description
I	Unilateral involvement.
II	Bilateral involvement with no postural abnormalities.
III	Bilateral involvement with mild postural imbalance; the patient leads an independent life.
IV	Bilateral involvement with postural instability; the patient requires substantial help.
V	Severe, fully developed disease; the patient is restricted to bed and chair.

Preoperative evaluation should provide information on disease severity, associated disorders, drug therapy, complications of therapy, and consequences of delaying therapy. Dysphagia is common in patients with Parkinson's disease but is often unrecognized. It may increase the risk of pulmonary aspiration perioperatively, and thus administration of antacids and prokinetic agents should be considered. The use of metoclopramide, a dopamine receptor antagonist, should be avoided, however, and medications such as cisapride, which has no effect on dopaminergic balance, should be selected. Parkinson's disease can also produce restrictive lung disease secondary to chest wall rigidity and hypokinesis, and obstructive sleep apnea and upper airway obstruction have been described. Although the preoperative history and physical examination should attempt to identify these problems if they exist, further workup, such as pulmonary function tests, are rarely necessary.

Because no cure exists, the goal of drug therapy for Parkinson's disease is simply to minimize symptoms. In general, treatment is intended to restore the balance in the basal ganglia between acetylcholine-mediated excitatory neurotransmission and the inhibitory effects of dopamine. Levodopa (L-dopa), the metabolic precursor of dopamine, is the cornerstone of such therapy and often produces dramatic improvement. A limitation of L-dopa is its short half-life (1 to 3 hours) and propensity to produce side effects such as nausea, vomiting, orthostatic hypotension, and cardiac irritability. The dopamine receptor agonists bromocriptine mesylate (Parlodel) and pergolide mesylate (Permax) have significantly longer half-lives than L-dopa and are effective in many cases; however, they can produce orthostatic hypotension, hallucinations, and confusion. Another approach, which is particularly useful in the early course of the disease, is to inhibit degradation of dopamine by inhibiting the enzyme monamine oxidase (MAO). Selegiline hydrochloride, which has greater affinity for MAO B than MAO A, increases dopamine levels in the basal ganglia but does not affect metabolism of epinephrine or norepinephrine (which are metabolized by MAO A). However, meperidine hydrochloride may produce stupor, rigidity, agitation, and hyperthermia in patients taking selegiline. Benztropine mesylate, an anticholinergic agent, blocks cholinergic transmission and has a modest antiparkinsonian action but is associated with side effects such as dry mouth, urinary retention, blurred vision, constipation, sedation, and delirium. Finally, some patients are treated with amantadine hydrochloride, an antiviral agent thought to alter dopamine release and uptake at presynaptic sites. Amantadine hydrochloride is useful as initial therapy in cases of mild Parkinson's disease or as an adjunct in patients on levodopa with dose-related fluctuations. Side effects include dizziness, lethargy, sleep disturbances, and nausea and vomiting. Due to the potential for altered catecholamine levels and proarrhythmic effects of some of the drugs used to treat Parkinson's disease, an abnormal rhythm detected on clinical examination should be confirmed with an ECG.

An important consideration during the preoperative evaluation of a patient with Parkinson's disease is to develop a plan for maintenance and restoration of drug therapy. This is especially true for patients treated with L-dopa, because the drug has a short half-life and abrupt withdrawal of this and other dopamine agonists is associated with neuroleptic malignant syndrome as well as acute exacerbation of the motor symptoms. Neuroleptic malignant syndrome is a life-threatening emergency characterized by autonomic instability, extrapyramidal dysfunction (pseudoparkinsonism), and hyperthermia. Exacerbations of Parkinson's disease can lead to severe chest wall rigidity and swallowing impairment and predispose to respiratory failure and pulmonary aspiration. Intravenous administration of L-dopa is not optimal because conversion of L-dopa to dopamine in the periphery produces cardiac and hemodynamic instability (carbidopa, the decarboxylase inhibitor that prevents conversion of levodopa to dopamine, is not available in intravenous form). Consequently, the patient with Parkinson's disease should receive the usual dose of antiparkinson medication orally just before surgery, and the need for enteral feeding should be anticipated if postoperative oral intake is impossible. Indeed, for very long surgeries or prolonged gastrointestinal malfunction, a duodenal feeding tube should be considered.

Surprisingly few anesthetic agents and anesthetic adjuncts are reported to produce adverse effects in the patient with Parkinson's disease. Rigidity has been exacerbated by droperidol, a dopamine antagonist, and by butyrophenones and phenothiazines. Metoclopramide should be avoided. In patients with Parkinson's disease, acute dystonia has been reported after administration of alfentanil hydrochloride, but opioid-induced rigidity cannot be excluded. Finally, despite a single case report of succinylcholine chloride–induced hyperkalemia in a patient with Parkinson's disease, the response to depolarizing and nondepolarizing muscle relaxants is thought to be normal.

MYASTHENIA GRAVIS

Myasthenia gravis[5,22–25] is an antibody-mediated autoimmune disease affecting the neuromuscular junction. It occurs in 1 of every 20,000 adults. Clinical manifestations result from a decrease in the number of functional postsynaptic acetylcholine receptors due to their inactivation or destruction by circulating antibodies, which are present in 90% of patients with the disease. The trigger for the autoimmune response is unknown, but a strong association is found with hyperplasia of the thymus and thymomas. Eaton-Lambert syndrome is pathophysiologically similar to myasthenia but usually occurs in association with small cell carcinoma of the lung. The diagnosis of myasthenia gravis is based on both clinical and laboratory data. Patients with myasthenia have a higher incidence of other autoimmune diseases such as rheumatoid arthritis, hypothyroidism, and systemic lupus erythematosus (see Chapters 6 and 10).

Myasthenia is characterized by skeletal muscle weakness and is marked by unpredictable periods of exacerbation and remission. The weakness is typically exacerbated by exercise and resolves partially with rest. Muscles innervated by cranial nerves are particularly susceptible. Diplopia and ptosis, due to ocular muscle weakness, are the most common initial clinical complaints and occur in most patients during the first year of the disease. The disease becomes generalized in the majority of patients and peaks over a 2- to 3-year period. Bulbar involvement leading to weakness of pharyngeal and laryngeal muscles presents as respiratory insufficiency or difficulty with swallowing and clearance of secretions. Peripheral muscle involvement may be asymmetric and can occur in any distribution. An acetylcholine receptor antibody assay detects antibodies in 90% of patients, but titer levels do not correlate with clinical status. The Tensilon test involves intravenous administration of the acetylcholinesterase inhibitor edrophonium chloride; a positive test is marked by objective and subjective signs of improvement in muscle strength. The regional curare test involves injection of a small dose of curare into a tourniquet-restricted arm; the test is positive if administration of this subtherapeutic dose induces marked muscle weakness. The EMG shows a rapid reduction in the amplitude of the evoked response with repetitive stimulation.

Preoperative evaluation of patients with myasthenia gravis should include assessment of disease severity (Table 11A-2), associated conditions, effectiveness of treatment, and complications of therapy.

Pulmonary and cranial nerve involvement are prominent features of the disease. Patients should be questioned about a history of upper airway incompetence, inability to clear secretions, and aspiration, because bulbar involvement is common and such patients are particularly vulnerable to perioperative airway obstruction and aspiration. Diaphragmatic and intercostal mus-

Table 11A-2. Classification of myasthenia gravis

Stage	Description
I	Only ocular signs and symptoms
IIA	Mild but generalized muscle weakness
IIB	Moderate, generalized muscle weakness, with or without bulbar dysfunction
III	Acute fulminating symptoms with or without respiratory dysfunction
IV	Generalized myasthenia gravis that is chronic and severe

cle involvement leads to shallow breathing and inadequate vital capacity, often resulting in hypoventilation, atelectasis, and hypoxia. Functional status and pulmonary function tests help delineate the extent of pulmonary impairment, but normal preoperative pulmonary status does not preclude postoperative pulmonary complications. Accordingly, regardless of preoperative status, the myasthenic patient should be informed of the possibility of postoperative mechanical ventilation. Risk factors for postoperative mechanical ventilation have been determined for transsternal thymectomy. These include disease duration longer than 6 years, a history of chronic respiratory disease, pyridostigmine bromide dosage greater than 750 mg per day, and a preoperative vital capacity of less than 2.9 L. These risk factors are less reliable in cases of transcervical thymectomy, and their predictive value for myasthenic patients undergoing other surgical procedures is unknown.

Treatment approaches are many. Anticholinesterases such as pyridostigmine bromide and neostigmine are the first-line therapies. These agents inhibit degradation of endogenous acetylcholine and hence increase the amount available at the neuromuscular junction. Because they are relatively short acting, frequent dosing is required. Accordingly, although some controversy exists because of the possibility of side effects such as bradycardia and salivation, patients probably should take their usual anticholinesterase medications on the day of surgery. This seems especially appropriate for severely disabled patients; those with milder symptoms can receive less than the normal dose.

Other approaches to treatment include the use of steroids, immunosuppressants, and plasmapheresis. Corticosteroids, especially prednisone, promote improvement in most patients, probably by interfering with the production of antibodies. One should evaluate for complications of prolonged steroid administration such as infection, peptic ulcer disease, hyperglycemia, and hypertension and should consider providing perioperative steroid coverage (see Chapter 15). Azathioprine (Imuran) improves function in 45% of patients; however, because it can produce bone marrow suppression and abnormalities of liver function, a CBC and liver function tests should be obtained preoperatively in patients taking this medication. Cyclosporine is usually reserved for patients who are resistant to other therapeutic modalities. Because complications of cyclosporine include hypertension, hepatotoxicity, and nephrotoxicity, measurement of blood urea nitrogen and creatinine levels and liver function tests are indicated. Plasmapheresis, which decreases antibody titers, can produce marked improvement in muscle strength that lasts several days to months. It has been used during myasthenic crises and before surgery, but improvement in muscle strength may require 1 to 2 weeks of treatment. Finally, thymectomy is recommended for patients with drug-resistant myasthenia gravis. Muscle strength improves significantly in nearly all patients undergoing thymectomy, and 50% achieve a complete remission. However, patients in remission remain sensitive to drugs known to exacerbate myasthenia, and caution should be used in prescribing them.

Rapid deterioration of neuromuscular function can occur at any time perioperatively as a result of a myasthenic or cholinergic crisis. Myasthenic crisis is an acute, severe exacerbation of muscle weakness. Perioperative factors that can exacerbate myasthenia gravis include stress, infection, electrolyte disturbances, and medications such as magnesium sulfate, aminoglycosides, local anesthetics, β-blockers, and calcium channel blockers. Cholinergic crisis is due to an overdosage of anticholinergics and is differentiated from myasthenic crisis by the presence of salivation, miosis, and bradycardia. The response to anticholinesterases is unpredictable in myasthenic patients. In some cases, transient improvement in muscle strength results, whereas in others weakness is accentuated. Resolution of motor symptoms in cholinergic crisis requires metabolism of excess anticholinesterase, but vagal effects can be effectively antagonized with glycopyrrolate or atropine sulfate. These patients should be managed in an intensive care unit because they often require intubation and mechanical ventilation while precipitating factors are sought and treated.

Several important perioperative implications should be considered with regard to patients with myasthenia gravis. These include the responses to sedatives and hypnotics, general anesthetics, and muscle relaxants. Preoperative anxiety reduction is important because stress can exacerbate myasthenia, but bulbar and respiratory compromise mandate cautious and conservative use of respiratory depressants. The response to succinylcholine chloride is unpredictable and ranges from resistance to blockade to development of phase II block. The duration of succinylcholine chloride–induced motor blockade is markedly prolonged in patients taking anticholinesterases. Patients with myasthenia are exquisitely sensitive to nondepolarizing muscle relaxants. Short- to medium-acting drugs in reduced dosage are recommended, with careful monitoring of neuromuscular function. Alternatively, inhalation agents that have muscle relaxant properties can be used alone. One should note that residual weakness can occur from the use of inhalational agents alone.

DEMENTIA

Dementia[5,26–32] is a chronic and progressive acquired alteration in intellectual function that is distinct from normal age-related memory decline or delirium. Although the differential diagnosis is extensive, most cases are of the Alzheimer's type. This chapter focuses on the preoperative evaluation of patients with Alzheimer's disease, both because it is the most prevalent type of dementia and because little evidence exists that the form of dementia alters perioperative considerations.

Definitive diagnosis of Alzheimer's disease requires demonstration of neurofibrillary tangles and neuritic plaques in the brain at postmortem examination. However, the clinical diagnosis is often based on standardized criteria as described in the *Diagnostic and Statistical Manual of Mental Disorders, Fourth Edition*. In general, dementia is a slowly progressive disease notable for a decline in cognitive function without alteration of consciousness. It affects memory, language, judgment, reasoning, decision making, and the ability to manage complex tasks. Behavioral and psychological abnormalities such as depression, hallucinations, delusions, anxiety, aggression, and agitation are common. Although dementia is unlikely to present before age 65 years, 30% of the elderly are affected by age 90. Alzheimer's disease progresses until death, which usually occurs from 2 to 16 years after onset. It is the fourth leading cause of death in the United States.

Alzheimer's disease, like other forms of dementia, is probably the end result of a number of biological and environmental factors. Genetic involvement is suggested by linkage studies of rare mutations in the amyloid precursor protein and presenilin genes, as well as an increased incidence of Alzheimer's disease among carriers of the apolipoprotein gene E4 allele. Genetic predisposition is neither necessary nor sufficient to cause Alzheimer's disease.

The CNS alterations associated with Alzheimer's disease are distinct from normal age-related changes in the CNS. Loss of brain mass among patients with Alzheimer's disease is 2.5 times that of age-matched controls. At the molecular level, a reduction is seen in the number of nicotinic cholinergic receptors as well as in acetylcholine synthesis in areas of the brain associated with memory and cognition. Alterations in other neurotransmitter systems, complement-mediated inflammatory responses, oxidative stress, and alterations in the hormonal milieu have been hypothesized to play a role.

Alzheimer's disease has several implications for preoperative evaluation. First, one must often rely heavily on information from sources other than the patient, and it may be difficult to obtain informed consent.

Second, dementia is typically a slowly progressive disease, but sudden and reversible deterioration in mental status is known to occur in association with acute, and often treatable, disease processes such as urinary tract and respiratory tract infections. Thus, any patient with known dementia who presents with an acute decline in mental status should be evaluated for a coexisting disease process before elective surgery.

Third, one must be aware of the implications of drug therapy for Alzheimer's disease. Medical therapy for Alzheimer's disease primarily involves the use of anticholinesterases such as tacrine hydrochloride and donepezil hydrochloride to treat deficiencies in central cholinergic activity. These drugs have a variety of side effects, including reversible hepatotoxicity, gastrointestinal symptoms (nausea, vomiting, diarrhea, dyspepsia, abdominal pain), and dermatitis. Thus, in some cases based on the history and clinical picture, evaluation of liver function may be appropriate. Because both tacrine hydrochloride and donepezil hydrochloride are degraded in the liver, potential interactions with other hepatically metabolized drugs such as cimetidine and warfarin sodium should be anticipated. The potential for altered responses to neuromuscular blocking agents can be encountered in patients taking tacrine hydrochloride. Intravenous administration prolongs the action of succinylcholine chloride, whereas oral administration has no effect on succinylcholine chloride but may cause resistance to nondepolarizing muscle relaxants.

Finally, there is a higher risk of postoperative delirium in a patient with dementia. Potential cases include cerebral hypoxia or hypoperfusion, endocrine or ionic imbalances, postoperative pain, sepsis, bowel or bladder distension, and drugs with known adverse CNS effects, are important. Medications used during the perioperative period that can precipitate or exacerbate delirium include high-dose steroids, neuroleptics, benzodiazepines, ketamine hydrochloride, tertiary anticholinergics, opioids, H_2 blockers, and droperidol. It is reasonable to speculate that the demented patient is more sensitive to physiologic and pharmacologic interventions such as these, but this is an assumption, not a fact. Perhaps the most important aspect of dementia is that such patients often require additional medical resources perioperatively because of confusion, inability to cooperate, and difficulties in comprehending a new environment.

In conclusion, patients with neurologic disease are a diverse group, and they present many challenges for the anesthesiologist. Complete preoperative evaluation and preparation is the first step to ensuring satisfactory perioperative care.

CASE STUDY

A 50-year-old woman with multiple sclerosis and recurrent urinary tract infections secondary to renal calculi is to undergo cystoscopy, transureteral lithotripsy, and stent placement. She has had progressive multiple sclerosis for the past 20 years and walks with a cane.

On review of systems, she denies any history of cardiac or pulmonary disease but does not exercise due to lower extremity weakness, spasticity, and ataxia, which are the primary manifestations of her disease. She has had recent exacerbations requiring steroid treatment in association with urinary tract infections. She denies a history of syncope, cranial nerve deficits, or seizures, but complains of bladder dysfunction. She denies the use of alcohol, tobacco, or illicit drugs. She was given an uncomplicated general anesthetic for an appendectomy 4 years before this hospitalization. She had ataxia and difficulties in walking before that surgery which worsened afterward, and she has since walked with a cane. She is concerned that she may have a similar exacerbation after this surgery. She has no known drug allergies, and her only medication is prednisone, with dosages of 20 to 50 mg per day over the past 6 months.

Physical examination reveals that she is 5 ft 4 in., weighs 120 lb, and has normal airway anatomy. Vital signs, including temperature, are normal. No orthostatic blood pressure change is noted when the patient is in the sitting or standing position. Cardiac and pulmonary examinations are normal. Cranial nerves, upper extremity reflexes, and motor strength are normal. She has hyperreflexia, decreased motor strength, and marked sensory abnormalities in both lower extremities. Her gait is ataxic, and she falls toward the left when not using her cane.

Preoperative diagnostic tests reveal normal levels of electrolytes and blood urea nitrogen but a slightly elevated creatinine level. CBC, including white blood cell count, and ECG are normal.

Important anesthetic considerations include the possibility of (a) adrenal suppression due to chronic steroid use, (b) autonomic insufficiency as demonstrated by bladder dysfunction, (c) perioperative exacerbation of the disease process, and (d) altered responses to muscle relaxants.

Because of the potential for adrenal suppression associated with chronic steroid administration, perioperative stress doses of steroids should be considered and unquestionably administered in the event of hemodynamic instability (see Chapter 15). Similarly, the potential for autonomic insufficiency and exaggerated hemodynamic responses to anesthetic agents and altered responses to vasopressors should be anticipated. Although at present no evidence exists of an infectious process, any infection should be treated aggressively because even small elevations in temperature can exacerbate MS. Along these same lines, care should be taken with perioperative warming devices so as to avoid even mild hyperthermia.

This procedure can be performed under regional or general anesthesia, and the risks and benefits of each should be discussed. Evidence that regional anesthesia can exacerbate MS is entirely anecdotal. No basis exists for recommending any particular general anesthetic technique and, although the patient's concerns about postoperative exacerbation may be valid, no evidence supports this possibility. Because of the lower extremity muscle weakness and atrophy, a risk of hyperkalemia may be present with the use of succinylcholine chloride, so a nondepolarizing muscle relaxant may be preferable. The patient should be instructed to take her usual medications with clear liquids on the day of surgery.

REFERENCES

1. Culley DJ, Crosby G. Impaired central nervous system function. In: Benumof JL, Saidman LJ, eds. *Anesthesia and perioperative complications*, 2nd ed. Philadelphia: Mosby, 1999:357–376.
2. Goldstein LB, Matchar DB. Clinical assessment of stroke. *JAMA* 1994;271:1114–1120.
3. Kim J, Gelb AW. Predicting perioperative stroke. *J Neurosurg Anesthesiol* 1995;7:211–215.
4. Easton J, Hauser SL, Martin JB. Cerebrovascular diseases. In: Fauci AS, Braunwald E, Isselbacher KJ, et al., eds. *Harrison's principles of internal medicine*, 14th ed. New York: McGraw-Hill, 1998:2325–2342.
5. Rusa R, Ulatowski JA. Preoperative evaluation in an era of cost containment: the patient with a neurologic disorder. *Probl Anesth* 1997;9:221–234.
6. Biller BMK, Daniels GH. Neuroendocrine regulation and diseases of the anterior pituitary and hypothalamus. In: Fauci AS, Braunwald E, Isselbacher KJ, et al., eds. *Harrison's principles of internal medicine*, 14th ed. New York: McGraw-Hill, 1998:1972–1999.
7. Kilibanski A, Zervas NT. Diagnosis and management of hormone-secreting pituitary adenomas. *N Engl J Med* 1991;21:822–831.
8. Lamberts SW, Vam der Lely AJ, de Herder WW, Hofland LJ. Octreotide. *N Engl J Med* 1996;334:246–254.
9. Razis PA. Anesthesia for surgery of pituitary tumors. *Int Anesthesiol Clin* 1997;35:23–34.
10. Brodie MJ, Dichter MA. Antiepileptic drugs. *N Engl J Med* 1996;334:168–175.
11. Kofke WA, Tempelhoff R, Dasheiff RM. Anesthetic implications of epilepsy, status epilepticus, and epilepsy surgery. *J Neurosurg Anesthesiol* 1997;9:349–372.
12. Scheuer ML, Pedley TA. The evaluation and treatment of seizures. *N Engl J Med* 1990;323:1468–1474.
13. Albers JW, Wald JJ. Neuroanesthesia and neuromuscular diseases. In: Albin MS, ed. *Textbook of neuroanesthesia: with neurosurgical and neuroscience perspectives*. New York: McGraw-Hill, 1997:456–461.

14. Farrell PT. Anaesthesia–induced rhabdomyolysis causing cardiac arrest: case report and review of anaesthesia and the dystrophinopathies. *Anaesth Intensive Care* 1994;22:597–601.
15. Mendell JR, Griggs RC, Ptácek LJ. Diseases of muscle. In: Fauci AS, Braunwald E, Isselbacher KJ, et al., eds. *Harrison's principles of internal medicine*, 14th ed. New York: McGraw-Hill, 1998:2473–2478.
16. Russell SH, Hirsch NP. Anesthesia and myotonia. *Br J Anaesth* 1994;72:210–216.
17. Hauser SL, Goodkin DE. Multiple sclerosis and other demyelinating diseases. In: Fauci AS, Braunwald E, Isselbacher KJ, et al., eds. *Harrison's principles of internal medicine*, 14th ed. New York: McGraw-Hill, 1998:2409–2419.
18. Rudick RA, Cohen JA, Weinstock-Guttman B, et al. Management of multiple sclerosis. *N Engl J Med* 1997;27:1604–1611.
19. Solomon D, Solomon D, Albin M. Neurologic syndromes and disorders with their anesthetic implications. In: Albin MS, ed. *Textbook of neuroanesthesia: with neurosurgical and neuroscience perspectives*. New York: McGraw-Hill, 1997:409–451.
20. Aminoff MJ. Parkinson's disease and other extrapyramidal disorders. In: Fauci AS, Braunwald E, Isselbacher KJ, et al., eds. *Harrison's principles of internal medicine*, 14th ed. New York: McGraw-Hill, 1998:2356–2363.
21. Calne DB. Treatment of Parkinson's disease. *N Engl J Med* 1993;329:1021–1027.
22. Albers JW, Wald JJ. Neuroanesthesia and neuromuscular diseases. In: Albin MS, ed. *Textbook of neuroanesthesia: with neurosurgical and neuroscience perspectives*. New York: McGraw-Hill, 1997:461–467.
23. Baraka A. Anesthesia and myasthenia gravis. *Can J Anaesth* 1992;39:476–486.
24. Barrons RW. Drug-induced neuromuscular blockade and myasthenia gravis. *Pharmacotherapy* 1997;17:1220–1232.
25. Drachman DB. Myasthenia gravis. In: Fauci AS, Braunwald E, Isselbacher KJ, et al., eds. *Harrison's principles of internal medicine*, 14th ed. New York: McGraw-Hill, 1998:2469–2472.
26. Bird TD. Memory loss and dementia. In: Fauci AS, Braunwald E, Isselbacher KJ, et al., eds. *Harrison's principles of internal medicine*, 14th ed. New York: McGraw-Hill, 1998:142–150.
27. Crismon ML. Pharmacokinetics and drug interactions of cholinesterase inhibitors administered in Alzheimer's disease. *Pharmacotherapy* 1998;18:47–54.
28. Duncan BA, Siegal AP. Early diagnosis and management of Alzheimer's disease. *J Clin Psychiatry* 1998;59[Suppl 9]:15–21.
29. Moller JT, Cluitmans P, Rasmussen LS, et al. Long-term postoperative cognitive dysfunction in the elderly: ISPOCD1 study. *Lancet* 1998;351:857–861.
30. O'Keeffe ST, Ni CA. Postoperative delirium in the elderly. *Br J Anaesth* 1994;73:673–687.
31. Whitehouse PJ. The cholinergic deficit in Alzheimer's disease. *J Clin Psychiatry* 1998;59:19–22.
32. Williams-Russo P, Sharrock NE, Mattis S, et al. Cognitive effects after epidural vs general anesthesia in older adults. A randomized trial. *JAMA* 1995;274:44–50.

11B Neurosurgical Disease

Joseph M. Hughes

BRAIN TUMORS

This section discusses brain tumors,[1-6] with the exception of pituitary adenomas (which are addressed in Chapter 11A). In the United States, the incidence of all brain tumors is 46 in 100,000. More than 75% of central nervous system tumors are metastases from systemic cancer. Metastases to the brain and meninges occur in approximately 25% of all cancers.

Brain tumors (including malignancies, meningiomas, acoustic neuromas, schwannomas) cause symptoms by growing within a fixed volume and displacing blood and cerebrospinal fluid or compressing and destroying brain tissue. Initially, changes in tumor volume cause only small changes in intracranial pressure (ICP); once the limit of compensatory changes is reached, however, the ICP rises. Increased ICP impairs optic nerve axonal transport and venous drainage and results in papilledema. Some slow-growing tumors, such as meningiomas, can cause large indentations of brain tissue without raising ICP or causing papilledema. Once a certain size is reached and compensatory mechanisms fail, increased ICP begins to displace remote tissues. This causes the false localizing signs seen in transtentorial herniations, including paradoxical corticospinal signs (caused by the compression of normal tissue on the side opposite the lesion due to herniation), cranial nerve III and IV palsies, and secondary hydrocephalus.

Brain edema is caused by the increased permeability of vascular endothelial cells and vasogenic edema due to tumor proteases. Hydrocephalus can occur if tumors obstruct the flow or absorption of cerebrospinal fluid. Some tumors present only with raised ICP. Certain tumors cause specific intracranial tumor syndromes that allow the clinical diagnosis even before computed tomography (CT) or magnetic resonance imaging (MRI). CT and MRI scans have greatly helped to identify tumor-related causes of nonlocalizing symptoms, often before the onset of focal signs.

Headaches are an early symptom in 30% of patients and often are of a deep, constant character. They range from sharp to dull and slight to intense. The most common feature is occurrence at night. None of these features excludes migraine, vascular, or hypertensive headaches. Initially, tumors cause localized pain by local edema and traction of blood vessels. Later, the ICP increase leads to bifrontal or bioccipital headaches.

Certain tumors predispose to elevated ICP with symptoms of mental inertia, unsteady gait, vomiting, and urinary and fecal incontinence. Vomiting usually is associated with headaches. In some patients, it may be projectile (sudden and without nausea), but in others nausea is a prominent feature. It may occur independent of meals, particularly before breakfast. Patients with brain tumors may present with nonlocalizing signs such as changes in mental function, dizziness, and seizures and only later develop focal signs. Mental status changes include decreased attention, increased irritability, poor judgment, poor memory, decreased mental activity, and decline in adherence to common social customs. Early signs are lethargy, nonrotational dizziness, and weakness. As tumor growth progresses, delays in answering questions increase, and patients may become confused or demented. With increasing ICP, mental dullness and sleepiness progress to stupor or coma. Tumors causing these symptoms are frequently centrally located and impinging on the thalamocortical areas responsible for alertness and attention.

Generalized or focal seizures occur in 20% to 50% of patients. Seizures may be the heralding symptom in adults with brain tumors. The pattern of the seizure may help localize the tumor. Standard anticonvulsants and surgery often decrease seizure frequency. Seizures are discussed in greater detail in Chapter 11A.

Brain tumors and elevated ICP can result in autonomic dysfunction, which manifests as bradycardia, arrhythmias, and changes on the electrocardiogram (ECG). (See Aneurysms and Arteriovenous Malformations, below, for further discussion.) Patients with brain tumors may have been treated with radiation therapy. Three syndromes of radiation damage are described. The acute syndrome may occur during or shortly after the final treatments. Acute effects of radiation include lethargy, loss of appetite, alterations of mental status, seizures, signs of increased ICP, and exacerbation of previous symptoms and signs. These changes usually are due to worsening cerebral edema and can be treated by increasing the dose of glucocorticoids. These symptoms usually resolve over days to weeks. The acute delayed syndrome occurs soon after treatment and involves an increase in the severity of symptoms caused by the tumor. The last syndrome is late delayed radiation injury. Structures adjacent to the tumor, particularly the white matter and brainstem, undergo coagulation necrosis. Radiation necrosis may occur if the total dose exceeds 6,000 rads to the brain. Late delayed injury appears 3 to 18 months after treatment and does not respond to glucocorticoid therapy.

Chemotherapy for primary brain tumors usually consists of nitrosoureas and is well tolerated. Nitrosoureas may cause confusion, depression, seizures, and ataxia. Chemotherapeutic complications occur more often when systemic malignancies are treated (see Chapter 15). High-potency glucocorticosteroids reduce tumor-induced edema within hours of administration by decreasing endothelial cell permeability and shrinking normal tissue. Patients with large tumors and large amounts of cerebral edema may benefit from higher doses of steroids but at the cost of steroid-induced side effects. Steroids can interfere with the metabolism of anticonvulsants, so that decreased doses may be required to avoid toxicity. Steroid use may cause hyperglycemia, which can worsen neurologic outcome after hypoxic insults. Treatment of hyperglycemia requires close monitoring because severe untreated hypoglycemia can result in rapid neurologic deterioration as the brain has no energy stores.

Preoperative embolization via intraarterial catheters can decrease intraoperative blood loss with vascular tumors. Temporary occlusion of feeder vessels in tumors near vital areas such as speech or vision centers is performed in awake patients to assess the effects before permanent embolization or surgery. Embolization is typically carried out in the radiology suite.

History and Physical Examination

A detailed neurologic examination highlighting those areas of particular importance to anesthesia is important. If raised ICP is suspected, the fundi should be examined for signs of papilledema. The level of consciousness and the integrity of the gag reflex help to predict the patient's ability to protect the airway. Sensory and motor deficits and asymmetric reflexes should be carefully documented preoperatively because these areas are tested on emergence from anesthesia. The presence of new deficits postoperatively may require emergent imaging studies and re-exploration. The gait can be assessed simply by observing the patient walk from the waiting area to the examination rooms.

The hydration status of any patient who has been vomiting should be assessed. This assessment includes examination of the mucus membranes, orthostatic blood pressures, and skin turgidity.

Embolization of vascular tumors may require manipulations of blood pressure, which necessitates thorough preoperative evaluation of the patient's cardiovascular status (see Chapters 3 and 4).

Diagnostic Testing

Preoperative glucose evaluation is needed if patients are taking steroids. Evaluation of an ECG is indicated. If the patient has had seizures of recent onset or they are poorly controlled, then anticonvulsant levels should be checked. Other studies are directed by clinical findings.

Implications for Anesthetic Management

Anesthetic issues that must be dealt with preoperatively include planning for postoperative intensive care unit admission and arterial line placement in patients who are having resection of brain tumors. "Stress-dose" steroid coverage should be addressed (see Chapter 15). If the patient has been taking anticonvulsants for some time and seizures are well controlled, then no further action is necessary. If the seizures are not well controlled and anticonvulsant levels are subtherapeutic, doses should be increased or new medications added. Correction of fluid deficits may be necessary to avoid excessive hypotension on induction.

Intravenous solutions containing free water should be avoided in favor of hypertonic solutions such as normal saline. Hypotonic solutions can increase vasogenic edema, further compromising neurologic function. Glucose solutions should be avoided because of worsened neurologic outcome after hypoxic insults in the presence of hyperglycemia. Administration of a hypertonic solution such as 25% mannitol at a dose of 0.5 to 1.0 g per kg over 10 minutes can shift water from brain tissue into the plasma and thereby reduce brain volume and ICP. Diuretics (furosemide, acetazolamide) are used to create a hyperosmolar state and to decrease cerebrospinal fluid formation. Hyperventilation produces respiratory alkalosis with resulting vasoconstriction and decreased cerebral blood flow. This decreases brain volume and is useful during surgery and in the management of tumors causing coma due to mass effect.

Patients should be prepared for the possibility of being awake during certain procedures (e.g., embolization, biopsy) if neurologic testing is necessary. Spinal anesthesia is contraindicated in patients with an elevated ICP.

ANEURYSMS AND ARTERIOVENOUS MALFORMATIONS

Patients with aneurysms and arteriovenous malformations (AVMs)[7–14] range from neonates to the elderly, and many have concomitant diseases. In North America, 28,000 aneurysms rupture each year. Of these patients whose aneurysms rupture, 18,000 have morbidity and mortality. Ninety percent of aneurysms are diagnosed after they rupture. Occasionally, aneurysms are found incidentally on MRI or CT. Asymptomatic aneurysms rupture at the rate of 1% to 2% per year. Symptomatic aneurysms rupture at the rate of 5% per year. Once rupture occurs, patient morbidity and mortality are high. The worst prognosis is for patients with giant intracranial aneurysms.

One-third of patients experience warning signs and symptoms before a major subarachnoid hemorrhage (SAH). These symptoms may be due to minor SAHs (sentinel bleeding) or aneurysm growth. Symptoms are due to compression of surrounding structures or emboli from an intraluminal thrombus. The time between a sentinel and a major SAH averages 2 to 3 weeks. If the aneurysm is clipped early after the sentinel SAH, the patient has an excellent prognosis; if not, the prognosis is poor because rehemorrhage may intervene before clipping. The diagnosis of an SAH is usually confirmed with CT (which is positive in 90% of patients soon after SAH) or MRI, although occasionally the diagnosis is provided by lumbar puncture (this carries the risk of herniation if a large mass lesion effect is present). The anatomy is subsequently defined by angiography.

Any but the smallest aneurysms (smaller than 3 mm) are at risk of rupture. Most neurosurgeons choose to clip unruptured aneurysms or embolize them to decrease surgical risk or if the patient's medical condition precludes surgery and anesthesia. The risk of rupture increases with age, with most occurrences between the fourth and sixth decades. Women have a higher incidence than men, with an overall ratio of 1.6:1 and an even higher incidence after age 40. Although hypertension is not a risk factor for development of SAH, once SAH occurs, patients with hypertension have a poorer prognosis. In first-degree relatives of a patient with SAH, the incidence of aneurysmal SAH is 6.7%. Rupture in such relatives tends to occur at a younger age and with smaller aneurysms. Systemic disorders predisposing to SAH include Ehlers-Danlos syndrome, coarctation of the aorta, polycystic kidney disease, and fibromuscular dysplasia (patients with the latter have a 20% to 40% incidence of intracranial aneurysms). Tobacco, alcohol, and cocaine abuse predispose to aneurysmal rupture. The incidence of rupture is increased with

Table 11B-1. Fisher's scale for the grading of aneurysms revealed by computed tomography

Grade	Definition
0	No hemorrhage
1	No subarachnoid blood
2	Diffuse or vertical layers <1 mm thick
3	Localized clot or vertical layers ≥1 mm
4	Intracranial or intraventricular clot

pregnancy and is highest in the final weeks of gestation and in the first several weeks postpartum. Certain intracranial vascular abnormalities predispose to aneurysmal rupture. These include all types of carotid-basilar anastomoses, an incomplete circle of Willis, ligations of the carotid artery, and AVMs with aneurysms on the feeder vessels.

Various clinical scales are used to grade aneurysms and aid in predicting outcome. Fisher's scale is based on the density of the clot (Table 11B-1). Hunt and Hess described clinical grades of intracranial aneurysms (Table 11B-2). Ogilvy and Carter[12] have proposed a new grading system using the scales of Fisher, and Hunt and Hess, as well as aneurysm- and patient-specific factors (Table 11B-3). When this new grading system was applied to 434 SAH patients, 100% of patients with grade 0 aneurysms were found to have an excellent or good outcome, whereas this proportion fell to 49% for those with grade 3 aneurysms and 18% for those with grade 4 aneurysms. Conversely, the incidence of poor outcome or mortality was 34% for those with grade 3 aneurysms and 64% for those with grade 4 aneurysms.

AVMs are congenital vascular lesions associated with high blood flows and very low cerebral vascular resistance. AVMs produce symptoms from mass effects, ischemia, or SAH. AVMs hemorrhage at a rate of 4% per year, although this is an infrequent presenting symptom. The major risk factors for SAH are older age and initial presentation with SAH. Temporal and occipital lobe AVMs are thought to have a greater incidence of bleeding than AVMs in other locations. The size and depth of an AVM do

Table 11B-2. Hunt-Hess clinical grading scale for intracranial aneurysms

Grade	Definition
0	Unruptured
I	Minimal headache, nuchal rigidity
II	Moderate to severe headache, nuchal rigidity, ± cranial nerve palsy
III	Drowsiness, confusion, or mild focal deficit
IV	Stupor, hemiparesis, early decerebrate rigidity, vegetative disturbances
V	Deep coma, decerebrate rigidity, moribund
+1	For vasopressin or systemic disease vasospasm

Table 11B-3. Ogilvy and Carter grading scale for intracranial aneurysms

Factors	Points
Aneurysm-specific	
Size ≤10 mm	0
Size >10 mm	1
Giant (≥2.5 cm) posterior circulation lesions	1
Patient-specific	
Age ≤50 yr	0
Age >50 yr	1
Density of SAH blood	
Fisher scale grade of 0–2	0
Fisher scale grade of 3–4	1
Clinical condition	
Hunt-Hess scale grade of 0–III	0
Hunt-Hess scale grade of IV–V	1

SAH, subarachnoid hemorrhage.
The final grade is equal to the total number of points. The higher the grade, the worse the prognosis.

not relate to the risk of SAH. Patients older than 50 years appear to have a higher annual rate of SAH, but younger patients face a significant cumulative risk of SAH. The annual mortality rate is 1% per year. With each SAH, the risk of death is 10% to 15%. The annual neurologic morbidity is 2% to 3%. Deep cerebral AVMs of the posterior fossa frequently present with SAH, whereas superficial AVMs more frequently present with seizures. Patients with SAH from an AVM develop seizures at the rate of 1% per year. Some of these seizures will become medically intractable and require surgical resection. Younger patients are at greater risk for seizure disorders. High-flow AVMs can cause chronic hypoperfusion and ischemia in surrounding tissues. Progressive ischemic neurologic deficit resulting from "steal" is a syndrome seen in older patients with large, high-flow AVMs.

Anatomic factors of importance to AVMs include the nidus, feeding arteries, draining veins, and blood flow. Large nidus size, complex flow pattern, proximity to important brain regions, deep location, presence of daughter nidi, and a diffuse AVM can complicate resection. A larger number and diameter of feeding arteries and the presence of multiple connections of anterior, middle, and posterior cerebral arteries make for a more difficult operation. Deep-draining veins are thought to be important. Large-caliber veins indicate a high-flow shunt and increase the risk of acute brain edema during the final stages of surgery.

Angiographic vasospasm can be demonstrated in 70% of patients with SAH, and 30% of these patients have ischemia and clinical deterioration. The cause of cerebral vasospasm is unclear. The treatment and prevention of vasospasm is of particular importance after an SAH. Once the aneurysm has been clipped or embolized to prevent rebleeding, hemodilution, hypervolemia, and efforts to increase blood pressure can be instituted to control vasospasm. Not infrequently, large doses of vasopressors may be required to elevate systolic blood pressure into a target range (i.e., 180 to 200 mm Hg). This increase in afterload can compromise patients with underlying heart disease. Calcium channel blockers (e.g., nimodipine) are an important part of vasospasm therapy. It is not unusual for patients in vasospasm to receive repeated endovascular treatment with papaverine hydrochloride or angioplasty.

The syndrome of inappropriate antidiuretic hormone secretion (SIADH) often occurs after an SAH. It should be suspected in the presence of serum hyponatremia in the face of hypertonic urine. If allowed to progress, the hyponatremia causes decreased alertness and leads to confusion and then coma, often with seizures. Clinical signs directly correlate with the speed of the sodium decline. Most patients respond to fluid restriction of 800 to 1,000 mL per day; this intake is usually less than urine output plus insensible losses. This negative water balance gradually increases serum sodium level and osmolality, reduces weight, and improves symptoms. Fluid restriction should be continued until the serum sodium concentration reaches 135 mEq per L.

In patients with convulsions, severe confusion, or coma, sodium chloride can be infused based on the following calculation: infused sodium (mEq) = (target sodium – starting sodium) × 0.6 × weight in kilograms. Normal saline has 154 mEq per L of sodium. Hypertonic or 3% saline has 462 mEq per L of sodium. If hypertonic saline is given, intravascular volume usually must be reduced using furosemide, starting with 0.5 mg per kg and increasing until a diuresis occurs. The speed of correction of hyponatremia must be limited (less than 10 mEq per L in the first 24 hours) to prevent central pontine myelinosis. SIADH may continue for weeks or months. Particularly in patients with SAH, one must distinguish SIADH from cerebral salt wasting that results in hyponatremia and decreased blood volume. In the latter syndrome, fluid restriction is dangerous.

ECG changes are common with SAH. The pathophysiology of these changes is controversial, but evidence exists that structural myocardial lesions may occur after SAH. Wall motion abnormalities demonstrated by echocardiography have been reported. Assuming that ECG changes are merely secondary to SAH may be erroneous. Raised ICP, cerebral edema, and the techniques used to treat these problems are discussed in detail in the previous section on brain tumors.

The treatment of aneurysms and AVMs has changed markedly with the use of preoperative embolization to devascularize these lesions (see Brain Tumors, above). Use of this approach over one or more sessions can simplify surgical resection.

Of the factors affecting outcome after aneurysm surgery, the most important are neurologic status on admission (level of consciousness or clinical grade), the patient's age, and the presence of vasospasm. Patients with aneurysms smaller than 12 mm have a better outcome. Hypertension and hyperglycemia worsen the outcome. Wide distribution of subarachnoid clot implies a worse prognosis. The greater the number and severity of comorbid medical conditions, the worse the prognosis. Nonsurgical treatment of aneurysmal SAH carries a 60% mortality at 12 months.

History and Physical Examination

See Brain Tumors, above, for details. Briefly, all neurologic deficits must be carefully documented preoperatively. Signs and symptoms of SAH include severe headache, nuchal rigidity, focal neurologic deficits, and an altered level of consciousness. Large hemorrhages can cause an elevated ICP and papilledema. Preexisting cardiac disease must be evaluated and optimized because of the use of hypervolemic and hypertensive therapies to prevent and treat vasospasm. Autonomic dysfunction occurs and can cause fever and vomiting, which result in dehydration. Bradycardia and arrhythmias may be present.

Diagnostic Testing

The evaluation for all patients should include an ECG and measurement of glucose and electrolyte levels. In SAH, ECG changes include bradycardia, many types of arrhythmias, ST segment elevation and depression, a prolonged QT interval, peaked and deeply inverted T waves and even Q waves. These changes are similar to those seen in ischemic heart disease, and if ECG abnormalities are present, further evaluation may be necessary (see Chapters 3 and 4.) When the patient has neurogenic pulmonary edema or has been intubated to protect the airway, measurement of arterial blood gases is indicated and a chest radiograph may be necessary to rule out pulmonary edema, infection, or aspiration.

Implications for Anesthetic Management

Preoperative anesthetic issues are much the same as for brain tumors (see Brain Tumors, above). The need for postoperative intensive care unit admission and intraoperative invasive monitor placement should be discussed with the patient. Ensuring that patients continue antihypertensives, including on the day of surgery, is critical. Significant hyponatremia should be corrected (see discussion of SIADH in the section on Aneurysms and Arteriovenous Malformations, above). Treatment of raised ICP includes administration of glucocorticoids and mannitol, hyperventilation, and avoidance of free water and hyperglycemia. The overlying principles of management include maintaining cerebral blood flow, optimizing cerebral perfusion pressure, and minimizing the risk of hemorrhage, ischemia, neurologic injury, and hypoperfusion.

REFERENCES

1. Adams RD, Victor M, Ropper AH. Intracranial neoplasms and paraneoplastic disorders. In: Adams RD, ed. *Principles of neurology*, 6th ed. New York: McGraw-Hill, 1997:642–694.
2. Black S, Cucchiara RF. Tumor surgery. In: Cucchiara RF, ed. *Clinical neuroanesthesia*, 2nd ed. New York: Churchill Livingstone, 1998:343–365.
3. Lanier WL, Stangland KJ, Scheithauer BW, et al. The effects of dextrose infusion and head position on neurologic outcome after

complete cerebral ischemia in primates: examination of a model. *Anesthesiology* 1987;66:39–48.

4. Levy ML, Rabb C, Couldwell WT, et al. Protection of the neuronal pool. In: Apuzzo MLJ, ed. *Brain surgery: complication avoidance and management.* New York: Churchill Livingstone, 1993:857–889.

5. Roizen MF. Oncologic disease. In: Miller RD, ed. *Anesthesia,* 4th ed. New York: Churchill Livingstone, 1994:986–987.

6. Sagar SM, Israel MA. Tumors of the nervous system. In: Fauci AS, Braunwald E, Isselbacher KJ, et al., eds. *Harrison's principles of internal medicine,* 14th ed. New York: McGraw-Hill, 1998:2398–2409.

7. Adams RD, Victor M, Ropper AH. Spontaneous subarachnoid hemorrhage and arteriovenous malformations. In: Adams RD, ed. *Principles of neurology,* 6th ed. New York: McGraw-Hill, 1997:841–873.

8. Black S, Sulek CA, Day AL. Cerebral aneurysm and arteriovenous malformation. In: Cucchiara RF, Black S, Michenfelder JD, eds. *Clinical neuroanesthesia,* 2nd ed. New York: Churchill Livingstone, 1998:265–318.

9. Garretson HD. Vascular malformations and fistulas. In: Wilkins RH, Rengachary SS, eds. *Neurosurgery,* 2nd ed. New York: McGraw Hill, 1996:2433–2442.

10. Kassell NF, Shaffrey ME, Shaffrey CI. Cerebral vasospasm following aneurysmal subarachnoid hemorrhage. In: Apuzzo MLJ, ed. *Brain surgery: complication avoidance and management.* New York: Churchill Livingstone, 1993:857–889.

11. Mayberg MR. Intracranial arterial spasm. In: Wilkins RH, Rengachary SS, eds. *Neurosurgery,* 2nd ed. New York: McGraw-Hill, 1996:2245–2254.

12. Ogilvy CS, Carter BS. A proposed comprehensive grading system to predict outcome for surgical management of intracranial aneurysms. *Neurosurgery* 1998;42:959–970.

13. Samson DS, Batjer HH. Preoperative evaluation of the risk/benefit ratio for arteriovenous malformations of the brain. In: Wilkins RH, Rengachary SS, eds. *Neurosurgery,* 2nd ed. New York: McGraw-Hill, 1996:2443–2446.

14. Sugita K, Takayasu M. Arteriovenous malformations. In: Apuzzo MLJ, ed. *Brain surgery: complication avoidance and management.* New York: Churchill Livingstone, 1993:1113–1117.

Psychiatric Disease and Substance Abuse

James B. Mayfield and Michael E. Henry

This chapter describes the symptoms associated with the most common psychiatric disorders and discusses their effects on history taking and the preoperative and postoperative management of the patient.

Most patients, including those with psychiatric illnesses, are motivated to provide their physicians with information that leads to positive outcomes. The physician should use this interview time not only for medical fact finding but to establish the appropriate trust and rapport with the patient, even if someone else is to manage the anesthesia. An empathetic and caring anesthesiologist can have tremendous influence on the preoperative emotional state of most patients. A good rapport can have a significant influence on the type and amount of preoperative psychoactive medication needed to provide a smooth and comfortable induction of anesthesia.[1]

Despite the best efforts of the caregiver and the patient, a patient who is depressed, delusional, or combative may be unable to provide an accurate history or cooperate with procedures. In such cases, obtaining historical information from collateral sources, such as the patient's primary care physician, a family member, or staff from a group home, can be informative. When obtaining such information, the physician should remember that the medical care of psychiatric patients often is fragmented, and many family members may have distanced themselves from the patient or are estranged from the patient. A simple strategy that optimizes the formulation and implementation of an anesthetic plan is to include the patient in discussions of his or her physical health when possible or, at a minimum, to verify information obtained from outside sources with the patient. Even combative and highly agitated patients may be able to cooperate with focused questions.

When presented with a patient with obvious psychiatric symptoms, the physician should remember that many diseases and certain medications can cause symptoms often associated with psychiatric illnesses (Table 12-1). For example, symptoms of major depression can be the result of clinically significant hypothyroidism.[2] Patients with brain tumors can present with personality changes, delusions, and social impairment similar to those associated with the disorganized subtype of schizophrenia.[3] Approximately 50% of patients with acquired immunodeficiency syndrome develop a neuropsychiatric syndrome that can present as a dementia, delirium, or mood or personality disorder.[4] Age of onset, family history, and time course of the symptoms, as well as information from collateral sources, can be helpful in focusing the differential diagnosis.

Table 12-1. Medical problems that can cause psychiatric symptoms

Hypothyroidism and hyperthyroidism
Cushing's syndrome
Acquired immunodeficiency syndrome
Seizure disorders
Brain tumors
Encephalitis
Nutritional deficiency
Toxic substance poisoning
Drug dependency

MOOD DISORDERS

Mood disorders are among the most common psychiatric disorders. Major depression has a point prevalence of 2% to 4% in the adult population and is one of the leading causes of disability in the world.[5] During the course of their lifetimes, approximately 20% of women and 10% of men develop major depression.[6] The etiology of mood disorders is currently unknown; however, a combination of genetic and environmental factors clearly seem to be involved.[7] On the molecular level, dysfunctional regulation of several neurotransmitter systems has been implicated in the pathophysiology of depression.[7]

The diagnosis of major depression requires the presence of a depressed mood or anhedonia, and a disturbance in vegetative symptoms (such as insomnia or hypersomnia, anorexia, or hyperphagia) for a minimum of 2 weeks[8–10] (Table 12-2). The symptoms must also be of sufficient severity that they impair interpersonal, social, or occupational functioning. A major depression may be part of a bipolar illness, in which the patient can have episodes of mania as well as depression. This is an important differential diagnosis to make because manic episodes can be triggered by sleep deprivation. Because bipolar patients appear to have a predisposition toward substance abuse,[11] the anesthesiologist should carefully assess the patient's substance use history and take appropriate precautions to avoid withdrawal syndromes and narcotic abuse.

The medications used most commonly to treat major depression are the selective serotonin reuptake inhibitors (SSRIs). These drugs act by blocking the uptake of serotonin from the synaptic cleft. As their name implies, they are selective for serotonin and essentially have negligible activity on other neurotransmitter systems.[7,12] Paroxetine hydrochloride (Paxil), with its weak anticholinergic effects, may be an exception to this general rule.

In terms of anesthetic management, the most important effect of the SSRIs may be their potent inhibition of the cytochrome P-450 enzymes in the liver, especially the 2D6 isoenzyme.[7] Another important consideration postoperatively is that abrupt discontinuation of these agents has been associated with a unique discontinuation syndrome characterized by dizziness, irritability, headache,

Table 12-2. Diagnostic characteristics of major depression*

Depressed mood
Diminished pleasure or interest in activities
Significant weight loss or gain
Insomnia or hypersomnia
Psychomotor agitation or retardation
Fatigue or loss of energy
Feelings of worthlessness
Diminished ability to think or concentrate
Recurrent thoughts of death
Symptoms in the absence of delusions or hallucinations

*At least five of the symptoms must be present for at least a 2-week period.
Reprinted with permission from American Psychiatric Association. *Diagnostic and statistical manual of mental disorders*, 4th ed. Washington, DC: American Psychiatric Association Press, 1994.

nausea, visual disturbance, and electric shock sensations. The frequency and severity of the syndrome appear to be related to the elimination kinetics of the drug, so that drugs with short half-lives and no active metabolites are associated with a higher incidence of the syndrome.[13] Fluoxetine hydrochloride, with its relatively long half-life and long-acting active metabolite, appears to be associated with a significantly lower incidence of the syndrome. When the syndrome occurs, resumption of therapy usually results in quick resolution of the symptoms.[13]

Other classes of drugs used in the treatment of major depression include the heterocyclic antidepressants, monoamine oxidase inhibitors (MAOIs), and the "atypical" antidepressants. Of the heterocyclic compounds, the tricyclic antidepressants are the most common. These compounds are thought to exert their antidepressant effects by blocking the reuptake of norepinephrine and serotonin from the synaptic cleft. Their blockade of alpha$_1$-adrenergic, muscarinic, and histamine receptors, as well as their quinidine-like slowing of cardiac conduction, account for the majority of their side effects and potential interactions with anesthetic agents.[7,12]

MAOIs irreversibly block the oxidative deamination of catecholamines, thereby increasing the presynaptic concentration of serotonin, norepinephrine, and dopamine. The agents used to treat depression are phenelzine sulfate (Nardil), isocarboxazid (Marplan), and tranylcypromine sulfate (Parnate). The use of these drugs has been limited because of the dietary restrictions necessary to avoid a hypertensive crisis from dietary vasoactive amines, such as tyramine. From the anesthesiologist's point of view, the important issue to remember is that combining meperidine hydrochloride (Demerol) with an MAOI can lead to a "serotonin syndrome" that can progress to death. The use of sympathomimetics with indirect action (such as ephedrine) can lead to severe hypertension and is potentially fatal. Newer agents that are reversible inhibitors of MAO and transdermal preparations are currently under development. The use of these agents avoids the dietary restrictions but probably not the potential for dangerous interactions with other drugs as noted above. Once the patient stops taking an MAOI, up to 2 weeks can be required before the inactivated enzyme is replaced with newly synthesized, active MAO.[12]

The atypical antidepressants include bupropion hydrochloride, nefazodone hydrochloride, trazodone hydrochloride, and mirtazapine. They are an eclectic group of medications whose receptor-binding and side-effect profiles should be reviewed when they are encountered. Bupropion hydrochloride, under the trade name Zyban, is also approved as an aid to smoking cessation. This drug has been found to be associated with a dose-dependent increase in the incidence of seizures in patients with a history of head trauma, prior seizure, or central nervous system tumor, or concomitant use of medications that lower seizure threshold.[14] Otherwise, its favorable cardiac and side effect profile makes it useful in the treatment of bipolar depression and depression in elderly patients.

Mania, which is often considered the opposite of depression,[9] is usually managed by the use of mood-stabilizing drugs. Most frequently, the drug is lithium or an antiepileptic medication. With regard to anesthesia, lithium has three effects that should be kept in mind. First, lithium impairs renal concentrating ability, producing a nephrogenic diabetes insipidus[14] that can result in unusually large fluid requirements. Second, lithium has been shown to impair thyroid hormone production and produce hypothyroidism and goiters.[14] Third, discontinuation of lithium has been associated with increased incidence of suicidal behavior.[15] Psychiatric consultation should be considered in almost all cases of bipolar disorder. The antiepileptic drugs are frequently used to treat patients with bipolar disorder. The kindling hypothesis of the natural history of mood disorders led to their discovery as mood stabilizers.[16] Their therapeutic efficacy has been demonstrated in controlled double-blind trials. The four most commonly used drugs are valproate sodium, carbamazepine, lamotrigine, and gabapentin. With the exception of gabapentin, which is cleared unmetabolized by the kidney, these drugs are metabolized by the liver.[14] Because of this, their effects on the metabolism of other medications may be variable. For example, valproate sodium tends to slow the metabolism of other drugs, whereas carbamazepine induces the production of hepatic enzymes and speeds up metabolism of itself and other drugs.[14] Although the effects of most anesthetics wear off by redistribution of the agents from the brain to other tissues, anesthetics that require hepatic metabolism for termination of their effects may have their rates of clearance significantly altered by the mood-stabilizing drugs. In addition, these drugs may have significant bone marrow effects that result in anemia or thrombocytopenia.[14] The preoperative evaluation of patients taking these medications should include liver function tests and a complete blood cell count. Another important consideration in the management of patients taking these medications is that abrupt discontinuation of these drugs can result in withdrawal seizures.[14] Lamotrigine is unique among these drugs in that a too-rapid escalation of the dose increases the risk of rash, which can progress to Stevens-Johnson syndrome and can be fatal.[14] To the authors' knowledge, no data exist on the management of treatment interruption of several days' duration. In the absence of such data, depending on the time interval since the last dose, titrating back to the preoperative dose may be best.

Finally, severe depression may affect patients' judgment. For example, depressed patients have been known to consent to high-risk procedures as part of a suicide attempt. Physically, severely depressed patients may have extremely poor oral intake that leads to hypotension and electrolyte abnormalities. Sometimes postponement of an elective procedure until the patient can be properly managed and is feeling better may be the best option.

ANXIETY AND PANIC DISORDERS

Anxiety is a normal human emotion for patients confronted with the prospect of undergoing a medical or surgical procedure. Anxiety disorders can be subdivided into generalized anxiety, panic disorder, obsessive compulsive disorder (OCD), and post-traumatic stress disorder (PTSD).[9] The differentiation of an anxiety disorder from the expected situational anxiety of the evaluation rests primarily on past history and the severity of the response.

Patients with generalized anxiety disorder are chronic worriers, whereas patients with panic disorder describe discrete episodes of very intense anxiety during which they are convinced that something catastrophic is about to happen. Panic disorder usually develops in young adulthood, with a mean age of onset of approximately 25 years and an equal incidence among men and women.[9] Patients with panic disorder may comprise as many as 15% of those who consult a cardiologist, 25% of those who consult an internist for psychiatric symptoms, and 10% to 15% of patients in outpatient psychiatric practices.[17,18] Many of these patients develop concurrent agoraphobia, which may make it difficult for them to come to the preoperative interview.

OCD is characterized by obsessions, which are intrusive recurrent thoughts, and by compulsions, which are repetitive actions designed to alleviate the anxiety caused by the obsessions.[19] Patients with PTSD have a history of undergoing some traumatic event and expend a great deal of energy avoiding anything that reminds them of the event. Depending on where they are in the course of their illness, these patients may also experience flashbacks in which they relive the traumatic event.[9] Incest survivors commonly experience PTSD and may have difficulties in turning over control of their bodies to the anesthesia and surgical teams. Knowledge of the gender of the abuser can be helpful in formulating the anesthesia treatment plan.

The principal treatment for anxiety disorders is a combination of antidepressant medications and psychotherapy.[12,19] Behavioral techniques such as meditation and relaxation taught during psychotherapy[12,19] can be very effective during the perioperative period in helping the patient with an anxiety disorder. The clinician can have a positive influence by inquiring as to which techniques are useful for the patient and then encouraging the patient to apply these relaxation techniques throughout the perioperative process.[20,21] Judicious use of benzodiazepines and β-blockers can greatly improve the patient's experience and clinical outcome.

SCHIZOPHRENIA

Schizophrenia is a chronic condition that affects approximately 1% of the population.[9] The symptoms, which usually begin before age 25 years, are seen in all socioeconomic classes and persist throughout life.[3,22] The disease is marked by acute exacerbations with progressive deterioration between episodes. Schizophrenia appears to include a variety of disorders with somewhat similar behavioral symptoms. Psychotic episodes manifested by hallucinations, delusions, and inappropriate affect comprise most of the acute clinical presentation. The inappropriate affect may reflect a poverty of thought or excessive involvement with psychotic internal dialogue.

When the clinician approaches the preoperative assessment of an acutely ill schizophrenic patient, speaking with the patient's caregivers before meeting with the patient is advisable. This gives the clinician an opportunity to understand the patient's delusional system and determine the best way to approach the patient for the interview and physical examination, so that the anesthesiologist avoids becoming entrapped in the patient's psychosis.

One finding that has been fairly consistently noted across several studies is the decrease of frontal lobe function in these patients.[23] Therefore, they are unable to read social cues, often appear unkempt, and have difficulty getting organized to take action. The frontal dysfunction also has been hypothesized to be responsible for the high incidence of cigarette smoking in these patients.[24] Because of the stimulant properties of nicotine, smoking is thought to be an attempt to self-medicate the decreased frontal lobe function. As a result, these patients have a high incidence of smoking-related illnesses, chronic obstructive pulmonary disease, and coronary artery disease.

Drug treatment of schizophrenia is with antipsychotic medications. In addition to dopamine blockade, these drugs also cause alpha blockade, which may result in exaggerated hypotensive responses to anesthesia.[25] Antipsychotics also affect cardiac conduction and electrocardiogram (ECG) wave morphology and may increase the risk of sudden death.[26] These drugs are classified as either typical (haloperidol, Thorazine) or atypical (risperidone, chlozapine). The most common side effects of typical antipsychotics are extrapyramidal symptoms, orthostatic hypotension, and sedation.[26] Atypical antipsychotics have fewer dopamine receptor blocking abilities and are less likely to cause parkinsonism, akathisia, and tardive dyskinesia. Preoperatively, these patients need evaluation of an ECG and, if they are chronic smokers, a chest radiograph.

SUBSTANCE ABUSE

Substance abuse in its many forms exists throughout the general population without regard to economic or social status. It tends to be more prevalent in the young adult population (ages 17 to 30) than among other age groups and remains more common among urban men than women.[27] Substance abuse may be defined as the use of any substance that alters consciousness or state of mind, that deviates from accepted medical or social use, and can lead to physical or psychological dependence. Dependence is diagnosed when a patient exhibits three or more of the characteristic symptoms listed in Table 12-3 during a given 12-month period.

Table 12-3. Criteria for psychoactive substance dependence

Increasing tolerance to substance effects

Characteristic withdrawal symptoms or substance use to avoid withdrawal symptoms

Substance taken in larger amounts than intended

Unsuccessful attempts to decrease substance intake

Increased time obtaining substance or recovering from effects

Reduced social or occupational activities due to substance use

Continued substance use despite substance-related social or medical problems

Reprinted with permission from American Psychiatric Association. *Diagnostic and statistical manual of mental disorders*, 4th ed. Washington, DC: American Psychiatric Association Press, 1994.

In this section, the preoperative evaluation of patients with the three most common substance abuse disorders—abuse of alcohol, cocaine, and opioids—is discussed. Barbiturates, benzodiazepines, hallucinogens, and marijuana all have significant abuse potential and should be considered in any preoperative evaluation.[27] Usually, the combination of these less common drugs with alcohol in the acute setting is what may require the clinician to prepare for unusual responses to anesthesia. Polysubstance abuse is common. Preoperative knowledge of a patient's substance abuse may prevent serious drug interactions and predict the need for an alteration in anesthetic agents. Unusual postoperative symptoms may be attributable to substance withdrawal syndromes that, if unknown and untreated, can be life-threatening.

A nonjudgmental, compassionate approach to individuals who use substances of abuse is most successful. A desirable preoperative objective is anxiolysis without producing a conscious euphoria that could reactivate prior behaviors. Buspirone (BuSpar) and hydroxyzine (Vistaril) have small abuse potential. Patients should receive enough narcotics to manage pain. Use of nonopioid analgesics (nonsteroidal antiinflammatory drugs) or regional anesthesia/analgesia are preferable. The risk of relapse is real but manageable. Consultation with an addictionist or pain specialist may be helpful.

Alcohol Abuse

Alcoholism is a common term defined as a disease manifested by the chronic and excessive consumption of alcohol that causes social, psychological, and medical problems. The major risk factors for developing alcoholism are a family history of alcohol abuse and male gender.[28] Alcohol abuse appears to be widespread throughout most cultures worldwide and affects at least 10 million to 15 million Americans.[29] The diagnosis of excessive alcohol intake is difficult to determine during a preoperative evaluation. The clinician can have a high index of suspicion, however, from a detailed history and physical examination. Although the patient may admit to daily alcohol intake, suggestive evidence comes from a history of alcohol-related medical problems.

Medical complications of excessive alcohol intake involve every organ system. Central nervous system effects include cerebral atrophy and cerebellar degeneration with associated amnestic black-outs and tremor. The cardiovascular system may show signs of a dilated cardiomyopathy, dysrhythmias, peripheral vascular insufficiency, and hypertension.[27] Gastritis, esophagitis, esophageal varices, gastric ulcers, pancreatitis, hepatitis, and hepatic cirrhosis are common among chronic alcohol abusers. Nutritional and metabolic effects include Wernicke-Korsakoff syndrome, hypoalbuminemia, hypomagnesemia, pellagra, and beriberi.[28] The majority of alcoholics are heavy smokers. Currently, no laboratory test exists that is specific for alcohol abuse or dependence, but elevated liver enzymes[30] and red blood cell mean corpuscular volume greater than 94 fL[31] can be suggestive of chronic alcohol ingestion.

As for screening tools available, the CAGE questionnaire can be helpful in eliciting a history of alcohol dependence. Specifically, patients are asked if they have ever tried to *c*ut down on their drinking, become *a*nnoyed by criticism of their drinking habits, felt *g*uilty about the amount they drink, or needed an *e*ye opener in the morning. Two or more positive answers to these four questions have a 60% to 95% sensitivity and a 40% to 95% specificity for lifetime alcohol problems.[28]

The primary treatment for alcohol abuse and dependence is active participation in Alcoholics Anonymous (AA) or one of the other groups that are similar to AA but are not based on the concept of a higher power. Pharmacotherapy for alcoholism is not common, but disulfiram (Antabuse) is used in refractory cases. Disulfiram therapy inhibits alcohol metabolism at the level of aldehyde dehydrogenase, and it occasionally causes hepatotoxicity.[27]

Delirium tremens is a medical emergency that occurs in 5% of patients who experience alcohol withdrawal symptoms. It is manifested as altered consciousness, confusion, hallucinations (usually visual and tactile), hypertension, hyperthermia, and grand mal seizures. It is potentially fatal. Once symptoms are under control, benzodiazepine dosage should be gradually tapered. The use of β-blockers is controversial because these drugs can mask symptoms of inadequate benzodiazepine coverage. Management of withdrawal or delirium tremens is with lorazepam, 2 mg (or an equivalent dose of another benzodiazepine), orally or intramuscularly every 1 to 2 hours until symptoms are suppressed. Thiamine, 100 mg, and folate, 1 mg, intravenously or intramuscularly should be given.

Preoperatively, these patients need an ECG and chest radiograph. Prothrombin time, hematocrit, albumin, glucose, bilirubin, serum alanine aminotransferase, aspartate aminotransferase, and alkaline phosphatase levels should be determined. Acutely intoxicated patients need a serum alcohol level determination.

One should anticipate withdrawal or delirium tremens and treat appropriately. Acutely intoxicated patients have delayed gastric emptying and should be treated with histamine$_2$ blockers, sodium citrate, and metoclopramide. They also have a decreased requirement for anesthesia and, because of alcohol-induced vasodilation, are prone to hypotension. Patients being treated with disulfiram may require less anesthetic medication because of disulfiram sedation. They are acutely sensitive (experiencing flushing, nausea, tachycardia) to small amounts of alcohol (skin preparations, medications). See Chapter 9 for a discussion of the patient with hepatitis or cirrhosis.

Patients in recovery in a 12-step program should intensify their therapy preoperatively and arrange for postoperative visits with their sponsor.

Cocaine Abuse

The prevalence of cocaine abuse is a public health problem. Estimates are that 20 million to 30 million Americans have used cocaine, and up to 5 million use it regularly.[32]

The acute effects of cocaine use include dramatic enhancement of sympathetic nervous system activity due to inhibition of catecholamine reuptake and direct stimulation of dopamine receptors. Patients with acute intoxication present with marked hypertension, tachycardia, mydriasis, elation, euphoria, and heightened self-esteem. These effects are self-limited, and full recovery occurs within 48 hours. As the effects wear off, dysphoria, agitation, and fatigue are common. Chronic use of cocaine is characterized by continual irritability, impaired judgment, and aggression.[33] Although uncommon, cocaine psychosis, which may occur after short-term cocaine exposure, may be quite debilitating. Cardiac effects, including acute myocardial infarction and arrhythmias, can be seen in both chronic and first-time users.

Diagnosis of cocaine abuse begins with suspicion arising from clinical observation, both physical and psychological.[29] Obtaining a complete history may be difficult in a patient with postcocaine dysphoria or sociopathic tendencies. Patients may be more cooperative if they are reassured about doctor-patient confidentiality and the clinician maintains a nonjudgmental approach.

The mode of ingestion is an important determinant of the sequelae of cocaine use. The nasal mucosa may be damaged or even necrotic in patients who snort cocaine powder, so that placement of a nasogastric or nasotracheal tube is risky. Intravenous administration may be associated with limited access for intravenous catheter placement and, more important, with hepatitis B and human immunodeficiency virus (HIV) infection (see Chapter 15).

Preoperatively, these patients need an ECG, a chest radiograph, and further studies based on complications resulting from their substance abuse (Table 12-4).

Neuroleptics and benzodiazepines are useful for cocaine-induced paranoia. Acute ingestion of cocaine increases anesthesia requirements. One should anticipate the need for central intravenous catheters. Comorbidities may require additional planning.

Opioid Abuse

Opioids produce both physical and psychological dependence. Morphine and heroin are the most frequently abused drugs in this class. Not uncommonly, however, patients are dependent on codeine, hydromorphone hydrochloride, meperidine hydrochloride, and methadone hydrochloride. The number of opioid addicts in the United States is unknown. The number of heroin addicts, who comprise the majority of those abusing drugs in this class, is estimated at 500,000.[34]

Anesthetic requirements for patients who are long-term users of high-dose opioids may vary significantly from those for normal patients, depending on the duration of use and acquired comorbid medical illnesses[35] (see Table 12-4).

The intravenous route of opioid use is associated with cutaneous infections such as cellulitis, thrombophlebitis, and skin abscesses. Systemic infections such as tetanus, hepatitis, and HIV are common in the long-term opioid abuser. Endocarditis and pulmonary

Table 12-4. Common medical problems encountered in chronic opioid and cocaine abusers

Infections
   Septic thrombophlebitis
   Cellulitis
   Skin abscesses
   Tetanus
   Hepatitis
   Human immunodeficiency virus infection
Cardiovascular problems
   Endocarditis and valvular insufficiency
   Septic emboli and infarctions
   Severe hypotension after overdose
Pulmonary problems
   Pulmonary emboli
   Aspiration pneumonitis
   Hypoventilation after overdose
   Hypoxic pulmonary edema after overdose
Hepatic problems
   Hepatic insufficiency
   Hepatitis
Central nervous system problems
   Dysphoria
   Unconsciousness after overdose
   Seizures after overdose
Malnutrition
   Iron-deficiency anemia

Data from Kaplan H, Sadock B. *Synopsis of psychiatry behavioral sciences/clinical psychiatry,* 8th ed. Baltimore: Williams & Wilkins, 1998:419–425; Mendelson JH, Mello NK. Management of cocaine abuse and dependence. *N Engl J Med* 1996;334:965–972.

emboli may complicate the cardiopulmonary system. Other major diseases that may lead to possible anesthetic complications include hepatic insufficiency and chronic pain syndromes.

As with all suspected substance abusers, the clinician should obtain a complete history, including duration of abuse, time and amount of last dose, route of administration, and associated medical problems. For a variety of reasons, including substance-induced personality changes and cognitive changes, patients may be unable or unwilling to provide an accurate history. In these cases, a thorough physical examination in which the clinician seeks evidence of medical problems associated with substance abuse minimizes surprises in perioperative anesthetic management.

For preoperative diagnostics and anesthetic implications, see Cocaine Abuse, earlier. Acute opioid ingestion delays gastric emptying (see Alcohol Abuse) and decreases anesthetic requirements. Chronic use produces a tolerance to anesthetics. Patients in methadone programs should receive their usual daily dose preoperatively. Care providers should check with the clinic to confirm the dose and notify them of the hospitalization so the patient is not dropped from the program.

CASE STUDY

The patient is a 62-year-old man with a history of abdominal pain and vomiting of blood and material resembling coffee grounds. He is scheduled for an upper gastrointestinal endoscopy and heat ablation of a bleeding gastric ulcer. The patient is a long-time resident of a nursing facility and has a history of mild mental retardation, a seizure disorder, a gastric ulcer, and catatonic schizophrenia. This information was obtained from the gastroenterologist, who has asked that an anesthesiologist help in evaluating and managing this complex case.

Before approaching this patient, as much information as possible should be found out about him from the current nursing staff, friends, family members, the local nursing facility where he resides, and his primary care physician. Important aspects that should be known before this patient is visited include (a) how he reacts to new people or physicians, (b) how he communicates with people, (c) whether he is prone to aggressive behavior, (d) whether he will tolerate a physical examination, and (e) whether the patient has a legal guardian with whom to discuss issues of informed consent for the procedure.

Conversations with others reveal that the patient does not communicate beyond simple yes or no answers. He is subdued and not prone to aggressive behavior, but he has pulled out several intravenous catheters. He does become frustrated with prolonged visits from or examinations by physicians, but he tolerates new people.

Review of his record should include his current hospital course, treatment, and allergies; his old record, with history of previous treatments and surgery; and, if possible, a summary of his nursing facility care and treatment. In particular, records of previous anesthesia and surgery and how induction was tolerated would be helpful. Information in his record reveals that he has a history of recurrent gastric bleeding but never required transfusions. He was diagnosed with schizophrenia at the age of 25 and has been in a local nursing facility for 12 years. He has had endoscopy procedures in the past under monitored anesthesia care without problems. He was not intubated for these previous procedures. His medications include clonazepam (Klonopin), carbamazepine (Tegretol), thioridazine hydrochloride, benztropine mesylate (Cogentin), cisapride (Propulsid), and docusate sodium (Colace). He has an allergy to haloperidol (Haldol).

With this information, the physician meets the patient with his nurse. He is shy and reserved but tolerates a brief examination. His blood pressure is 110/70 mm Hg and heart rate is 98 beats per minute while supine, and blood pressure is 88/50 mm Hg and heart rate is 98 beats per minute while standing. Respirations are 16 per minute. The patient has an edentulous oral cavity and decreased breath sounds due to poor inspiratory effort. The rest of his examination is normal. Laboratory tests should be performed only as indicated by the patient's medical problems and current condition. This patient has several issues that call for laboratory evaluation, including his age of 62 years, history of vomiting and bleeding, history of gastric ulcer, and seizure disorder. Results include a hematocrit of 38 and normal electrolyte levels, coagulation studies, and ECG.

Before surgery, the patient should receive his medications at the regular time. No reason usually exists to discontinue psychiatric medications before surgery. The antipsychotic medication thioridazine hydrochloride may have effects on the heart, with T wave flattening, ST segment depression, and prolongation of the PR and QT intervals. Thioridazine hydrochloride is a D_2 dopamine antagonist. Mild alpha-adrenergic blockade and anticholinergic activity may manifest as orthostatic hypotension and dystonic reactions. The patient needs an intravenous line for preoperative hydration. This may be difficult in uncooperative patients; however, induction of general anesthesia in a dehydrated patient may cause significant hypotension.

Anxious or uncooperative patients may need preoperative medications before going to the operating room. If the medication is given orally, sufficient time should be allowed for maximum drug effect. The patient has a bleeding gastric ulcer, which can interfere with gastric emptying. Administration of a nonparticulate antacid, metoclopramide, and a histamine$_2$ blocker are indicated.

In patients with a long history of psychiatric problems, tolerance to the effects of hypnotic agents may make judging the patient's dose requirements difficult. Significantly higher doses of anesthetic agents may be needed with such patients. In these cases, a bispectral analysis monitor can be useful to determine the adequacy of hypnotic effects.

REFERENCES

1. Klafta JM, Roizen MF. Current understanding of patient's attitudes toward and preparation for anesthesia: a review. *Anesth Analg* 1996;83:1314–1321.
2. Hale AS. ABC of mental health. Depression. *BMJ* 1997;315:43–46.
3. Turner T. ABC of mental health. Schizophrenia. *BMJ* 1997; 315:108–111.
4. Kaplan H, Sadock B. *Synopsis of psychiatry behavioral sciences/ clinical psychiatry*, 8th ed. Baltimore: Williams & Wilkins 1998: 456–491.
5. Murray CJL, Lopez AD. Alternating visions of the future: projecting mortality and disability, 1990–2020. In: Murray CJL, Lopez AD, eds. *The global burden of disease*. Cambridge, MA: Harvard University Press, 1996.
6. Depression Guideline Panel. Depression in primary care. Rockville, MD: U.S. Department of Health and Human Services, Agency for Health Care Policy and Research, 1993. Detection and Diagnosis, vol 1. Clinical Practice Guideline, no 5. AHCPR publication 93-0550.
7. Gruenberg AM, Goldstein RD. Depressive disorders. In: Tasman A, Kay J, Lieberman JA, eds. *Psychiatry*. Philadelphia: WB Saunders, 1997:990–1019.
8. Lebowitz BD, Pearson JL, Schneider LS, et al. Diagnosis and treatment of depression in late life. Consensus statement update. *JAMA* 1997;278:1186–1190.
9. American Psychiatric Association. *Diagnostic and statistical manual of mental disorders*, 4th ed. Washington, DC: American Psychiatric Association Press, 1994.
10. Meagher D, Murray D. Depression. *Lancet* 1997;349[Suppl]: 17sl–20sl.

11. Frank E, Thase ME. Natural history and preventative treatment of recurrent mood disorders. *Ann Rev Med* 1999;50:453–468.
12. Kellar MB, Boland RJ. Antidepressants. In: Tasman A, Kay J, Lieberman JA, eds. *Psychiatry.* Philadelphia: WB Saunders, 1997:1606–1639.
13. Rosenbaum JF, Fava M, Hoog SL, et al. Selective serotonin reuptake inhibitor discontinuation syndrome: a randomized clinical trial. *Biol Psychiatry* 1998;44:77–87.
14. *Physicians' desk reference.* Montvale, NJ: Medical Economics Co, 1999.
15. Tondo L, Baldessarini RJ, Hennen J, et al. Lithium treatment and risk of suicidal behavior in bipolar disorder patients. *J Clin Psychiatry* 1998;59:405–414.
16. Post RM, Denicoff KD, Frye MA, et al. A history of the use of anticonvulsants as mood stabilizers in the last two decades of the 20th century. *Neuropsychobiology* 1998;38:152–166.
17. Kaplan H, Sadock B. *Synopsis of psychiatry behavioral sciences/ clinical psychiatry,* 8th ed. Baltimore: Williams & Wilkins, 1998: 623–628.
18. Mintzer O, Lydiard RB. Generalized anxiety disorders. In: Tasman A, Kay J, Lieberman JA, eds. *Psychiatry.* Philadelphia: WB Saunders, 1997:1100–1116.
19. Jenkusky SM, Reeve A, Uhlenhuth EH. Anxiolytic drugs. In: Tasman A, Kay J, Lieberman JA, eds. *Psychiatry.* Philadelphia: WB Saunders, 1997:1640–1649.
20. Wolfe BE, Maser JD, eds. *Treatment of panic disorder.* Washington, DC: American Psychiatric Press, 1994.
21. Spiegel DA, Bruce TJ. Benzodiazepines and exposure-based cognitive behavior therapies for panic disorder: conclusions from combined treatment trials. *Am J Psychiatry* 1997;154:773–781.
22. Kane JM. Drug therapy: schizophrenia. *N Engl J Med* 1996;334: 34–41.
23. Pinals DA, Breier A. Schizophrenia. In: Tasman A, Kay J, Lieberman JA, eds. *Psychiatry.* Philadelphia: WB Saunders, 1997:927–965.
24. Dalack GW, Healy DJ, Meador-Woodruff JH. Nicotine dependence in schizophrenia: clinical phenomena and laboratory findings. *Am J Psychiatry* 1998;155:1490–1501.
25. Pinals DA, Breier A. Schizophrenia. In: Tasman A, Kay J, Lieberman JA, eds. *Psychiatry.* Philadelphia: WB Saunders, 1997:927–951.
26. Marder SR. Antipsychotic drugs. In: Tasman A, Kay J, Lieberman JA, eds. *Psychiatry.* Philadelphia: WB Saunders, 1997:1569–1585.
27. Larson MJ, Samet JH, McCarty D. Managed care of substance abuse disorders. Implications for generalist physicians. *Med Clin North Am* 1997;81:1053–1069.
28. O'Connor P, Schottenfeld R. Patients with alcohol problems. *N Engl J Med* 1998;338:592–601.
29. Schorling JB, Buchsbaum D. Screening for alcohol and drug abuse. *Med Clin North Am* 1997;81:845–865.
30. Holt S, Skinner HA, Isreal Y. Early identification of alcohol abuse. II. Clinical and laboratory indicators. *Can Med Assoc J* 1981;124:1279–1295.
31. Peach HG, Bath NE, Farish S. Predictive value of MCV for hazardous drinking in the community. *Clin Lab Haematol* 1997;19: 85–87.
32. Kaplan H, Sadock B. *Synopsis of psychiatry behavioral sciences/ clinical psychiatry,* 8th ed. Baltimore: Williams & Wilkins, 1998: 419–425.
33. Mendelson JH, Mello NK. Management of cocaine abuse and dependence. *N Engl J Med* 1996;334:965–972.
34. Woody GE, McNichols LF. Opioid-related disorders. In: Tasman A, Kay J, Lieberman JA, eds. *Psychiatry.* Philadelphia: WB Saunders, 1997:867–878.
35. Warner EA, Kosten TR, O'Connor PG. Pharmacotherapy for opioid and cocaine abuse. *Med Clin North Am* 1997;81:909–925.

The Pediatric Patient

Lynne R. Ferrari

The objective of the preoperative evaluation of the pediatric surgical patient is to gather medical information and alleviate the fear and anxiety that exist for the patient and family. Parents are often more concerned with the risks and administration of anesthesia when their children are receiving anesthesia than they would be if they were receiving the anesthesia themselves. The preoperative visit should be viewed as an opportunity for the anesthesiologist to evaluate the child's psychological status and family interactions.

PSYCHOLOGICAL PREPARATION

Diseases carry with them a psychosocial aspect that is different in children than in adults. For many healthy children undergoing elective surgery, the emotional disruption may surpass the medical issues.[1] Children respond to the prospect of surgery in a varied and age-dependent manner, and the anesthesiologist must address this during the preoperative interview.

The understanding of and response to illness is affected by a child's maturity. The medical practitioner should anticipate the child's needs and concerns and be able to interpret the child's nonverbal expressions and actions when communication skills are not highly developed. The toddler's greatest fear is the loss of control of actions and choices. Helping a child make choices in the health care setting is important. A choice as simple as, "What flavor air would you like in the mask?" puts the toddler in control of this aspect of the situation. The preschooler fears injury, loss of control, the unknown, and abandonment. The preschooler interprets words literally and is unable to differentiate between what is heard and what is actually being implied. The words adults use with children are as important as the messages they try to convey. Telling a preschooler that he or she is going to be "put to sleep" for an operation may be scary and confusing for a child whose pet was recently put to sleep. Because preschoolers are unable to distinguish between reality and fantasy and exist in a world of magical thinking, they are unable to recognize the difference between the safe kind of sleep from anesthesia and the kind of sleep from which their animal did not awaken. The school-aged child fears loss of control, injury, inability to meet the expectations set by adults, and death. Between the ages of 6 and 12, children begin to think more logically; they may nod with understanding and listen intently, when in fact they do not fully grasp the explanation. These children may fail to ask questions or admit a lack of knowledge because they feel that

Table 13-1. Minor anesthesia-related risk in pediatric patients

Event	Risk
Laryngospasm	
0–9 years of age	17:1,000
Concomitant respiratory infection	96:1,000
Previous anesthetic complications	55:1,000
Bronchospasm	
0–9 years of age	4:1,000
Concomitant respiratory infection	41:1,000
Abnormal ECG	24:1,000
ASA physical status score ≥3	24:1,000
Aspiration pneumonia	1.7:1,000

ASA, American Society of Anesthesiologists; ECG, electrocardiogram.

they should know the information. Adolescents fear loss of control, an altered body image, and segregation from peers. They are usually convinced that the anesthesiologist will not be able to put them to sleep and that, if the anesthesiologist does succeed, they will never wake up.[2]

RISKS OF ANESTHESIA

Parents may ask about the risks of anesthesia for their child. As with all patients, this matter must be considered on an individual basis, with the child's age, type of surgery, and other confounding factors taken into account. Minor risks that occur more frequently in pediatric patients include laryngospasm, bronchospasm, and croup (Table 13-1). Parents are most concerned with the risk of death, which occurs at a rate of 1 in 185,000 healthy children. Most deaths that are due entirely to anesthesia occur in the first week of life.[3]

HISTORY AND REVIEW OF SYSTEMS

The medical history for pediatric patients begins with a description of the prenatal period. Events during pregnancy and delivery may influence the current state of health (Table 13-2). If a patient has a history of having been admitted to the neonatal intensive care unit after birth, specific conditions should be ruled out[4] (Tables 13-3 and 13-4). Previous surgical experiences or medical admissions to the hospital should be noted. A complete review of systems should be completed, with particular attention to the items listed in Table 13-5.[5]

The child's prior anesthetic experience should be explored during the preoperative visit. The child's reaction to previous anesthetics is important and may predict the response to this anesthesia and indicate which techniques to use or avoid. Was anesthesia induced with a mask? Was the parent present during

Table 13-2. Neonatal problems commonly associated with maternal history

Neonatal problem	Maternal history
Hemolytic anemia Hyperbilirubinemia Kernicterus	Rh-ABO incompatibility
Small for gestational age	Toxemia
Small for gestational age Drug withdrawal	Drug addiction
Sepsis Thrombocytopenia Viral infection	Maternal infection
Anemia Hypotension Shock	Hemorrhage
Hypoglycemia Birth trauma Large for gestational age	Maternal diabetes mellitus
Tracheoesophageal fistula Anencephaly Multiple anomalies	Polyhydramnios
Renal hypoplasia Pulmonary hypoplasia	Oligohydramnios
Birth trauma Hyperbilirubinemia Fractures	Cephalopelvic disproportion
Hypoglycemia Congenital malformations Fetal alcohol syndrome Small for gestational age	Alcoholism

Adapted with permission from Cote C, Ryan J, Todres ID, Goudsouzian N, eds. *A practice of anesthesia for infants and children.* Philadelphia: WB Saunders, 1993.

induction? Was the induction difficult? Were any sequelae noted after the hospital experience, such as nightmares, bad dreams, regression to earlier behavior, or new fears of odors? Will the child probably require premedication?

Family history regarding anesthesia-related events should be explored. Because halothane may be chosen for inhalation induction in children, a history of halothane hepatitis or liver problems after anesthesia should be sought. Malignant hyperthermia is always a concern in the pediatric age group, and high fevers or unusual events in the operating room (OR) or in family members should be investigated (see Chapter 14). Although most pediatric anesthesiologists refrain from using succinylcholine, questions should be asked about prolonged paralysis or mechanical ventilation after general anesthesia in family members. If a history of pseudocholinesterase deficiency is possible, a simple blood test can be performed to

Table 13-3. Problems encountered in the premature infant

Problem	Anesthetic concern
Intraventricular hemorrhage	Presence of VP shunt
Retinopathy of prematurity	Strict attention to inspired oxygen concentration
Patent ductus arteriosus	Need for prior surgical intervention
Bronchopulmonary dysplasia	Respiratory compromise
Necrotizing enterocolitis	Ostomy/malabsorption
Anemia	Perioperative oxygen-carrying capacity
Hypoglycemia	Choice of intravenous fluid
Hyperbilirubinemia	Possibility of prior transfusion
Sepsis	Hemodynamic instability, respiration compromise, multiorgan failure
Hypothermia	Adjustment of OR environment
Apnea and bradycardia	Postanesthetic monitoring
Social problems	Parental concerns

OR, operating room; VP, ventriculoperitoneal.

determine if that child is at risk (see Chapter 14). Succinylcholine and mivacurium should be avoided in patients with enzyme deficiencies. Families should be asked about any history of unexpected death, sudden infant death syndrome, genetic defects, or familial conditions such as muscular dystrophy, cystic fibrosis, sickle cell disease, bleeding tendencies, or human immunodeficiency virus infection.

Table 13-4. Potential medical problems associated with admission to the neonatal intensive care unit

Condition	Potential problem
Esophageal atresia	Tracheoesophageal fistula
	Esophageal dysmotility
Diaphragmatic hernia	Pulmonary hypertension
	Hypoplastic lungs
	Congenital heart disease
Myelodysplasia	Hydrocephalus
	Urogenital disease
	Latex allergy
Omphalocele/gastroschisis	Associated midline defects
	Congenital cardiac abnormalities
	Small abdominal cavity
	Poor body temperature maintenance
Tracheoesophageal fistula	Cardiac defects
	Musculoskeletal abnormalities

Adapted with permission from Badgwell JM, ed. *Clinical pediatric anesthesia.* Philadelphia: Lippincott–Raven Publishers, 1997.

Table 13-5. Systems approach to questioning

System	Focus of questions	Possible anesthetic concerns
Respiratory	Cough, asthma, recent cold	Irritable airway, broncho-spasm, atelectasis, pneumonia
Cardiovascular	Murmur, cyanosis, history of squatting, hypertension, rheumatic fever, exercise intolerance	Avoidance of air bubbles in IV, right-to-left shunt, tetralogy of Fallot, coarctation, renal disease, congestive heart failure, cyanosis
Neurologic	Seizures, head trauma, swallowing problems	Medication interactions, metabolic derangement, increased intracranial pressure, aspiration, neuro-muscular relaxant sensitivity, hyperpyrexia
Gastrointestinal/hepatic	Vomiting, diarrhea, malabsorption, black stool, gastroesophageal reflux, jaundice	Electrolyte imbalance, dehydration, full stomach considerations (rapid-sequence induction), anemia, hypovolemia, hypoglycemia
Genitourinary	Frequency, time of last urination, frequency of urinary tract infections	Infection, hypercalcemia, hydration status, adequacy of renal function
Endocrine-metabolic	Abnormal development, hypoglycemia, steroid therapy	Endocrinopathy, hypothyroidism, diabetes mellitus, hypoglycemia, adrenal insufficiency
Hematologic	Anemia, bruising, excess bleeding	Transfusion requirement, coagulopathy, thrombocytopenia, hydration status, possible exchange transfusion
Allergy	Medications	Drug interactions
Dental	Loose teeth, carious teeth	Aspiration of loose teeth, SBE prophylaxis

SBE, subacute bacterial endocarditis.
Adapted with permission from Cote C, Ryan J, Todres ID, Goudsouzian N, eds. *A practice of anesthesia for infants and children*. Philadelphia: WB Saunders, 1993.

MEDICATIONS AND ALLERGIES

Currently prescribed and previously ingested medications can have significant effects on the outcome of general anesthesia. Many nonprescription cold remedies contain aspirin or aspirin-like compounds that interfere with platelet function and coagulation. The use of nonsteroidal antiinflammatory drugs should be investigated. In children who have been treated for a malignancy, specific chemotherapeutic regimens should be determined. The anthracycline drugs [doxorubicin hydrochloride (Adriamycin) and daunomycin] cause myocardial dysfunction, which may require further preoperative investigation with an echocardiogram. Use of mitomycin and bleomycin sulfate may result in pulmonary dysfunction, which may need further evaluation with pulse oximetry and pulmonary function tests and avoidance of high inspired oxygen concentrations. Nonprescription therapies such as the use of herbal remedies should be documented. The use of herbal substances such as St. John's wort and weight-loss agents such as fenfluramine hydrochloride, phentermine hydrochloride, and dexfenfluramine hydrochloride may produce altered physiology, which may complicate the course of a general anesthetic (see Chapter 15).

Children should be questioned regarding allergies to antibiotics. Sensitivity to bananas, the rubber dam used by dentists and oral surgeons, or latex balloons strongly suggests latex allergy, and this requires further investigation and additional anesthetic planning[6] (see Chapter 15). Some evidence suggests that children with long-term exposure to tobacco smoke experience an increased incidence of airway complications under general anesthesia. Exposure to tobacco smoke should be investigated during the preoperative interview and should be documented.[7,8]

PHYSICAL EXAMINATION

The respiratory, cardiovascular, and neurologic systems and the system that is the focus of the surgical procedure, as well as the airway evaluation, are of primary importance. One of the key features of the physical examination in children is simple observation, because approaching the child may cause inconsolable crying. The color of the skin and the presence of pallor, cyanosis, rash, jaundice, unusual markings, birthmarks, and scars from prior operations should be noted. Abnormal facies might be an indication of a syndrome or constellation of congenital abnormalities (Table 13-6). One congenital anomaly often is associated with others.

The rate, depth, and quality of respirations should be evaluated. Nasal and upper respiratory obstruction are indicated by noisy or labored breathing. The color, viscosity, and quantity of nasal discharge should be documented. If the child is coughing, the origin of the cough (upper airway versus lower airway) and the quality (dry or wet) can be evaluated even before auscultation of the lungs. Is wheezing or stridor audible, or are retractions visible? The airway should be evaluated for ease of intubation (see Chapter 14). If the child will not open his or her mouth, a manual estimation of the thyrohyoid distance should be made. Children with micrognathia, as in Pierre Robin syndrome or Goldenhar's syndrome, may be especially difficult to intubate. Notation of loose teeth should be made.

The child with a heart murmur or a history of a murmur warrants special consideration. Is the murmur innocent (a flow murmur or a murmur noted during a growth spurt) or is it pathologic? Is hemodynamic compromise apparent? Innocent or nonpathologic heart murmurs can be identified by four charac-

Table 13-6. Craniofacial deformities and associated conditions

Name	Deformity	Associated conditions	Anesthetic implications
Apert's syndrome	Craniosyn- ostosis, hypo- plastic midface	Polysyndactyly, possible mental compromise	Difficult intra- venous access
Crouzon's disease	Craniosyn- ostosis, hypo- plastic max- illa, hyper- telorism, exophthalmos	Conductive hearing loss, possible mental compromise	Possible upper airway obstruction
Goldenhar's syndrome	Unilateral mandibular hypoplasia, cleft palate, micrognathia	Vertebral anomalies	Possible difficult intubation
Hemifacial microsomia	Unilateral ear anomalies, unilateral mandibular hypoplasia	None	Possible difficult intubation
Möbius' syndrome	Micrognathia, limited mandibular mobility	Possible cranial nerve VI and VII palsy, ptosis, limited tongue move- ment	Difficult intubation
Pfeiffer's syndrome	Brachycephaly, hypoplastic maxilla	Broad thumbs and toes, syndactyly, possible mental compromise	Difficult intubation
Pierre Robin syndrome	Mandibular hypoplasia, micrognathia, glossoptosis, cleft palate	None	Difficult intubation
Treacher Collins syndrome	Mandibular hypoplasia, zygomatic arch hypopla- sia, ear mal- formations	Compromised hearing	Difficult intubation

Adapted with permission from Badgwell JM, ed. *Clinical pediatric anesthesia.* Philadelphia: Lippincott–Raven Publishers, 1997.

teristic findings: the murmur is early systolic to midsystolic; it is softer than grade III of VI; the pitch is low to medium; and the sound has a musical, not harsh, quality[9] (see Chapter 4). Is the child at risk for paradoxic air embolus? Is prophylaxis for sub-acute bacterial endocarditis required[10]? (See Chapter 16.) The child with significant or active cardiac disease might require an evaluation by a cardiologist before general anesthesia. Cardiac catheterization data and recommendations should be included in the preoperative evaluation.[11]

Neurologic status should be assessed by noting associated congenital syndromes, neurologic deficits, seizure disorders, and current or prior increases in intracranial pressure manifested by nausea, vomiting, difficulty concentrating, headaches, and inability to protect the airway. Children with metabolic disorders, hypotonia, or an increase in head circumference may have neurologic impairment. The physical examination should include an evaluation of the level of consciousness, ability to swallow, intactness of the gag reflex, and an adequate cervical spine range of motion. Hypotonia, spasticity, flaccidity, and any sign of increased intracranial pressure (gait disorders, altered mental status) should be noted.

DIAGNOSTIC TESTING

Few, if any, diagnostic laboratory tests are routinely necessary in the pediatric population (see Chapter 2). Diagnostic studies should be individualized to the patient's medical condition and the surgical procedure being performed. Determination of hemoglobin level before elective surgery is unnecessary for most healthy children.[12] Mild abnormalities in white blood cell and platelet counts have no significant impact on the perioperative outcome in healthy children. Hemoglobin determination is indicated for premature infants and infants younger than 6 months, and when significant surgical blood loss is anticipated.

The routine measurement of coagulation parameters is controversial, and a history of "excess bruising" is subjective. A history of abnormal coagulation, prolonged epistaxis, bleeding from a circumcision or a tooth extraction, and the presence of hematomas and large bruises are better predictors of abnormal coagulation. If an otherwise healthy child has a negative history for bruising, no further testing is required, because commonly used screening tests such as bleeding time, activated partial thromboplastin time, prothrombin time, and platelet count do not reliably predict surgical bleeding[13] (see Chapter 7). Coagulation screening may be indicated in children who have a history of abnormal bleeding or are undergoing surgery in which abnormal coagulation might be induced (cardiopulmonary bypass) or procedures in which adequate hemostasis is essential (tonsillectomy, neurosurgical procedures).

A urinalysis is not needed before surgery for most children. Serum chemistry measurements are indicated only to confirm a *suspected* abnormality. Serum medication levels are measured when specifically indicated (e.g., for seizure medications). Chest radiographs (CXRs) and electrocardiograms (ECGs) are taken only when abnormalities are suspected.

Pregnancy testing has caused a great deal of controversy. A *confidential* interview with a postmenarchal female of childbearing age should disclose current sexual activity, the use of birth control, or the possibility of pregnancy. Often parents refuse pregnancy testing for their child because it assumes that the child either is sexually active or is not truthful about her activities. The legality of such testing is not clear.

In summary, because most laboratory examinations are painful and distressing to children, an attempt should be made to minimize psychological and physical pain. A child who has been traumatized preoperatively may show more problematic behavior during the anesthetic induction.

SPECIAL CIRCUMSTANCES

Upper Respiratory Infection

The child with a recent, full-blown, or early upper respiratory infection (URI) poses a clinical dilemma for the anesthesiologist. Because most children can have up to six URIs per year, this is a common problem for which no absolute rules exist. Several potential risks are encountered in the perioperative period in the child who has an active cold or is recovering from a recent one. These include atelectasis, oxygen desaturation, bronchospasm, croup, and laryngospasm.[14] Most of these children may be anesthetized for short procedures; however, the decision to perform a lengthy or invasive procedure must be made with caution. Decisions to cancel or postpone surgery should be made in conjunction with the surgeon and should be based on the type of procedure, the urgency of the procedure, and the child's overall medical condition. Bronchial hyperreactivity may exist for up to 7 weeks after the resolution of URI symptoms, and delaying surgery for this length of time is often impractical. Most practitioners would agree that surgery may be scheduled after the acute symptoms have resolved and no sooner than 2 weeks after the initial evaluation.

When a child with symptoms of a URI is examined, the presence of secretions and their color should be noted. Clear secretions usually indicate a viral illness, whereas green or yellow secretions are more suggestive of a bacterial infection. Cough is a sign of lower respiratory involvement and should be evaluated for origin (upper airway or bronchial) and quality (wet or dry). Most children have clear breath sounds during quiet respirations. Crackles are best detected during coughing and crying.

Premature Birth

Former premature infants present for a variety of surgical procedures, some seemingly minor. The anesthetic management can be challenging, however. The extent of chronic lung disease and the possibility of postoperative apnea are of concern and require planning for appropriate monitoring. Documentation of coexisting conditions, such as gastroesophageal reflux, patent ductus arteriosus, and hydrocephalus, is important.

The degree of respiratory compromise in former premature infants may range from no residual lung disease to serious bronchopulmonary dysplasia. The presentation of bronchopulmonary dysplasia is variable and ranges from mild radiographic changes in an asymptomatic patient to pulmonary fibrosis, emphysema, reactive airway disease, chronic hypoxemia and hypercarbia, tracheomalacia or bronchomalacia, and increased pulmonary vascular resistance with cor pulmonale. If pulmonary hypertension and cor pulmonale are suspected, an ECG is useful to confirm the diagnosis and guide medical therapy. Diuretics, bronchodilators, and corticosteroids—medications that many of these patients require—should be continued up to and including the day of surgery. Measurement of serum electrolyte levels to evaluate hypokalemia and compensatory metabolic alkalosis may be valuable, especially if therapy has been altered recently. A hematocrit and CXR are useful in evaluating these infants. Administration of pharmacologic "stress doses" of steroids should be considered in infants receiving steroid treatment (see Chapter 15).

Postoperative apnea after anesthesia has been reported in preterm and full-term infants.[15,16] No agreement exists on which infants are at risk. Reports are not consistent in identifying the postconceptional age or gestational age of at-risk patients, the methods used to detect apnea or periodic breathing, the surgical procedure, other confounding medical conditions, or even the definition of apnea. One review has summarized available information.[16] The definition of apnea used in this analysis was cessation of breathing or no detection of air flow for 15 seconds or more or for 15 seconds or less with bradycardia (heart rate less than 80 beats per minute). The cause of apnea is central in 70% of cases, obstructive in 10%, and mixed in 20%. The risk of apnea is less than 5% for infants whose gestational age is more than 35 weeks until they reach 48 weeks postconceptual age and for infants of 32 to 35 weeks postconceptual age until they are 50 weeks postconceptual age. Infants with anemia, apnea in the recovery room, apnea at home (as measured with home apnea-monitoring equipment), and a prior history of apnea and bradycardia are at increased risk. Any child considered to be at risk for postoperative apnea should be admitted for overnight observation and monitoring. A recent hematocrit or hemoglobin determination is required for the former preterm infant because anemia is associated with an increased incidence of postanesthesia apnea that is unaffected by postconceptional age. Of note is the finding that apnea of prematurity and postanesthetic apnea have no relationship to sudden infant death syndrome, as had previously been considered.

Asthma

The management of children with asthma is similar to that of adult patients with asthma (see Chapter 5). Their asthma treatment and medical management should be optimized. All medications, both oral and inhaled, should be continued up to and including the day of surgery . Oral medications may be taken with clear fluids up to 2 hours before the induction of anesthesia. Patients with particularly severe asthma may benefit from short-term corticosteroid therapy for several days before surgery (see Chapter 15). Therapy should be optimized with their pulmonologist.

Surgery should generally be postponed for children with an acute exacerbation of asthma or those who have an acute URI superimposed on chronic asthma. Asthmatic children are at increased risk of bronchospasm during general endotracheal anesthesia. The incidence of bronchospasm in asthmatic patients during anesthesia is between 8.4 and 71.0 per 1,000, compared with 0.2 to 8.0 per 1,000 in the general population. This incidence is further increased during acute exacerbations.

Cystic Fibrosis

Children with cystic fibrosis have a multisystem disease, and each of these systems should be addressed during the preoperative period. Pulmonary function should be optimized through the use of antibiotic and bronchodilator therapy and vigorous chest physical therapy to clear secretions and enhance airflow. Many children have some degree of malnutrition and may need parenteral or supplemental enteral nutrition before undergoing general anesthesia and surgery (see Chapter 16). Many cystic fibrosis patients should be admitted to the hospital for medical management before their surgical procedures. All medications should be continued up to and including the day of surgery.

Cardiac Disease

Children with cardiac disease can be divided into two categories: those who have structural congenital heart disease (corrected and uncorrected) and those who have a heart murmur (previously diagnosed or new). The child who is followed regularly by a cardiologist should be evaluated in the preoperative period to detect and document any interval change. When the child has had a surgical repair of congenital heart disease, a description of the repair and current anatomy should be made available to the anesthesia team. If a defect still exists, management recommendations should be requested from the cardiologist. All current cardiac catheterization data should be reviewed.

Heart murmurs in children should be identified as innocent or pathologic. A screening ECG may be necessary. If a murmur is pathologic, the degree of physiologic and hemodynamic compromise should be determined. The need for antibiotic prophylaxis should be assessed during the preoperative visit; current guidelines are outlined in Chapter 16.

Central Nervous System Disorders

Myelomeningocele

Most children who are born with a myelomeningocele have other abnormalities, and a thorough investigation is necessary. Many of these children return to the OR frequently, so the current perioperative management may influence patients' future behavior and concerns. Myelomeningocele patients may have associated urogenital and musculoskeletal system dysfunction that may result in frequent urinary tract infections, ureteral reflux, scoliosis, and respiratory compromise. Patients and families should be questioned regarding abnormalities in these organ systems. A high incidence of latex sensitivity is seen and can range from anaphylaxis to mild reactions. For this reason, an attempt is made to minimize exposure to latex in myelomeningocele patients. The notation "Latex Alert" or "Latex Allergy" should be written on the chart of every myelomeningocele patient going to the OR.

Seizure Disorders

A description of the type, frequency, and characteristics of seizure activity should be part of the preoperative evaluation. Current medications and, if applicable, serum levels of anticonvulsant medications should be noted. Information regarding medications that were ineffective in controlling seizure activity should be included. All seizure medications should be taken up to and including the day of surgery. Oral medications may be taken with clear fluids up to 2 hours before the time of surgery.

Cervical Spine Instability

Several groups of pediatric patients are at risk for cervical spine instability. Children with Hurler's syndrome and Morquio's syndrome as well as other mucopolysaccharidoses may have abnormalities of the odontoid process, which may result in cervical spine instability. Atlantoaxial instability and superior migration of the odontoid process can occur in patients with rheumatoid arthritis. Approximately 15% of children with Down syndrome are likewise affected. Although no uniform guidelines exist regarding preoperative testing in these children, the suggestion has been made that children who are symptomatic (e.g., have gait disturbances, incontinence problems) should undergo flexion-extension radiography of the cervical spine and should have a neurologic consultation.[17] If cervical abnormalities are noted, intubation in a neutral head position or somatosensory evoked potential monitoring of the upper extremities may be required.[18]

Hematologic Disorders

Sickle cell disease is one of the most common hematologic diseases in children in the United States. Sickle cell disease is a genetically transmitted autosomal recessive disease that occurs in the heterozygous form with a frequency of 8% in African Americans and in the homozygous form in 0.16% of patients who are susceptible. Heterozygous sickle cell trait does not influence anesthetic management or perioperative outcome, but homozygous sickle cell disease, sickle cell–hemoglobin C disease, and hemoglobin S-thalassemia disease carry implications for anesthetic management. Acute chest syndrome, stroke, myocardial infarction, and sickle cell crises are of concern to the anesthesiologist. To minimize these risks, patients are vigorously hydrated preoperatively and the OR temperature is kept elevated to optimize vascular flow. In severe cases, partial exchange transfusion is performed in an attempt to decrease the level of hemoglobin S to less than 40% or transfusion to a hemoglobin of 10 g per dL is performed (see Chapter 7). Consultation with a hematologist for management of these patients is recommended. Coordination of care among the anesthesiologist, surgeon, pediatrician, and hematologist is essential and must begin in the preoperative period.

Diabetes Mellitus

The incidence of diabetes mellitus in the pediatric population is approximately 1.9 in 1,000 school-aged children, with age of onset peaking at 5 to 7 years and again at puberty. Consultation with the pediatrician and pediatric endocrinologist is advisable. Information regarding the typical range of serum glucose control and medication regimen should be included in the preoperative evaluation. Any suggestions for perioperative glucose management (insulin infusion, split-dose insulin injection) should be documented. Patients with diabetes mellitus should be scheduled for surgery early in the morning, and a fasting serum glucose measurement should be obtained in the immediate preoperative period before insulin or glucose administration.

Oncologic Disease

Children with malignant disease—either active, in remission, or cured—may have received radiation or chemotherapy that will directly affect the anesthetic outcome. Information regarding the course of the disease, prior surgery, and a list of chemotherapeutic agents and doses should be included in the preoperative evaluation. Children suspected of having an anterior mediastinal mass require flow volume loop examination in the supine and upright positions before anesthetic induction. Clinical findings should dictate the need for other laboratory examinations, such as an ECG, hemoglobin measurement, and platelet count.

PREOPERATIVE MEDICATIONS AND BEYOND

Fasting Guidelines

Fasting guidelines for children before general anesthesia have been modified extensively during the 1990s. Restricting children to fasting after midnight is no longer common practice.[19] Liberalization of oral intake results in a less anxious child, calmer parents, better maintenance of hemodynamic parameters, and less risk of intraoperative hypoglycemia.

Gastric volume and gastric emptying times are age related, and most surgical facilities have age-specific guidelines. In general, most institutions allow the ingestion of clear fluids until 2 to 3 hours before the time of surgery. These include water, electrolyte solutions (Pedialyte), glucose water, apple juice, white grape juice, frozen pops without fruit pulp, and gelatin. Clear fluids are defined as any fluid through which a newspaper can be read. Frozen pops that contain fruit solids, ciders, nectar juices that contain pulp and particulate material, and clear broth, which may contain animal proteins, are not considered clear liquids. No evidence exists that volume has an impact on gastric emptying time or residual volume; therefore, the quantity of clear fluids is not limited.

Formula and breast milk are not clear fluids. Breast milk is usually considered to be intermediate between clear fluids and formula. Some institutions consider formula to be less restricted than a solid, whereas other institutions consider it to have solid-like properties. Anesthesiologists and surgeons should establish clear policies regarding formula, breast milk, and solids.

Induction Choices

The preoperative interview offers a good opportunity to expose the child and family to the options that are available for the induction of general anesthesia. It must be made clear that the choice is the ultimate responsibility of the attending anesthesiologist and that the input of the child and family members will be considered.

For children younger than 8 years, anesthesia is best induced with a volatile anesthetic agent administered by mask. The reason is that the onset of unconsciousness is rapid using this method, and most children are needle phobic. When the child is calm and cooperative, increasing concentrations of anesthetic are administered by mask until unconsciousness is achieved. The anxious or uncooperative child is best treated with a "single-breath" inhalation induction technique in which a high concentration of anesthetic is delivered; although this is less pleasant for the child because of the pungent odor of the anesthetic, it is much faster. Children older than 8 years occasionally are anesthetized by mask induction, and cooperative children may choose a single-breath induction technique. The choices are based on the most appropriate method for each child and situation.

Anesthesia is usually induced in older children in the same manner as in adult patients, via an intravenous route. EMLA cream is a *e*utectic *m*ixture of *l*ocal *a*nesthetic that is applied to intact skin and covered with an impervious dressing (Tegaderm), providing analgesia to the underlying skin. EMLA cream is often applied in the pediatric population and allows an intravenous line to be inserted without pain. Explaining the procedure to children in advance so that they are prepared is important.

For mentally challenged children who are uncooperative and difficult to reason with, anesthesia may be induced with an intramuscular injection of ketamine hydrochloride, midazolam hydrochloride, or a combination of the two. This is a fast and effective means of bringing these children into the OR, and discussion of this option is reassuring to parents who are concerned about an uncooperative or combative child.

Parent-Present Induction

When patients and families are prepared for anesthesia, a common concern of many parents and caretakers is, "How will my child be taken into the OR?" The presence of the parents is often the most effective premedication for a young child, especially a toddler, because the separation from parents is eliminated. A parent may accompany the child into the OR, and this should be an accepted practice.

Parents are most effective if they have been well prepared and usually are not helpful when the child is younger than 8 months. The clinician must remember that most parents have not been in an OR, and the sounds of surgical instruments being prepared and of anesthesia monitors are new and can be frightening to both parents and children. The parents should be told that they may remain with the child until he or she is unaware of their presence. Parents should be warned that the child might not look as he or she does during natural sleep. Parents should be given a *brief* description of eye and body movements during stage 2 of anesthesia. Excitement may be seen, which consists of rolling back of the eyes, random body movements, and vocalization. This is normal and expected. When a parent-present induction is unsuccessful, the cause often is inadequate preparation of parents. Parents may express their desire *not* to accompany their child into the OR. This sentiment should be respected. Alternatives to parent-present induction include the use of rectal methohexital sodium, so that the child falls asleep in the parent's arms or on a stretcher. Oral, intranasal, or rectal midazolam may be used as premedications. Parents should be cautioned that children usually do not fall asleep after administration but have a "drunken sailor" appearance and relief of anxiety. Fentanyl Oralet (fentanyl citrate; an opioid-laced lollipop) is useful in certain patients.

When presenting options for anesthetic induction, the clinician must not promise that a specific technique or medication will be used unless he or she is actually going to administer the anesthetic and can ensure that the plan is followed. Alternatively, an acceptable course is to explain that the final decision will be made by the anesthesiologist on the day of surgery and that all factors and requests will be taken into consideration.

SPECIAL ANESTHETIC CONSIDERATIONS

One phrase that the OR team shudders to hear is, "By the way, the patient is . . ." The sentence may be completed with phrases such as "Jehovah's Witness" or "do not resuscitate (DNR)." These circumstances have complicated ethical and legal ramifications for the anesthesiologist and require careful preoperative planning among the surgeon, anesthesiologist, pediatrician, family, parents or guardian, hospital administrators, and attorneys. Frequently, medical decisions are influenced by nonmedical considerations. Therefore, planning must take place before arrival in the OR, and all parties must be in agreement to prevent cancellation of surgery.

Jehovah's Witness Patients

Although adult Jehovah's Witness patients may choose to refuse lifesaving blood transfusions, pediatric patients are minor children and do not have that right. The anesthesiologist, the surgeon, and hospital officials are responsible for developing a plan with the parents in the event that blood is required. The anesthesiologist and surgeon should explore the particular beliefs of the family, because some Jehovah's Witness individuals allow the use of blood conservation in an attempt to minimize intraoperative blood loss and transfusion requirements. Perioperative volume expanders (albumin, hydroxyethyl starch), hemodilution, and blood salvage are acceptable to some individuals, depending on their interpretation of biblical passages.[20,21] In an emergency, most medical personnel agree that for a parent to make a decision that could result in a minor child's death is unacceptable. In such a case, appropriate medical therapy, including transfusion of blood and blood products, is administered against the wishes of the family. In most circumstances, the courts have intervened to allow blood transfusions over the religious objections of the parents. No child of Jehovah's Witness parents should die for lack of transfused blood without the physician seeking a court order to administer the blood. A petition to the appropriate court is made for judicial declaration that the minor is a "neglected child" and that a guardian be appointed, usually the hospital or hospital administrator. Evidence in support of the need for blood transfusion is made to the judge, either in person or by telephone, and may be presented by the pediatrician, surgeon, anesthesiologist, or all of them. If the petition is granted, the new guardian consents to transfusion of blood or blood products, and this is followed by a formal petition to the court.

"Do Not Resuscitate" Orders for Children

DNR orders are implemented to prevent long-term dependence on life-support systems when no reversal or resolution of a disease process is anticipated and to avoid prolongation of death when it is inevitable. The issue arises of what to do when a child with a DNR order comes to the OR, because general anesthesia is a continuous state of cardiopulmonary resuscitation. Determining where anesthesia ends and resuscitation begins often is difficult. Orders directing DNR status outside the OR are not applicable during surgery and anesthesia unless the family has specifically indicated that they should continue. If they have done so and the anesthesiologist chooses to ignore their wishes, the physician may be accused of battery.[22]

Each institution should have a policy regarding suspension of DNR orders during surgery, and that policy should be understood and agreed on by all involved parties. This matter should be discussed with the family before surgery, and written documentation of the plan either to maintain or to suspend DNR orders should be made. A distinction exists between goal-directed resuscitation and procedure-directed resuscitation.[23] Most determinations of DNR outline the specific interventions that may or may not be carried out. Because these procedures often are part of the normal administration of general anesthesia, the definition becomes meaningless. Perhaps more useful is an understanding of outcome expectations. The anesthesiologist can decide what intervention will result in the desired postoperative outcome and determine which therapy is acceptable and in keeping with parental wishes. If a child requires emergency surgery and the parent or legal guardian is unavailable, the recommendation is that the DNR status be suspended.

CASE STUDY

A 6-year-old girl with a history of asthma is scheduled for a tympanomastoidectomy. The patient has had several admissions to the emergency department for acute bronchospasm but has never been hospitalized for complications of asthma. She has had three sets of myringotomy tubes placed under general anesthesia without incident. Current medications are cromolyn sodium (Intal) and albuterol (Ventolin), both administered by nebulizer. She has had a URI, including a cough, for 5 days. On the day before her preoperative visit, she was evaluated by her pediatrician, who found her lungs clear to auscultation, noted no wheezing, and cleared her for surgery.

On physical examination in the preoperative clinic, the patient is afebrile and has scant, clear rhinorrhea. She appears pale and lethargic. On auscultation, she has mild end-expiratory wheezing. She is asked to cough, and auscultation at this time reveals bilateral crackles, which are worse on the right side. The wheezing has cleared. A CXR is ordered and is remarkable for a small area of atelectasis in the right lower lung field. Her white blood cell count is 10,000 per cubic millimeter with a slight left shift.

This child has an acute illness, probably of viral origin, with slight exacerbation of her asthma. She is at risk for intraoperative hypoxemia, intrapulmonary shunting, bronchospasm, laryngospasm, and postoperative pneumonia. The surgeon is informed of these findings, and the surgery is postponed for 3 weeks. The patient is instructed to continue the nebulizer treatments and, if the URI does not improve in 3 days, to return to her pediatrician for further evaluation.

On return to the preoperative clinic on the day before her rescheduled surgery, she is less pale and her activity has returned to a normal level. She is no longer coughing, and her lungs are clear to auscultation during quiet respiration and after a forced cough. After discussion with the parents and the child, plans are outlined for a mask induction with the mother present in the OR. The patient is instructed to avoid food after midnight but is told she may have clear fluids until 3 hours before surgery. The parents are told to administer an albuterol nebulizer treatment before coming to the hospital on the day of surgery.

REFERENCES

1. McGraw T. Preparing children for the operating room: psychological issues. *Can J Anaesth* 1994;41:1094–1103.
2. Moynihan R, Kurker C. Bridging the gap to the operating room and beyond. In: Ferrari LR, ed. *Preoperative evaluation and pain management of pediatric patients*. Baltimore: The Johns Hopkins University Press, 1998.
3. Holzman RS. Morbidity and mortality in pediatric anesthesia. *Pediatr Clin North Am* 1994;41:239–256.
4. Means LJ. Preoperative evaluation. In: Badgwell JM, ed. *Clinical pediatric anesthesia*. Philadelphia: Lippincott–Raven Publishers, 1997.
5. Cote CJ, Todres ID, Ryan JF. Preoperative evaluation of pediatric patients. In: Cote CJ, Ryan JF, Todres ID, Goudsouzian NG, eds. *A practice of anesthesia for infants and children*, 2nd ed. Philadelphia: WB Saunders, 1993.

6. Means LJ, Fescorla FJ. Latex anaphylaxis: report of occurrence in two pediatric surgical patients and review of the literature. J *Pediatr Surg* 1995;30:748–751.

7. Skolnick ET, Vomvolakis MA, Buck KA, et al. Exposure to environmental tobacco smoke and the risk of adverse respiratory events in children receiving general anesthesia. *Anesthesiology* 1998;88:1144–1153.

8. Koop CE. Adverse anesthesia events in children exposed to environmental tobacco smoke. *Anesthesiology* 1998;88:1141–1142.

9. Harris JP. Evaluation of heart murmurs. *Pediatr Rev* 1994;15: 490–493.

10. Dajani AS, Taubert KA, Wilson WW, et al. Prevention of bacterial endocarditis. Recommendations by the American Heart Association. *JAMA* 1997;277:1794–1801.

11. Means LJ, Ferrari LR, Fisher QA, et al. American Academy of Pediatrics. Evaluation and preparation of pediatric patients undergoing anesthesia. *Pediatrics* 1996;98:502–508.

12. Baron MJ, Gunter J, White P. Is the pediatric preoperative hematocrit determination necessary? *South Med J* 1992;85: 1187–1189.

13. Burk CD, Miller L, Handler SD, Cohen AR. Preoperative history and coagulation screening in children undergoing tonsillectomy. *Pediatrics* 1992;89:691–695.

14. Rolf N, Cote CJ. Frequency and severity of desaturation events during general anesthesia in children with and without upper respiratory infections. *J Clin Anesth* 1992;4:200–203.

15. Noseworthy J, Duran C, Khine HH. Postoperative apnea in a full term infant. *Anesthesiology* 1988;97:879–880.

16. Cote CJ, Zaslavsky A, Downes JJ, et al. Postoperative apnea in former premature infants after inguinal herniorrhaphy. A combined analysis. *Anesthesiology* 1995;82:809–822.

17. Williams JP, Somerville GM, Miner ME, Reilly D. Atlanto-axial subluxation and trisomy 21: another perioperative complication. *Anesthesiology* 1987;67:253–254.

18. Cunningham MJ, Ferrari LR, Kerse L, McPeck K. Intraoperative somatosensory evoked potential monitoring in achondroplastic dwarfs. *Paediatr Anaesth* 1994;4:129–132.

19. Cote CJ. NPO after midnight for children—a reappraisal. *Anesthesiology* 1990;72:589–592.

20. Benson KT. The Jehovah's Witness patient: considerations for the anesthesiologist. *Anesth Analg* 1989;69:647–656.

21. *Jehovah's Witnesses and the question of blood*. Brooklyn, NY: Watch Tower Bible and Tract Society, 1977:1–64.

22. *Beausoleil v. Providential Sisters of Charity*, 53 DLR 2d 65 (1964).

23. Truog R, Rockoff MA. Ethical issues in pediatric anesthesia. *Semin Anesth* 1991;10:187–194.

Anesthetic Issues

Joshua A. Bloomstone

This chapter discusses the preoperative evaluation and management of patients with **pseudocholinesterase deficiency, malignant hyperthermia,** and a **difficult airway.** The common thread of these issues is that they only pose a problem to individuals who have these conditions when anesthesia is administered to them. The chapter concludes with a case study of a preoperative encounter.

PSEUDOCHOLINESTERASE DEFICIENCY

Succinyldicholine is the only depolarizing muscle relaxant commonly used during general anesthesia. It is a relatively small quaternary ammonium compound with a fast onset and brief duration. It is metabolized by plasma cholinesterase (pseudocholinesterase) or, more specifically, by butyryl cholinesterase and by the liver. Only a small fraction (5%) of the injected dose reaches its site of action: the acetylcholine receptor within the synaptic cleft of the neuromuscular junction. Once there, muscle depolarization followed by relaxation occurs. The drug diffuses away from the synaptic cleft and is further metabolized to succinylmonocholine, then to succinic acid and choline, and spontaneous recovery from relaxation occurs. Onset ranges from 30 to 60 seconds and recovery usually occurs within 10 minutes. Acetylcholinesterase, cell-bound or true cholinesterase, plays no role in the metabolism of succinyldicholine.

Prolonged apnea may occur after the administration of succinylcholine chloride (succinyldicholine) if large doses (more than 7 to 10 mg per kg intravenously) are administered[1,2] or if the patient has quantitative or qualitative abnormalities in pseudocholinesterase.[3] Recovery from mivacurium chloride and ester-linked local anesthetics, which are also metabolized by pseudocholinesterase, may be a problem in patients with pseudocholinesterase abnormalities. Quantitative abnormalities in pseudocholinesterase (i.e., low levels of functioning enzyme) may occur naturally, in specific disease states, and after certain drug therapies (Table 14-1). Although patients with low absolute levels of functioning pseudocholinesterase are not symptomatic, prolonged apnea may occur in such patients after succinylcholine or mivacurium chloride administration.

Genetic analysis has demonstrated the existence of three allelic variants in addition to the wild type. The phenotypes that relate to these four alleles have been named differently by investigators and can be distinguished using plasma cholinesterase inhibitors such as chloride, fluoride, and dibucaine *in vitro*. Names include *atypical, dibucaine sensitive, fluoride sensitive,* and *silent gene.*[4,5] These four alleles give rise to ten genotypes. Pharmacogenetic

Table 14-1. Causes of decreased plasma cholinesterase activity

Disease states	Hepatic failure
	Uremia
	Malnutrition
	Myxedema
	Collagen vascular diseases
	Acute myocardial infarction
	Acute infection
	Carcinoma
	Tuberculosis
Drug therapies	Echothiophate iodide
	Neostigmine
	Chlorpromazine
	Oral contraceptives
	Cyclophosphamide
	Pancuronium bromide
	Phenylzine
	Trimethaphan camsylate
Expected alterations in enzyme activity	Third trimester of pregnancy
	Newborns and infants

Data from Whittaker M. Plasma cholinesterase variants and the anaesthetist. *Anaesthesia* 1980;35:175; Morgan GE, Mikhil MS. *Clinical anesthesiology*, 2nd ed. Norwalk, CT: Appleton & Lange, 1996:190.

studies suggest that allelic predominance differs with ethnicity.[6–9] Table 14-2 summarizes information on the common North American variants of pseudocholinesterase.

Davies et al. demonstrated that normal and variant pseudocholinesterase differed in at least two important ways.[10] The normal enzyme W-W has a much greater affinity for choline substrate, and cholinesterase activity in normal plasma is inhibited to a greater extent by cholinesterase inhibitors than in those with an abnormal enzyme. These researchers published a method for detecting individuals with atypical plasma cholinesterase using

Table 14-2. Genetic classification, frequency of occurrence, and response to succinylcholine chloride

Genotype	Phenotype	Frequency	Dibu-caine number	Expected apnea time (min)
W-W	Typical homozygote	96 in 100	80	10
W-A	Heterozygote	1 in 40	60	20–30
A-A	Atypical homozygote	1 in 2,000	20	480 (8 h)

A, atypical gene; W, wild-type gene.
Data from Barash PG, Cullen BF, Stoelting RK. *Clinical anesthesia*, 2nd ed. Philadelphia: JB Lippincott Co, 1992:605; Morgan GE, Mikhail MS. *Clinical anesthesiology*, 2nd ed. Norwalk, CT: Appleton & Lange, 1996:152, 154; Whittaker M. Plasma cholinesterase variants and the anaesthetist. *Anaesthesia* 1980;35:178; Thompson JS, Thompson MW. *Genetics in medicine*, 4th ed. Philadelphia: WB Saunders, 1980:104.

the local anesthetic dibucaine. Dibucaine (10^{-5} mol per L) inhibits the metabolism of a choline substrate by plasma cholinesterase *in vitro*. In individuals homozygous for the wild type, dibucaine causes inhibition of substrate metabolism by 80%. In those who are homozygous for the atypical genes, inhibition is only 20%. In individuals heterozygotic for the atypical genes, inhibition is approximately 60%. The percentage inhibition of plasma cholinesterase by dibucaine is termed the *dibucaine number*; normal individuals have a dibucaine number of 80.

The assessment of an individual thought to have a genetic variant of this enzyme should begin with the determination of a dibucaine number. This result yields important information regarding the *quality* of the individual's plasma cholinesterase. Inhibition of the enzyme *in vitro* by fluoride and chloride further delineate phenotypes.

In addition to the qualitative assessment obtained using dibucaine, a quantitative assessment of the enzyme can be obtained by determining the absolute cholinesterase activity. These tests help differentiate genetic from nongenetic causes for prolonged apnea after administration of succinylcholine or mivacurium chloride.

MALIGNANT HYPERTHERMIA

Malignant hyperthermia (MH) is a fulminant hypermetabolic state characterized by tachycardia, hypertension, hypercarbia, arterial hypoxemia, mixed venous oxygen desaturation, metabolic acidosis, hyperkalemia, muscle rigidity, hyperthermia, renal failure, disseminated intravascular coagulation, and death if the condition is untreated. Individuals are genetically predisposed to the development of MH and are asymptomatic until they are exposed to either potent volatile anesthetics or succinylcholine. The incidence of MH is three times higher in the pediatric population than in adults; MH occurs in 1 of every 12,000 pediatric anesthesia cases.[11] A number of neuromuscular diseases have been associated with the development of MH (Table 14-3). Sixty percent of susceptible individuals manifest MH when exposed to triggering drugs on first exposure, especially when succinylcholine is combined with potent volatile anesthetics.[12] Those in whom no response is triggered initially may develop MH with subsequent anesthetic administration.

MH results from the activation of skeletal muscle due to an increase in intracellular sarcoplasmic calcium concentration caused by the aforementioned triggers. Calcium-selective microelectrode studies have demonstrated that individuals who are susceptible to MH have increased resting levels of sarcoplasmic calcium and develop excessive levels when exposed to specific triggers.[13]

Excitation-contraction coupling with subsequent muscle contraction requires the rapid release of calcium from the sarcoplasmic reticulum. Electron micrographic studies of striated muscle demonstrate a protein structure linking the T tubule system with the sarcoplasmic reticulum, which mediates calcium release. With exposure to ryanodine, a toxin, a marked alteration occurs in excitation-contraction coupling in striated muscle, which leads to skeletal muscle contraction.[14] Extensive genetic studies have

Table 14-3. Conditions associated with susceptibility to malignant hyperthermia

Duchenne's muscular dystrophy
Becker's muscular dystrophy
King-Denborough syndrome
Central core disease
Carnitine palmityl transferase deficiency
Periodic paralysis
Myotonia congenita
Osteogenesis imperfecta
Schwartz-Jampel syndrome
Fukuyama type congenital muscular dystrophy
Mitochondrial myopathy
Possibly associated:
    Strabismus
    Scoliosis
    Burkitt's lymphoma
    Neuroleptic malignant syndrome
    Myelomeningocele
    Congenital hip dislocation

Based on data from Kaplan R. Malignant hyperthermia. *Refresher courses in anesthesiology*, vol 22. Philadelphia: JB Lippincott Co, 1994:177; Stoelting RK, Dierdorf SF. *Anesthesia and co-existing disease*, 3rd ed. New York: Churchill Livingstone, 1993:613.

been performed on family members susceptible to MH. Although mutations in the gene encoding for the ryanodine receptor have been identified in certain families, no single mutation segregates with all susceptible patients.[15,16] The inheritance pattern in humans appears to be autosomal dominant.

In vitro studies show that the slow sodium current in cultured human muscle cells is altered in cells from patients with MH; this finding implies that sodium channels, in addition to the ryanodine receptor, are defective.[17] These data suggest that susceptibility to MH is multifactorial.

Although a genetic test for MH susceptibility would be desirable, a number of patients with MH have not been shown to have disease linked to the ryanodine receptor gene or mutations.[18] In spite of the genetic basis for the disease, the diagnosis is still dependent on fresh muscle biopsy and *in vitro* testing with the halothane-caffeine contracture test. Although many tests for MH have evolved, the halothane-caffeine contracture test remains the gold standard and is performed at ten institutions in the United States. A positive result occurs when muscle biopsy tissue, usually taken from the quadriceps femoris, develops at least 200 mg tension when challenged with 0.2 mmol caffeine or 3% halothane.

Testing is usually performed on individuals who are thought to have experienced an episode of MH, have a family history of MH, had an anesthetic-related event that could have been MH, or have a disorder that puts them at higher risk for developing MH (see Table 14-3). Alternatively, one can prepare the anesthesia equipment, select a nontriggering anesthetic technique, have

Table 14-4. Anesthesia machine preparation for patients susceptible to malignant hyperthermia

Change the rubber bellows.
Change the carbon dioxide absorbent.
Use a new breathing circuit and bag.
Consider changing the fresh gas line.
Flush the new system with oxygen at 10 L/min for 15–20 min.
Consider removing potent volatile anesthetic vaporizers from the machine.

dantrolene sodium available, and proceed without testing (Tables 14-4 and 14-5).

Perhaps the most controversial aspect of MH concerns the occurrence of masseter muscle rigidity on induction of anesthesia. Most commonly, this rigidity occurs in children in whom anesthesia has been induced with a combination of halothane and succinylcholine. However, masseter muscle rigidity has been reported with succinylcholine alone. The most difficult aspect of this clinical presentation is the lack of a uniform definition for rigidity. Therefore, evaluation of the patient who reports a history of "tight jaw" with anesthesia is difficult. Obtaining prior anesthesia records for details is key in determining what might have occurred. Only those patients whose mouths could not be opened after the rest of the body was relaxed should be described as having masseter muscle rigidity. Fifty percent of children and 25% of adults who fall into this group are MH susceptible.[19,20] Although opinions differ as to how best to anesthetize these patients, the most conservative approach is to use a nontriggering technique.[21]

The management of MH crises includes supportive care, active cooling, and the administration of dantrolene sodium. The *pro-*

Table 14-5. Agents that do not trigger malignant hyperthermia

All local anesthetics
Anticholinergics
Anticholinesterases
Barbiturates
Benzodiazepines
Calcium
Digoxin
Droperidol
Epinephrine
Etomidate
Ketamine
Nitrous oxide
Nondepolarizing muscle relaxants
Opioids
Potassium
Procainamide hydrochloride
Propofol
Sympathomimetics

phylactic administration of dantrolene sodium is not recommended. Each vial of dantrolene sodium (a lyophilized mixture) contains 20 mg of dantrolene and 3 g of mannitol. At least 10 mg per kg of dantrolene sodium should be available. The effective dose in 90% of patients is a bolus intravenous injection of 2.5 mg per kg. The drug acts by inhibiting the release of calcium from the sarcoplasmic reticulum and is the specific therapy for MH.

The Malignant Hyperthermia Association of the United States maintains a 24-hour telephone hotline [at (209) 634-4917] for questions regarding the management of MH.

DIFFICULT AIRWAY

Adverse respiratory events remain the major cause of injury in anesthetic practice.[22] Caplan et al.[22] identified inadequate ventilation as the largest class of adverse events. Since his closed-claim analysis of adverse respiratory events in anesthesia, one hopes that this aspect of patient care has been improved, if for no other reason than the widespread acceptance of the difficult airway algorithm of the American Society of Anesthesiologists (ASA), championed by Benumoff.[23] Despite the lack of definitive research, preoperative evaluation, intraoperative preparation, and adherence to accepted guidelines can reasonably be assumed to lead to improved outcomes.

The goals of this section are to describe the key anatomic features of the adult and pediatric airways and to provide a systematic approach to airway evaluation based on history, physical examination, and commonly used airway classification systems. In addition, planning for the management of a patient with a suspected difficult airway is discussed. Recognition of a potentially difficult airway begins with an understanding of normal airway anatomy. A full description of the anatomic structures of the human airway is beyond the scope of this chapter but has been reviewed superbly by Roberts[24] and Moore.[25] A number of specific features play a role in the identification of patients at risk for failed intubation, which are reviewed below.

The human airway can be divided into upper and lower segments. Anatomic abnormalities in each of these segments present different problems for the anesthesiologist. The anatomic components of the upper airway form the basis of the popular Samsoon-Young modification of the Mallampati pharyngeal classification (Table 14-6) and of the Cormack-Lehane laryngeal grading system (Table 14-7).[26–29]

Table 14-6. Modified Mallampati classification*

Class	Oropharyngeal components visualized
I	Soft palate, uvula, tonsillar pillars.
II	Base of the tongue obscures the tonsillar pillars, but the posterior pharyngeal wall is visible below the soft palate.
III	Soft palate.
IV	Essentially nothing visualized, not even soft palate.

*The original Mallampati system had only three classes. The Samsoon and Young[28] modification includes the fourth class.

Table 14-7. Cormack-Lehane grading system of the glottic view during direct laryngoscopy

Grade	Glottic structures visualized
I	Entire glottic opening
II	Posterior glottic structures
III	Epiglottis
IV	Soft palate only

Reprinted with permission from Cormack RS, Lehane J. Difficult tracheal intubation in obstetrics. *Anaesthesia* 1984;39:1105–1111.

Sensory and motor innervation to the oral cavity and pharynx are reviewed in Table 14-8. Cranial nerve (CN) XI (the accessory nerve) provides motor innervation to the pharyngeal plexus. These fibers innervate all the muscular structures within the pharynx and soft palate with two exceptions: motor innervation to the tensor veli palatini is from the trigeminal nerve (CN V), and motor innervation to the stylopharyngeus is from the glossopharyngeal nerve (CN IX). Oropharyngeal sensory innervation is predominantly supplied by the glossopharyngeal nerve (CN IX). The mucous membranes of the nasopharynx are supplied by the maxillary nerve, a purely sensory branch of the second division of CN V.

The larynx derives its sensory and motor innervation from the superior and recurrent laryngeal nerves, both branches of the

Table 14-8. Major sensory and motor innervation to the nasal passages, oral cavity, and pharynx

Cranial nerve (CN)	Sensory	Motor
Trigeminal (CN V)	Nasal passages General sensation to the tongue	Tensor veli palatini (tenses the soft palate)
Glossopharyngeal (CN IX) lingual branch	Posterior one-third of the tongue, soft palate, epiglottis to the pharyngoesophageal junction	Stylopharyngeus (elevates pharynx and larynx)
Facial (CN VII) *chorda tympani*	Taste	
Vagus (CN X)		
Superior laryngeal nerve		
Internal branch	Epiglottis and vocal cords	
External branch		Cricothyroid (adducts vocal fold)
Recurrent laryngeal nerve	Vocal cords and trachea	All laryngeal muscles except cricothyroid
Hypoglossal (CN XII)		All intrinsic tongue muscles

vagus nerve (CN X). Specifically, the superior laryngeal nerve is divided into its motor (external) and sensory (internal) branches. The external branch innervates the cricothyroid muscle. This is the only muscle of the larynx not innervated by the recurrent laryngeal nerve. Cricothyroid muscle activity results in the adduction (tensing) of the vocal folds, which, clinically, allows a patient to say "E." The internal branch of the superior laryngeal nerve provides sensory input to the epiglottis and vocal cords. The recurrent laryngeal nerve, which supplies the remainder of the motor innervation to the larynx, results in the abduction (opening) of the vocal cords. Unilateral damage to the recurrent laryngeal nerve leads to hoarseness without difficulty in breathing. The affected vocal cord takes a more midline position when viewed. Bilateral recurrent laryngeal nerve damage is said to cause closure of the glottis due to the unopposed action of the external branch of the superior laryngeal nerve. Patients with this condition are aphonic and require reintubation or tracheostomy. In actual fact, although the vocal cords assume a midline position with this type of nerve injury, *tense* closure of the vocal cords does not occur because this is accomplished by muscles innervated by the recurrent laryngeal nerve. The lower airway, below the vocal cords, receives its sensory innervation from the recurrent laryngeal nerve.

As noted in Table 14-9, significant differences exist between pediatric and adult airways. Figure 14-1 reviews these and other differences. Appropriate airway management of the newborn and infant requires recognition of these important differences.

Difficulty with mask ventilation ranges from easy ventilation to impossible ventilation, even with two individuals (one "working the mask" and the other "working the bag") and appropriate use of naso- and oropharyngeal airways. The incidence of difficulty with mask ventilation is not known. Data do exist regarding the inability of the anesthesia provider to ventilate by mask or

Table 14-9. Key anatomic components of the adult and pediatric airway

Component	Description
Larynx	Cartilaginous and muscular structure housing the vocal apparatus
Vocal cords	Most narrow portion of the *normal* adult airway
Cricoid ring	Only complete cartilaginous ring in the airway; just below the thyroid cartilage; most narrow portion of the pediatric airway
Cricoid membrane	Membrane connecting the cricoid with the thyroid cartilage
Trachea	12 cm in length in the adult; 4–5 cm in the newborn
Carina	Tracheal bifurcation point; opposite the fourth thoracic vertebra

Data from Desoto H. Difficult airway recognition and management in childhood. *Refresher courses in anesthesiology,* vol 25. Philadelphia: JB Lippincott Co, 1997:31–33; Gaiser R. Airway evaluation and management. In: *Clinical anesthesia procedures of the Massachusetts General Hospital,* 4th ed. Boston: Little, Brown and Company, 1993:171.

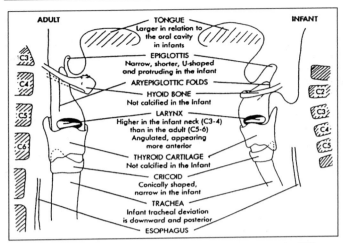

Fig. 14-1. Comparison of adult and infant airway anatomic differences. (Reprinted with permission from Ho M. The pediatric airway. In: Bell C, Hughes C, Oh T, eds. *The pediatric anesthesia handbook*. St. Louis: Mosby–Year Book, 1991:130.)

endotracheal tube.[30] The ability to predict difficulty with mask ventilation before the induction of anesthesia is important, so the anesthesia practitioner can have airway tools available should problems be encountered. Patient characteristics suggesting possible difficulty with mask ventilation include edentia; presence of a beard or mustache; significant underbite or overbite; facial deformity; and an enlarged tongue, tonsils, or adenoids.

Of the many anatomic features, three have been identified as helpful in predicting possible difficulty with laryngoscopy and tracheal intubation. These include tongue size relative to the pharynx, thyromental distance (the distance between the thyroid cartilage and the tip of the mandible), and atlanto-occipital extension.[29] The Mallampati and modified Mallampati airway classification systems are based on the extent to which the oropharyngeal structures are obscured by the patient's tongue. To assign a Mallampati class, the patient is examined in the upright and sitting position, mouth fully open with the tongue maximally protruding. The oropharyngeal structures identified with the patient in this position are the basis for the pharyngeal classes (see Table 14-6). The patient should not vocalize during the test, because vocalization raises the soft palate and alters the view.

In 1984, Cormack and Lehane[29] described four grades of the glottic view with direct laryngoscopy (see Table 14-7). The incidence of difficult tracheal intubation varies with the Cormack-Lehane laryngeal grade. Both Mallampati and Samsoon have published a correlation between Mallampati pharyngeal class and ease of laryngoscopy and tracheal intubation. In summary, patients found to have Mallampati pharyngeal class I airway examinations have Cormack-Lehane grade I laryngoscopic views 99% to 100% of the time. Those with Mallampati pharyn-

Table 14-10. Physical findings suggestive of possible difficulty with tracheal intubation

Trismus
Poor cervical spine mobility
Airway and maxillofacial trauma
Congenital facial and upper airway deformities
Facial and airway tumors and abscesses
Face and neck fibrosis (burns, radiation exposure)
Postsurgical facial and neck deformity
Large tonsils
Micrognathia
Macroglossia
Poor dentition or prominent incisors
Short neck
Large breasts
Morbid obesity

geal class IV airways have Cormack-Lehane laryngoscopic grades of III and IV up to 100% of the time.[27,28,31] Unfortunately, most patients present with Mallampati class II or III airways, and these patients have been found to have Cormack-Lehane laryngeal grades ranging from I through IV. Thus, the ability to rely on these airway classification systems as predictors of difficult laryngoscopy and tracheal intubation is faulty, at least for the majority of patients whose airways are Mallampati class II and III.

The likely explanation for the wide range in Cormack-Lehane laryngeal grade versus Mallampati pharyngeal class, at least for Mallampati class II and III airways, lies not only in interobserver variability[32] but also in specific anatomic features of the airway that are not included in the modified Mallampati airway classification, including atlanto-occipital extension, thyromental distance, and a number of other features (Table 14-10). Frerk[33] studied whether a combination of the modified Mallampati class and measurement of the thyromental distance could be used to predict difficult laryngoscopy and tracheal intubation. Specifically, he demonstrated the individual and combined sensitivities and specificities of these two easily performed bedside tests. He found that categorization into modified Mallampati class III or class IV had a sensitivity and specificity of 81.2% for predicting a difficult tracheal intubation. The finding of a thyromental distance of less than 7 cm alone showed 91% sensitivity and 81.5% specificity. Use of the two tests together had 81.2% sensitivity and 97.8% specificity. In summary, he found that patients whose airways were categorized as modified Mallampati class III or class IV and who had a thyromental distance of less than 7 cm could be expected to have difficult laryngoscopy and tracheal intubation. Of note, thyromental distance was measured with the patient's head in maximum extension. A major limitation of this study was the limited number of patients evaluated.

A number of disease states and craniofacial and cervical spine abnormalities are associated with difficult intubation. These can be identified by history (Table 14-11), physical examination (see Table 14-10), and radiographic techniques (chest radiography, neck and chest computed tomography, cervical spine imaging, tracheal tomogram).

In addition, obtaining previous operative records is critical. Little excuse exists for proceeding with an elective procedure in the absence of such documentation. This is especially true for patients who meet criteria for possible difficulty with tracheal intubation.

In summary, tongue size relative to the pharynx, atlanto-occipital extension, thyromental distance, craniofacial and cervical spinal deformities, and various disease states influence both prediction of possible difficult intubation and actual difficulty in intubating the trachea. No single factor, except perhaps a history of difficult intubation, has proven absolutely reliable in predicting difficulty. Preoperative evaluation is the key to optimizing the chance of successfully intubating a given patient. Once the patient is inside the operating room, optimizing head position and having access to a number of airway devices as outlined in the ASA difficult airway management algorithm (Fig. 14-2) further enhance successful intubation of the trachea.

How, then, should the anesthesia practitioner approach the induction of anesthesia when a difficult airway is suspected? First, the practitioner should become exceedingly familiar with the ASA difficult airway management algorithm. Second, a determination should be made as to whether mask ventilation will be easy to perform. If the practitioner recognizes the presence of a *potentially difficult airway* in association with the *possibility of inadequate mask ventilation*, then the most conservative approach would be to prepare the patient for an awake intubation. For this method of securing an airway to be successful, the practitioner must explain to the patient exactly what will occur and must coach the patient through the procedure. Judicious use of sedatives is indicated. Topically anes-

Table 14-11. History suggestive of possible difficulty with tracheal intubation

Congenital abnormalities	Down syndrome, Treacher Collins syndrome, Pierre Robin syndrome, Goldenhar's syndrome, Klippel-Feil syndrome
Endocrine disorders	Obesity, acromegaly, dwarfism, Cushing's disease
Infection	Epiglottitis, Ludwig's angina
Immune and collagen vascular disease	Scleroderma, rheumatoid arthritis, cervical spine degeneration, cervical disc disease
Burns, trauma, foreign body	—
Neoplasms	Cancer, lingual hemangioma, mucopolysaccharidoses

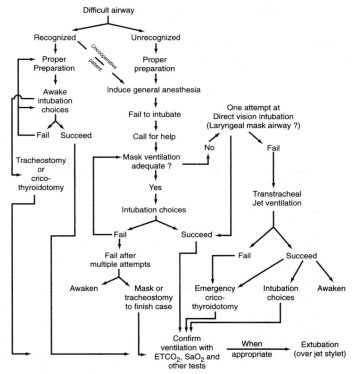

Fig. 14-2. The American Society of Anesthesiologists Task Force difficult airway management algorithm. (ETCO$_2$, end-tidal carbon dioxide concentration; SaO$_2$, oxygen saturation.)

thetizing of the airway with local anesthetics (Table 14-12) is the *key element* of successful "awake" intubation.

The already anesthetized patient who proves difficult to intubate presents a different set of challenges. First, the practitioner should request additional anesthesia help. The situation is not urgent if ventilation by mask is adequate. Optimization of head position,[34] change of laryngoscope blade, insertion of a laryngeal mask airway through which intubation may occur, intubation using a fiberoptic bronchoscope, and blind nasal attempts may all be performed. If intubation is required for an elective operative procedure, then the patient may be allowed to wake up and an awake intubation performed. If the patient cannot be ventilated by mask and tracheal intubation is difficult after the induction of anesthesia, the situation may become critical. In many ways, the patient who meets criteria for potential difficulty with tracheal intubation presents less of a challenge to the anesthesiologist than the patient with an unrecognized difficult airway.

Table 14-12. Methods of anesthetizing the upper and lower airways

Nebulized local anesthetic
Local anesthetic swish and swallow
Local anesthetic spray
Bilateral lingual nerve block
Superior laryngeal nerve block
Transtracheal local anesthetic injection
Judicious use of mucous membrane drying agent before topical anesthesia (glycopyrrolate)

From Gaiser R. *Clinical anesthesia procedures of the Massachusetts General Hospital*, 4th ed. Boston: Little, Brown and Company, 1993:180–181; Benumof JL. Management of the difficult airway: the ASA algorithm. *Refresher courses in anesthesiology*, vol 22. Philadelphia: JB Lippincott Co, 1994:39–44.

What this chapter demonstrates is that no simple test exists to identify a patient at risk for failed tracheal intubation. A clear understanding of and ability to implement the ASA difficult airway management algorithm and facility with all of the recommended instruments are of paramount importance. Careful history taking and physical examination and review of radiographic data and previous anesthetic records are critical to the preoperative evaluation. Finally, communication between the individual who performed the preoperative evaluation and the individual who is to perform the anesthetic is paramount if patients are to be cared for in an optimal way.

Any patient whose airway was difficult to manage, because of either poor mask ventilation or difficulty with tracheal intubation, should be encouraged to obtain a MedicAlert bracelet. MedicAlert can be reached at 2323 Colorado Avenue, Turlock, CA 95382, and at (800) 432-5378.

CASE STUDY

A 25-year-old woman with a lump in her neck is to undergo a partial thyroidectomy. She has no significant medical or surgical history and is on no medications. When asked whether anyone in the family has had problems with anesthesia, she presents a card containing the word *succinylcholine*. She says that her father had a bad "allergy" to this medication and previously had to stay in the intensive care unit after a surgical procedure. Unfortunately, she has no records.

Could he have had MH? Was he in need of ventilation due to pseudocholinesterase deficiency? Perhaps he had received too much succinylcholine and required ventilation for a phase II block? When pressed, she states that her father had received a single dose of this drug, and on completion of the operation he "could hear everything but could not move." He was ventilated in the intensive care unit for several hours with no other problems. She has never heard of MH but states that her father's anesthesiologist had said that no one in the family should receive succinylcholine.

With a likely family history of pseudocholinesterase deficiency, this patient and her children should be tested to determine whether they are at risk for prolonged apnea with use of succinylcholine and mivacurium chloride. Her dibucaine level should be determined. All close relatives should be evaluated. All affected persons need to be advised to obtain a MedicAlert bracelet and registration. She should be reassured that neither succinylcholine nor mivacurium chloride is necessary for anesthesia or surgery.

This case highlights the importance of obtaining medical records before elective surgery, because patients often are unaware of the specific details regarding medical care.

REFERENCES

1. Bevan DR, Donati F. *Muscle relaxants in clinical anesthesia*, 2nd ed. Philadelphia: JB Lippincott Co, 1992:484.
2. Donati F, Bevan DR. Long-term succinylcholine infusion during isoflurane anesthesia. *Anesthesiology* 1983;58:6–10.
3. Kalow W, Genest K. A method for the detection of atypical forms of human serum cholinesterase. Determination of dibucaine numbers. *Can J Biochem Physiol* 1957;35:339–346.
4. Viby-Mogensen J. Succinylcholine neuromuscular blockade in subjects homozygous for atypical plasma cholinesterase. *Anesthesiology* 1981;55:429–434.
5. Lehmann H, Lidell J. Pseudocholinesterase: genetic variants and their recognition. *Br J Anaesth* 1969;41:235–243.
6. Krause A, Lane AB, Jenkins T. Pseudocholinesterase variation in southern Africa populations. *S Afr Med J* 1987;71:298–301.
7. Hanel HK, Viby-Mogensen J, de Muckadell OB. Serum cholinesterase variants in the Danish population. *Acta Anaesthesiol Scand* 1978;22:505–507.
8. Gutsche BB, Scott EM, Wright RC. Hereditary deficiency in pseudocholinesterase in Eskimos. *Nature* 1965;215:322–323.
9. Rosenberg H, Fletcher J, Seitman D. *Pharmacogenetics in clinical anesthesia*, 2nd ed. Philadelphia: JB Lippincott Co, 1992:604.
10. Davies RO, Marton AV, Kalow W. The action of normal and atypical cholinesterase upon a series of esters of choline. *Can J Biochem Physiol* 1960;38:545–551.
11. Stoelting RK, Dierdorf SF. *Anesthesia and co-existing disease*, 3rd ed. New York: Churchill Livingstone, 1993:612.
12. Ording H. Incidence of MH in Denmark. *Anesth Analg* 1985;64:700–704.
13. Lopez JR, Alamo L, Caputo C, et al. Intracellular ionized calcium concentration in muscles from humans with malignant hyperthermia. *Muscle Nerve* 1985;8:355–358.
14. Hymel L, Inui M, Fleischer S, Schindler H. Purified ryanodine receptor of skeletal muscle sarcoplasmic reticulum forms calcium activated oligomeric calcium channels in planar bilayers. *Proc Natl Acad Sci U S A* 1988;85:441–445.
15. Lai FA, Erickson HP, Rousseau E, et al. Purification and reconstitution of the calcium release channel from skeletal muscle. *Nature* 1988;331:315–319.
16. Jenden DJ, Fairhurst AS. The pharmacology of ryanodine. *Pharmacol Rev* 1969;21:1–25.
17. Wieland SJ, Fletcher JE, Rosenberg H, Gong QH. Malignant hyperthermia: slow sodium current in cultured human muscle cells. *Am J Physiol* 1989;257:759–765.
18. Gillard EF, Otsu K, Fuji J, et al. Polymorphisms and deduced

amino acid substitutions in the coding sequence of the ryanodine receptor (RYR1) gene in individuals with malignant hyperthermia. *Genomics* 1992;13:1247–1254.

19. Rosenberg H, Fletcher J. Masseter muscle rigidity and malignant hyperthermia susceptibility. *Anesth Analg* 1998;65:161–164.

20. Allen GC, Rosenberg H. Malignant hyperthermia susceptibility in adult patients with masseter muscle rigidity. *Can J Anaesth* 1990;37:31–35.

21. Kaplan R. Malignant hyperthermia. *Refresher courses in anesthesiology*, vol 22. Philadelphia: JB Lippincott Co, 1994:169–180.

.22. Caplan RA, Posner KL, Ward RJ, Cheney FW. Adverse respiratory events in anesthesia: a closed claims analysis. *Anesthesiology* 1990;723:828–833.

23. Benumof JL. Management of the difficult airway. *Anesthesiology* 1991;75:1087–1110.

24. Roberts JT. *Clinical management of the airway*. Philadelphia: WB Saunders, 1994:3–17.

25. Moore KL. *Clinically oriented anatomy*, 2nd ed. Baltimore: Williams & Wilkins, 1984:1033–1062.

26. Mallampati SR. Clinical sign to predict difficult tracheal intubation (hypothesis). *Can Anaesth Soc J* 1983;30:316–317.

27. Mallampati SR, Gatt SP, Gugino LD, et al. A clinical sign to predict difficult tracheal intubation: a prospective study. *Can Anaesth Soc J* 1985;32:429–434.

28. Samsoon GLT, Young JRB. Difficult tracheal intubation: a retrospective study. *Anaesthesia* 1987;42:487–490.

29. Cormack RS, Lehane J. Difficult tracheal intubation in obstetrics. *Anaesthesia* 1984;39:1105–1111.

30. Benumof JL. Management of the difficult airway: the ASA algorithm. *Refresher courses in anesthesiology*, vol 22. Philadelphia: JB Lippincott Co, 1994:39–44.

31. Cohen SM, Zaurito CE, Segil LJ. Oral exam to predict difficult intubations: a large prospective study. *Anesthesiology* 1989;71:A937.

32. Charters P, Horton WA. Soft tissues and difficult intubation. *Anaesthesia* 1991;45:996–997.

33. Frerk CM. Predicting difficult intubation. *Anaesthesia* 1991;46:1005–1008.

34. Roberts JT, Ali HH, Shorten GD, Gorback MS. Why cervical flexion facilitates laryngoscopy with a Macintosh laryngoscope but hinders it with a flexible fiberscope. *Anesthesiology* 1990;73:A1012.

Miscellaneous Issues

Jeffrey Uppington

This chapter discusses the perioperative evaluation of patients with a number of different conditions and issues. The topics covered are evaluation of patients with **latex allergy**; patients who are **breast-feeding**; patients with **morbid obesity, sleep apnea, acquired immune deficiency syndrome**, or **cancer**; and **geriatric** patients, including those having **cataract surgery**. In addition, patients on **corticosteroid therapy**, patients for whom **"do not resuscitate"** orders are in effect, and those who **refuse blood transfusion** are discussed.

PATIENTS TAKING CORTICOSTEROID THERAPY

The recommendations for the perioperative management of patients taking corticosteroid therapy have historically been based on a relatively small number of published case reports of perioperative death and morbidity in patients taking corticosteroids and not on a systematic population study. One of the early case reports[1] concluded with a list of recommendations for perioperative glucocorticoid treatment that has formed the basis of therapy ever since. These recommendations roughly amounted to a fourfold increase in glucocorticoid administration and have often been generalized to indicate a fourfold increase in the daily dose. Much of the thinking related to this topic has approximated the dictum "Better safe than sorry" and reflects the feeling that very high dose steroids, administered for a short period, should not be harmful. An excess of glucocorticoids can lead to adverse clinical consequences, however. These include the catabolic effects of high doses of steroids on muscle and wound healing; the antiinsulin effects, which decrease glucose tolerance; and immune compromise, which can lead to increased susceptibility to infection or worsen infection if already present. Therefore, some rational system must be developed that minimizes the adverse consequences of glucocorticoids.

Glucocorticoid administration suppresses the normal hypothalamic-pituitary-adrenal (HPA) cortical system. The functioning of this system is the means by which serum corticotropin and cortisol concentrations increase during surgical procedures. Considerable individual variability is found in this response to surgical stress. Other variables include the effects of anesthetics, exogenous and endogenous opiates and analgesics, and antihypertensive agents, as well as age, sleep, and the presence of infection.[2] The magnitude of the increase in cortisol concentrations also is correlated with the extent of the surgery. For example, an increase of 84% over preoperative base values has been found after laparotomy compared with a 36% increase after less extensive procedures such as surgery involv-

Table 15-1. Symptoms and signs of hypoadrenalism

Unexplained circulatory instability

Discrepancy between the anticipated severity of the disease and the present state of the patient, including

Nausea

Vomiting

Orthostatic hypotension

Dehydration

Abdominal or flank pain (acute adrenal hemorrhage)

Fatigue

Weight loss

Reprinted with permission from Lamberts SWJ, Bruining HA, de Jong FH. Corticosteroid therapy in severe illness. *N Engl J Med* 1997;337:1285–1292.

ing the breast, neck, or joints. If a patient undergoing a surgical procedure is unable to generate these increases in cortisol, a state of acute adrenal insufficiency may occur.[3] The symptoms and signs that are suggestive of hypoadrenalism in critically ill patients are listed in Table 15-1.

The circulatory instability can mimic hypovolemic shock (decreased preload, depressed myocardial contractility, increased systemic vascular resistance) or can resemble hyperdynamic shock (high cardiac output and decreased systemic vascular resistance as in septic shock). Perioperative corticosteroid administration is designed to prevent these potential adverse consequences.

What is the reality of the risk of these potential consequences in patients taking corticosteroids? As mentioned before, much of the original data came from individual case reports. A careful review of these reports[4] showed that the majority of the early cases were inconclusive and lacked any biochemical confirmation of adrenal insufficiency. In addition, other factors were present that could have contributed to or caused the symptomatology reported. The same review, however, does support the concept that the problem is real and certainly can occur. However, many patients taking glucocorticoids have undergone major surgery without perioperative steroid coverage, and most of these patients have had uneventful clinical courses. These patients probably have normal HPA axis function despite glucocorticoid administration. Studies have also been done on patients receiving long-term prednisone therapy, showing that the vast majority of patients have normal or increased urinary cortisol concentrations. These results suggest that circulating cortisol concentrations were sufficient to meet patients' requirements during the time of surgical stress. None of these patients was given an increased dosage of glucocorticoids, and no symptoms that occurred were explainable purely as adrenal insufficiency.

The degree of HPA dysfunction depends on the duration and the dosage of glucocorticoid therapy. Medication history may be unreliable. Ideally, HPA function should be assessed preoperatively to determine the need for perioperative management. A number of tests are feasible. These include provocative tests measuring the plasma cortisone response to administration of adrenal corticotropin hormone (ACTH), corticotropin-releasing hormone, pyrogen, lysine vasopressin, and metyrapone, and to insulin-induced hypoglycemia. Although the insulin-tolerance and pyrogen tests have the advantage that their site of stimulation is central, the 30-minute ACTH test is the most convenient and accurate diagnostic tool for preoperative evaluation of HPA axis function. Synthetic ACTH in a dose of 250 mg is administered intravenously, and a blood sample is collected 30 minutes later to test plasma cortisone level. A plasma cortisone concentration equal to or higher than 500 nmol per L (18 to 20 mg per dL) indicates adequate adrenal function. In practice, however, perioperative testing of every patient who is on glucocorticoid therapy is not feasible, and thus some other rational approach must be used.

Adults are estimated to secrete 75 to 150 mg of cortisol per day in response to major surgery and 50 mg per day in response to minor procedures. Although large variation exists, cortisol secretion in the first 24 hours after surgery rarely exceeds 200 mg, and the secretion rate parallels the duration and extent of surgery. No data exist to support the concept that glucocorticoid administration exceeding this amount is beneficial.

A number of therapeutic strategies have been recommended in the past. One recommendation is to give 25 mg of intravenous cortisol or its equivalent with induction of anesthesia and 100 mg by continuous infusion over the next 24 hours. An alternative is to give 25 mg of cortisol equivalent intravenously every 4 hours. Another suggestion has been to provide minimal coverage, with supplementation only if postoperative hypotension occurs. Others have recommended 100 mg of intramuscular cortisone every 6 hours, and yet another recommendation is intramuscular injection of depot betamethasone, which has effects lasting up to 6 days from one injection.[2]

A multispecialty group has recommended glucocorticoid coverage that is dependent on the type of surgery.[2] Thus, for minor surgery (e.g., inguinal herniorrhaphy) the daily cortisone secretion rate and plasma cortisone measurement suggest that the glucocorticoid target is 25 mg of hydrocortisone equivalent. For example, a patient receiving 5 mg of prednisone every other day for asthma should receive 5 mg of prednisone preoperatively and should be watched carefully. If no complications occur, the patient can restart the usual steroid dosage the next day.

For moderate surgical stress (e.g., nonlaparoscopic cholecystectomy, abdominal hysterectomy, or total joint replacement), the glucocorticoid target is 50 to 75 mg of hydrocortisone a day for 1 or 2 days. Thus, a patient on 10 mg of prednisone a day should receive 10 mg of prednisone (or equivalent) preoperatively and 50 mg of intravenous hydrocortisone intraoperatively. Sixty milligrams of intravenous hydrocortisone may be given the next day, and the patient can be returned to the preoperative steroid dose on postoperative day 2.

For major surgical stress (e.g., esophagogastrectomy or cardiopulmonary bypass), the glucocorticoid target should be 100 to 150 mg of hydrocortisone equivalent per day for 3 days. For example, a patient who has been taking 40 mg of prednisone daily should receive 40 mg of prednisone (or equivalent) preoperatively and 50 mg of hydrocortisone intravenously every 8 hours for the first 48 to 72 hours after surgery. A patient on 5 mg of prednisone daily who is having major surgery should receive 5 mg of prednisone (or equivalent) preoperatively, 25 mg of hydrocortisone intraoperatively, and 25 mg every 8 hours for the next 2 days.

The advantages of these recommendations are that they are based on some reasonable studies, they limit the dose of steroids so that potential side effects are reduced, and they can be reasonably individualized. Monitoring all patients carefully for any sign of adrenal insufficiency remains important. A list of the relative potencies of some common corticosteroids is presented in Table 15-2.

PATIENTS WITH LATEX ALLERGY

Latex is derived from natural rubber, which is obtained from the tree *Hevea brasiliensis*. The milky fluid produced by special lactifer cells acts as a natural wound sealant for the tree. After harvesting, it undergoes a variety of chemical processes to produce the various latex products used in the medical field.

Reactions to rubber products have been known for many years, but these were of the contact dermatitis type. Only relatively recently have severe urticarial and systemic reactions been described. Although this may be due to better recognition and reporting of the problem, the greatly increased use of latex gloves after the adoption of universal precautions and, possibly, changes in the manufacturing process are more likely to have led to an increased incidence.[5] Many latex proteins act as allergens, and accelerators present in the rubber of protective gloves remain the most frequent source of allergy. Starch in the powder in many gloves can act as an airborne carrier and can cause asthma if inhaled.

Certain people are at an increased risk of developing latex allergy. These include health care workers, who have an increased exposure to latex, usually in the form of gloves. Others are patients with repeated or prolonged exposure to latex products such as urinary catheters. Patients with meningomyelocele or urologic problems are

Table 15-2. Relative antiinflammatory dose and potency of some common corticosteroids

	Equivalent anti-inflammatory dose (mg)	Equivalent anti-inflammatory potency
Cortisone acetate	37.5	0.8
Hydrocortisone	30	1
Prednisone	7.5	4
Prednisolone	7.5	4
Methylprednisolone	6	5
Triamcinolone	6	5
Paramethasone acetate	3	10
Betamethasone	1	30
Dexamethasone	1	30

The dose given for each drug is equivalent to the daily physiologic secretion rate of hydrocortisone.
Reprinted with permission from Calvey TN, Williams NE. *Principles and practice of pharmacology for anesthetists*, 3rd ed. Oxford: Blackwell, 1997:562.

particularly susceptible. Latex factory workers are at increased risk, especially if they have a history of atopy or hand eczema. Latex-allergic patients are more likely to have a history of asthma, rubber-contact allergy, food allergy (especially allergy to tropical fruits), or adhesive tape rash, and to have undergone nine or more surgical procedures. Immunoglobulin E (IgE) antibodies have been implicated as a major cause of latex-induced allergy and anaphylaxis. Susceptible patients may have increased latex-specific IgE or total IgE serum levels.

The diagnosis of latex allergy is made by history, examination and, if necessary, by *in vivo* and *in vitro* testing. The most sensitive and specific test is skin-prick testing, but systemic reactions are possible. Thus, this test should be restricted to those patients with a definite history but inconclusive serologic tests. A radioallergosorbent test for latex-specific IgE antibodies has been described but is less sensitive than the skin-prick test. Circulating levels of latex-specific IgE can be measured. A provocative latex challenge has been described in which the response of one dampened hand 15 minutes after placement in a latex glove is compared with the response of the other hand after placement in a vinyl glove. Again, this test should be avoided if severe systemic reactions have occurred.

Patients can be divided into those with definite latex allergies and those with a high likelihood of such allergy. Careful coordination among anesthesia, surgical, and nursing teams is necessary to identify such patients and avoid patient contact with the many latex products present in an operating room.

Holzman has provided a checklist for dealing with latex-allergic patients.[6] The following are included:

1. Solicit history of latex allergy or risk of latex allergy.
2. Consider allergy testing and consultation.
3. Minimize latex exposure for patients at risk; differentiate latex-alert patients who have significant risk factors but no overt symptoms from latex allergy patients, who have a positive history, signs, or symptoms of latex allergy.
4. Create a medical alert tag.
5. Place warning signs on chart and bed.
6. Have a list of latex products and nonlatex alternatives, and display latex allergy signs inside and outside the operating room.

PATIENTS WHO ARE BREAST-FEEDING

Little reliable information is available on the effects of maternal drug administration on the babies and infants of women who are breast-feeding. Much of the data on the physiochemical and pharmacokinetic factors of drug transfer into breast milk is derived from animal experiments, although increasing data from humans are becoming available. Many variables exist, including characteristics of the drug itself, the variability of the composition of human milk, and infant factors.[7]

Drug Factors

The pharmacokinetic profile of the drug—that is, how it moves from the blood to breast milk—is important. Wilson[8] has proposed a three-compartment model. A central compartment receives the drug directly after administration. A second compartment represents interstitial and intracellular water. The third compartment is breast milk. Movement of a drug from each compartment in both directions occurs at various rates. There is an elimination rate constant from the central compartment, and an infant-modulated rate constant for removal of drug from breast milk. The rate constants vary for different drugs, depending on a number of factors.

The degree of plasma protein binding of the drug affects its potential movement into breast milk, because only the unbound form crosses freely into the mammary cells. Fat solubility is important, because highly fat soluble drugs readily cross the lipid boundary of the mammary cell membrane. Milk contains a lipid phase that is lacking in plasma, and thus drugs that are highly lipid soluble can partition into milk fat and achieve higher concentrations in milk than in plasma.

The degree of ionization of the drug also affects transfer. Nonionized drugs are excreted in the milk more readily than are ionized ones. A pH difference exists between plasma (pH 7.4) and milk (pH 6.8 to 7.3, average 7.0). Thus, weakly acidic drugs are ionized to a greater extent in plasma than in milk, and the reverse is true for weak bases. Under normal pH conditions, the concentration of weak acids is lower in milk than in plasma, although the free concentration of basic drugs in milk may exceed that in plasma. Changes in plasma or milk pH affect this degree of drug ionization.

Molecular weight limits transfer of drugs into breast milk. However, most clinically useful drugs have molecular weights between 200 and 500 daltons and can pass into breast milk.

Breast Factors

The amount of blood flow into the mammary glands affects transfer of drugs. The metabolic activity of the mammary glands probably affects blood flow, as does the release of lactogenic hormones in response to suckling. Bulk flow of drugs, including water-soluble ones, can occur through pores between mammary cells. This mechanism accounts for the bulk of the fluid changes across the epithelium. These pores are completely open at delivery and gradually tighten over the next few days.

Infant Factors

After a drug has been excreted into breast milk, it must be absorbed by the infant's gastrointestinal tract. Transit time, which affects drug absorption, varies from the newborn to the adult. Ionization and lipid solubility of the drug, however, are the main variables governing transport of drugs across the gastrointestinal mucosa. The younger the infant and the younger the gestational age, the more likely that drugs will be poorly tolerated due to immature detoxification pathways in the infant liver. At birth, renal function is not fully developed, but the kidney matures rapidly so that glomerular filtration approaches adult levels by 2 months of age. Decreased rate of elimination may allow for the accumulation of plasma levels of drugs that may be present in only small quantities in breast milk.

Milk Factors

The pH and composition of milk vary over time, which can influence the amount of drugs that accumulate in the milk. In the first few days after delivery, the breast produces colostrum, which has a pH of 7.45, contains no fat, and is secreted in small volumes. After several days, and until approximately the third month, a transitional phase occurs in which the milk has a pH of 7.0 and contains fat. Mature milk has a rising pH and increasing lactose concentration.[9] Fat also increases, and thus an increase in lipophilic drug concentration can occur. The actual effects on infants of drugs ingested from breast milk are variable and for many drugs are not well defined.[10] The Committee on Drugs of the American Academy of Pediatrics has categorized medications in relation to the safety of their ingestion by breast-feeding mothers (Table 15-3).[11] Other drugs of interest for anesthesia are included in Table 15-4.[7]

Table 15-3. American Academy of Pediatrics classification of maternal medication use during lactation

Classification	Definition	Examples
Category 1	Medications that should not be consumed during lactation. Strong evidence exists that serious adverse effects on the infant are likely with maternal ingestion of these medications during lactation.	Ergotamine
Category 2	Drug whose infant effects in humans are unknown, but caution is urged.	Amitriptyline, desipramine, doxepin, fluoxetine, imipramine, trazodone
		Diazepam, lorazepam, midazolam
Category 3	Medications compatible with breast-feeding.	Carbamazepine, phenytoin, valproic acid
		Atenolol, propranolol, diltiazem
		Codeine, fentanyl, methadone, morphine, propoxyphene
		Butorphanol
		Lidocaine, mexiletine
		Acetaminophen
		Ibuprofen, indomethacin, ketorolac, naproxen
		Caffeine

Adapted from Committe on Drugs, American Academy of Pediatrics. The transfer of drugs and other chemicals into human milk. *Pediatrics* 1994;93:137–150.

Table 15-4. Passage of drugs into breast milk and effects on infants

Drug	Milk to plasma ratio	Amount in milk after therapeutic dose	Comments
Analgesics and antiinflammatory drugs			
Alfentanil	—	—	No data available
Aspirin	0.03–0.08	Aspirin is converted to salicylic acid, which is distributed in milk; infant receives 21% of maternal dose	Caution in early infancy; complications rare
Butorphanol	Oral dose, 1.9; i.m. dose, 0.7	4 μg in 1 L of milk	No adverse effects reported
Codeine	0.3–2.5	Milk peak at 1 h	No effect with therapeutic level and transient use; can accumulate; watch for neonatal depression
Diclofenac	0.02–0.07	—	No adverse effects reported
Fentanyl	>1	Milk peak at 45 min after 2 μg/kg i.v.	No adverse effects reported
Ibuprofen	0.01	Milk levels <0.5 mg/mL	No adverse effects reported
Indomethacin	>1	—	Convulsions in breast-fed infant; may be nephrotoxic
Ketoprofen	—	Trace amounts	
Morphine	2.46	Peak level, 19 ng/mL	Single doses have minimal effects; potential accumulation; elimination half-life in infant's plasma markedly increased
Paracetamol	0.2–1.9	Milk peak at 2 h; half-life in milk, 2.6 h; infant receives 1.85% of maternal oral dose of 1 g	Detoxified in liver; drug and metabolite found in infant's urine; well tolerated by the infant
	0.76	Maximum level, 3 μg/100 mL	No adverse effects reported
Pentazocine	—	Not excreted in milk	—
Pethidine	1.0–1.4	Trace <0.1 mg/mL; peak level at 2 h	Marked increase in half-life in neonate
Sufentanil	—	—	No data available

continued

Table 15-4. *Continued*

Drug	Milk to plasma ratio	Amount in milk after therapeutic dose	Comments
Antagonists			
Naloxone	—	Not known if excreted in breast milk	No adverse effects reported; no data available
Neostigmine	—	No data available	—
Anticholinergics and histamine$_2$-antagonists			
Atropine sulphate	—	0.1 mg/100 mL	Hyperthermia, tachycardia, constipation, urinary retention; decreased milk secretion in the mother
Cimetidine	4.6–11.7	Maximum amount, 6 mg/L	Suppression of gastric acidity and activity; inhibition of hepatic metabolism
Ranitidine	1.9–6.7	Peak levels, 1,000–3,000 ng/mL	Infant receives 1–3 mg per day
Benzodiazepines			
Chlordiazepoxide	—	Found in breast milk	No adverse effects reported
Clonazepam	0.33	Only one case reported in 7-day-old neonate who had 2.9 ng/mL in serum	No clinical data available
Diazepam	0.2–2.7	—	Can be detected in infant as long as 10 days after a single dose; when taken in multiple doses, has caused sleepiness, mild depression in the infant; tendency to accumulate in the neonate in the first week
Flunitrazepam	—	Milk level, 1–2 ng/mL after a 2-mg dose	Clinically insignificant for the infant
Lorazepam	—	Found in low concentrations in milk	Increased half-life in neonate
Oxazepam	0.10–0.33	Very small amounts in breast milk	No adverse effects reported
Intravenous anesthetics			
Etomidate	—	—	No data available
Ketamine	—	—	No data available

continued

Table 15-4. *Continued*

Drug	Milk to plasma ratio	Amount in milk after therapeutic dose	Comments
Propanidid	—	—	No data available
Propofol	—	Milk levels, 0.089–0.240 μg/mL after an induction dose of 2.5 mg/kg; milk levels, 0.04–0.74 μg/mL after an induction dose of 2.5 mg/kg and mainten-ance dose of 5 mg/kg/h)	No clinical effects reported
Thiopentone	0.39–0.50	Maximum levels, 0.034 mg/100 mL in colostrum and 0.090 mg/100 mL in mature milk	No clinical effects reported
Inhalation anesthetics			
Halothane	—	2 p.p.m. found in nursing mothers who worked in environment with halothane	No adverse effects reported
Local anesthetics			
Bupivacaine	—	Not found in breast milk	—
Lignocaine	—	Not found in breast milk	—
Muscle relaxants			No data available but no clinical adverse effects reported
Miscellaneous			
Adrenaline	—	—	Destroyed in gastro-intestinal tract of infant
Caffeine	0.48–0.82	Peak level in milk at 1 h	Irritability and poor sleeping patterns found
Ergot derivatives	—	—	No adverse effects reported
Magnesium sulfate	2	Only during 24 h after i.v. injection	Infant receives approximately 6.5 mg/100 mL; calcium levels remain stable
Metoclopra-mide	1.8	Mean amount in milk, 125 ng/mL	Sedation and poor feeding can be seen in neonates

Preoperative Management

Patients who are breast-feeding must be identified. As shown in Tables 15-3 and 15-4, a general or regional anesthetic regime can be found that should theoretically have little if any effect on the suckling infant. In an elective case, however, a conservative but safe approach is to advise the mother to pump the breast milk preoperatively and refrigerate it for later feeding. This milk, or formula, can be used to feed the baby in the first 24 hours after the surgical procedure. The breast milk produced during the 24-hour postoperative period should be pumped and discarded. After 24 hours, the maternal plasma levels of any anesthetic drug should be low enough so that no effective amount is found in breast milk, and normal breast-feeding can be resumed. For emergent surgery, selection of suitable anesthetic agents should be made, but discarding the first 24 hours of breast milk remains the conservative option.

PATIENTS WHO REFUSE BLOOD TRANSFUSION

Patients who refuse blood transfusion usually are discussed under the heading of Jehovah's Witness patients, and the majority of them are members of the Jehovah's Witness faith. However, other patients, for whatever reason, adamantly refuse blood transfusion, and whatever policies are put in place must include this nonreligious group.

The refusal of blood and blood products by Jehovah's Witnesses is based on a strict interpretation of certain passages in the Bible (Genesis 9:3–4, Leviticus 17:14). However one may wish to argue the interpretation of these passages, the true Jehovah's Witness is convinced that they forbid blood transfusion and is often well informed of the inherent dangers of blood transfusion and the alternatives.[12] The law surrounding this issue is based on the 1990 ruling of the Supreme Court of the United States in *Cruzan v Missouri*,[13] which affirmed the right of any individual to refuse medical therapy, although the court recognized that the state also has strong interests that need to be balanced against the individual's right to refuse medical treatment. Not only does the Constitution of the United States guarantee individuals personal autonomy, but the First Amendment guarantees the free exercise of religion. The state's interests in these cases have expanded from preserving life to protecting third parties, preventing suicide, and maintaining the integrity of the ethics of the medical profession.[14] Medical ethics, as discussed in the section on "do not resuscitate" orders, emphasize patient autonomy and self-determination. The balance among the patient's rights, state's rights, and the ethics of the medical providers pervades the issue of the refusal of blood transfusion.

In addition, different states may come to seemingly different conclusions. In 1989, the Florida Supreme Court[15] held that the state's interest in preserving a two-parent home for two minor children was not sufficiently strong to overcome the mother's right to privacy and religious freedom, and thus the state should not have forced her to accept a blood transfusion against her will. However, in the *Georgetown* case,[16] the court did uphold a court order to transfuse a Jehovah's Witness patient for the sake of her 7-month-old infant. Massachusetts does not allow injunctions to force transfusions on parents if it can be shown that the minor children have someone to look after them if the parent dies and thus will not be "abandoned."

Every institution and clinical department within that institution should have a policy that can guide clinicians in dealing with such patients and that is in accordance with the applicable state law. Some of the situations that should be addressed in such a document are outlined below.

Elective Procedures

Unlike in an emergency, with elective procedures time is available to discuss all the issues with the patient and clinicians involved. If an adult Jehovah's Witness (or any other person) refuses blood products, the patient should be interviewed in detail and in private. Each individual has a different level of commitment to the religion, and the individual should not be interviewed in the presence of relatives or church elders, who may, however inadvertently, influence the patient's decision. The physician must be sure the patient would rather die than receive blood. Although such a position may seem irrational to those who are not Jehovah's Witnesses, one must realize what is at stake for the true believer. Jehovah's Witness patients do not want to die and are not suicidal, but for them the consequences of receiving blood could include forfeiture of a chance for eternal life, severance of their individual relationship with God, and excommunication from their church and religious community.[17] Occasionally, patients' faith may not be sufficient for them to risk death, and they will accept blood. Each person has different beliefs regarding which blood alternatives will be accepted[18] (Table 15-5). Individuals within the department of anesthesia who are ethically comfortable dealing with Jehovah's Witnesses should be identified.

If the Jehovah's Witness patient has minor children, the patient should be asked who would be able and willing to look after them if the parent dies. The interviewer should document that a willing caregiver has been identified for the minor children, and a release of liability form should be signed. In the case of a patient who is a minor child of a Jehovah's Witness or a pregnant Jehovah's Witness with a viable child, most courts favor the state's interest in preserving the life of the child and will authorize blood transfusion. In these circumstances, legal opinion and a court order should be sought. To transfuse the child of a Jehovah's Witness is not an inconsequential thing, however, because some children who have had a blood transfusion have been rejected by their parents, so the transfusion should have definite lifesaving indications.

Emergent Procedures

In an emergency, when circumstances or time do not permit discussion with patients or relatives, most anesthesiologists would institute transfusions on the ethical principle of beneficence and worry about the legal position later. Some Jehovah's Witness individuals carry cards proclaiming their faith and describing their refusal of blood and blood products. In at least one case, a Jehovah's Witness patient who was carrying such a

Table 15-5. Perioperative therapies and techniques acceptable to Jehovah's Witnesses

Therapy
  Crystalloid solution
  Synthetic colloid solutions
  Dextran
  Aprotinin
  Aminocaproic acid
  Desmopressin
  Iron
  Erythropoietin*
  Human albumin*
  Perfluorocarbons
Technique
  Hypotensive anesthesia
  Induced hypothermia
  Continuous arterial blood gas monitoring
  In-line blood reserves
  Microchemistry blood analysis
  Extracorporeal circulation* (non–blood primed)
  Red blood cell salvage systems*
  Hemodilution*

*Potentially unacceptable to many Jehovah's Witnesses; therefore, these must be discussed with the individual patient.

card but was transfused anyway was awarded damages.[19] A legal opinion should be sought whenever any doubts exist with regard to an individual case. Court orders can be granted in a few hours if necessary and on a 24-hour basis.

GERIATRIC PATIENTS

The definition of *geriatric patients* is inevitably somewhat arbitrary but has been accepted to apply to those people older than 65 years. The chronologic age of a person is less important than the "physiologic" age, and the fact that many people age "better" than others—in other words, have a slower rate of biological decline—is well recognized. At whatever age it is defined, the geriatric or elderly population is the fastest growing segment of the population, not only in the United States but in all developed countries. Morbidity and mortality from surgical procedures increase as the individual ages, as evidenced by studies in vascular surgery.[20] One aim of preoperative evaluation of these patients is to identify the elements in each individual that might increase the risk of surgery, so that various techniques can be used to reduce this risk. An understanding of the pathophysiologic effects of aging on the various organ systems of the body is important to best choose preoperative laboratory tests. Whether age itself is a risk factor is also discussed in this section.

Table 15-6. Structural cardiovascular changes with age

Decrease in number of myocytes
Decrease in number of cells in sinoatrial node
Increase in fibrous tissue in internodal tracts
Gradual hypertrophy of left ventricle
Progressive stiffening of arterial system and increase in systemic vascular resistance
Increase in left atrial size
Fibrosis and calcification of heart valves

Cardiovascular System

As the individual grows older, structural changes occur in the heart and major arteries (Table 15-6). These anatomic changes lead to certain functional changes,[21] which are shown in Table 15-7.

Early diastolic filling is reduced in elderly people, due partly to left ventricular hypertrophy and partly to a defect in ventricular relaxation. Left ventricular end diastolic pressure may be elevated. This diastolic change may make the elderly patient more sensitive to the loss of atrial contraction and more prone to orthostatic hypotension, and may predispose to symptoms of congestive heart failure (CHF) even in the absence of abnormal systolic function. The cardiovascular system of the elderly is less sensitive to baroreceptor activity and also less responsive to beta-adrenergic stimulation during stress or exercise. Despite this response, or because of it, older people have higher basal levels of norepinephrine and epinephrine.

Anatomic changes in the conduction system can lead to cardiac arrhythmias, including sick sinus syndrome, which are more common in the elderly population. Coronary artery disease is more common as the individual ages, but whether it is part of the

Table 15-7. Cardiovascular changes in healthy older patients compared with healthy young adults

Cardiovascular parameter	Aging effect at rest	Aging effect with exercise
Heart rate	No change or slight decrease	Attenuated increase
Systolic blood pressure	Increased	Greater increase
Cardiac output	No change	Attenuated increase
Ejection fraction	No change	Smaller increase
Stroke volume	No change or slight increase	Greater increase

Reprinted with permission from Moore LE, Stiff JL. Evaluation of the geriatric patient. In: Longnecker DE, Tinker JH, Morgan GE Jr, eds. *Principles and practice of anesthesiology*, 2nd ed. St. Louis: Mosby–Year Book, 1998:473–486.

Table 15-8. Effects of aging on pulmonary function

Respiratory function test	Changes with normal aging
Vital capacity	Decreased (20 mL/yr)
Forced expiratory volume in 1 sec (FEV$_1$)	Decreased
FEV$_1$/forced vital capacity	Unchanged or small decrease
Closing capacity	Increased
Functional residual capacity	Unchanged or small increase
Residual volume	Increased
Total lung capacity	Unchanged or small decrease
Diffusing capacity	Decreased
Maximum minute ventilation	Decreased
Partial pressure of oxygen, arterial	Decreased

Reprinted with permission from Moore LE, Stiff JL. Evaluation of the geriatric patient. In: Longnecker DE, Tinker JH, Morgan GE Jr, eds. *Principles and practice of anesthesiology*, 2nd ed. St. Louis: Mosby–Year Book, 1998:473–486.

normal aging process or a concomitant disease remains open for debate. The incidence of "silent" myocardial infarction and ischemia increases with age, and these conditions should be identified in an individual patient.

Respiratory System

Anatomic and physiologic changes occur in the respiratory system. Lung and chest wall mechanics are altered by a decrease in intervertebral spaces, stiffening of the chest wall, loss of muscle strength, and decrease in the elastic recoil of the lungs. The reduction in elastic recoil leads to early airway closure, and thus closing volume increases with age. When closing volume exceeds functional residual capacity, airway closure occurs during normal breathing, and the resulting change in ventilation distribution causes a mismatch of ventilation to perfusion. Arterial oxygen tension is lower in the elderly and has been described as follows:

$$PaO_2 \text{ (mm Hg)} = 104 - (0.24 \times age)$$

where PaO_2 is the oxygen tension in arterial blood. Ventilatory drive decreases with age, and sensitivity to changes in both oxygen and carbon dioxide is reduced. Airway reflexes may also be less active in the elderly patient. The changes in pulmonary function tests that occur with age are summarized in Table 15-8.

Nervous System

Cortical neuronal loss occurs with aging, in both the brain and spinal cord. Normal changes of cognition with aging cannot be detected by the usual clinical methods, however, although detailed neuropsychological testing can reveal some changes in processing time and acquisition of new data. Cerebral blood flow regulation seems little affected by normal aging. A reduction in cerebral blood flow is seen that correlates with the reduction in gray matter. Cerebral autoregulation is intact, although it may be shifted upward in response to hypertensive changes. This adaptation in the elderly may be irreversible, and thus hypotension is poorly tolerated.

With age, beta-adrenergic activity declines as does the beta-adrenergic response to various physiologic changes. Thus, in theory, the elderly are more likely to respond to pain by hypertension than by tachycardia, and the tachycardic response to hypovolemia may be attenuated. Thermoregulation is affected as individuals age. Not only does temperature discrimination at the skin decrease, but the hypothalamic center is set at a lower thermal point. The intensity of shivering decreases, and the ability of the skin to close arteriovenous shunts is reduced. The elderly operative patient is thus more likely to develop hypothermia with all the possible consequences of a low temperature.

Delirium occurs frequently in the elderly in the postoperative period; interestingly, the incidence does not seem to be affected by either the type of anesthesia or regional block, or the mode of postoperative pain control. The onset may indicate an organic illness and is associated with an increase in mortality rate. A paucity of information exists on the anesthetic management of patients with Alzheimer's disease. Not much data are found on the effects of sedation and anesthesia, but a reduction of dosages would seem reasonable. A great deal of psychological support should be given to these patients in the perioperative period, because being in hospitals and the operating room must be a confusing and frightening experience for them (see Chapter 11A).

Renal System

Renal function decreases by approximately 1% per year. Creatinine clearance decreases at a predictable rate, but because of loss of muscle mass, serum creatinine levels usually remain in the normal range (see Chapter 8). Aging appears to affect the kidney's handling of sodium both by conserving it less well and by handling salt loading poorly. The elderly are therefore more susceptible to hypovolemia and volume overload.

Hepatic System

Liver size regresses as aging progresses, although hepatocellular function is reasonably preserved. Liver function tests are normal, and although plasma cholinesterase activity is reduced, little clinical effect is seen from this.

Drug Metabolism

Changes occur with age in both drug pharmacodynamics and drug pharmacokinetics. Drug clearance is reduced, which usually means that elderly patients need lower dosages of drugs than their younger counterparts. The changes in pharmacology with

Table 15-9. Altered drug effects with aging

Pharmacodynamic
    Decrease in receptor numbers
    Decrease in receptor sensitivity
    Increase in receptor sensitivity
Pharmacokinetic
    Decrease in cell absorption
    Change in distribution
    Decrease in muscle mass
    Increase in adipose tissue
    Increased bioavailability
    Decreased albumin
    Altered protein binding
    Reduced clearance
    Decreased hepatic blood flow
    Reduced oxidative metabolism

aging are summarized in Table 15-9. The minimum alveolar concentration of all volatile anesthetics decreases with age.

Perioperative Risk

An important question is whether increased age per se increases perioperative risk in the elderly. Some studies suggest that it does.[22,23] The American Society of Anesthesiologists Physical Status scale and risk classification places patients 70 years of age and older into class 2. In the original Goldman Cardiac Risk Index, age older than 70 was an independent weighted risk factor.[24] However, few studies have separated age and coexisting diseases and studied the effect of each separately. In one study that did attempt this distinction,[25] results indicated that in elderly patients with no comorbid conditions, the postoperative risk was not influenced by age independently. The most important factor affecting surgical risk in the elderly population would seem to be the number and severity of comorbid conditions; age itself is less important.

Preoperative assessment of the geriatric patient should concentrate on identifying and determining the severity of the comorbid conditions that are common in this age group. Good medical history taking and a physical examination have been demonstrated to be the best method for this.[26] The same principles apply as to all preoperative patients and are detailed in other parts of this book. Some preoperative screening tests are worthwhile, however, and should be performed (see Chapter 2).

Preoperative laboratory testing should be determined by the clinical need of each individual patient based on the history and physical examination. Nonselective screening tests are not cost effective, because borderline abnormalities and false-positives are pursued to no useful clinical effect. False-negatives add to the problems, and more medicolegal problems are likely to occur from the failure to evaluate apparent abnormalities than from not ordering the tests. The predictive values of screening tests have been reviewed elsewhere[27] (see Chapter 2). In the geriatric population (those older than 65 years), the routine tests that are likely to be cost effective are hemoglobin level or hematocrit; electrocardiogram (ECG); chest radiograph (CXR); and albumin, glucose (or hemoglobin A_{1c}), and blood urea nitrogen levels.

GERIATRIC PATIENTS UNDERGOING CATARACT SURGERY

Cataract surgery is, perhaps, a special category. The majority of patients are elderly and may have serious comorbid conditions. As discussed earlier, these comorbid conditions constitute the main risk to surgery and anesthesia for these patients. Balanced against this is the fact that cataract surgery is a low-risk procedure, with no blood loss, no appreciable third shifts, and little postoperative pain. Even though the surgical population is high risk, the mortality is far lower for those undergoing ophthalmic surgery than for the general surgical population,[28] even in patients with previous myocardial infarction.[29] Cataract surgery is easily and commonly performed with regional anesthesia. The benefits of the surgery are obvious and enormous for the patient. However, elderly high-risk patients having cataract surgery occasionally experience serious perioperative complications.

One approach is to evaluate the patient along the lines suggested earlier in this chapter. If a patient is found to have a reversible medical condition or a condition that can be optimized, then surgery should be postponed so that medical therapy can be undertaken. Patients who are optimized medically should be able to lie flat, or relatively flat, and still for the duration of the procedure. Patients who are so sick that they are unable to lie flat (e.g., short of breath from congestive heart failure or severe lung disease), or patients who are unable to be still (e.g., demented or with very frequent coughing from chronic lung disease), may be unsuitable for regional anesthesia. The risk/benefit ratio should be considered carefully before embarking on a course of general anesthesia. The majority of patients can undergo cataract surgery under regional anesthesia, and only the rare and severely ill patient does not tolerate the procedure.

PATIENTS WITH DO NOT RESUSCITATE ORDERS

Do not resuscitate (DNR) orders may be issued if, in the judgment of the attending physician, pursuing cardiopulmonary resuscitation (CPR) would be inappropriate. The physician should discuss this matter with the patient or surrogate.[30] The patient, or surrogate, may be the initiator of DNR orders. A number of these patients may come to surgery for palliative procedures or procedures to enhance comfort and nursing care (e.g., tracheotomy, gastrostomy). Because anesthesia involves many of the elements of CPR, (e.g., intubation and use of vasoactive drugs), confusion can arise as to what is and is not appropriate intraoperatively. A cardiac arrest occurring under anesthesia has a much higher likelihood of successful resuscitation than one that occurs spontaneously. Also, if a DNR order limits the anesthesiologist's normal armamentarium of techniques or drugs, the patient may not receive the best anesthetic available. For these reasons, the policy has evolved of automatically suspending DNR orders for some arbitrary period of time (usually 24 hours) for patients undergoing surgery.[31] The matter should be discussed with the patient or surrogate before DNR orders are suspended, the reasons given, and the patient's agreement sought.[32]

This revocation of DNR orders has been challenged, however. Patient autonomy and self-determination are now leading principles in modern medical ethics; the physician informs patients of their choices and enters into a process of mutual exchange of ideas and feelings.[33] Based on this principle of patient autonomy, the suggestion has been made that all DNR orders continue during the perioperative period.[34] Central to this concept is full and open discussion with the patient or patient's representative and surgeon as to what the anesthesia entails and establishing an understanding of the patient's wishes within this context.

Problems may lie with the anesthesiologist, who might believe that withholding resuscitation during anesthesia constitutes malfeasance, and with the institution, which fears a malpractice case from withholding care. Hence, establishment of an institutional policy may be necessary, and preoperative discussion is important. The Committee on Ethics of the American Society of Anesthesiologists reviewed this issue, and guidelines were approved by the House of Delegates on October 13, 1993[35] (Fig. 15-1).

PATIENTS WHO ARE MORBIDLY OBESE

A number of methods have been used to define obesity and determine what constitutes the extreme form, morbid obesity. Tables of "ideal" weight for height have been derived from actuarial data and, although standard in the insurance industry, may be biased to subgroups of the population. Morbid obesity can be defined as weight 100 pounds above the ideal body weight. Another method of determining morbid obesity, which has the benefit of simplicity, is body mass index. Body mass index is weight in kilograms divided by the square of the height in meters (wt/ht^2 or kg/m^2). Obese patients are those with a body mass index above 28, and the morbidly obese are those with an index above 35. The latter constitute 3% to 5% of the U.S. population. To properly evaluate these patients preoperatively, knowledge of the physiologic and pathophysiologic changes associated with obesity is necessary, as is an understanding of how these patients develop potentially morbid conditions.

Pulmonary System

Changes occur in resting lung volumes in obese patients. Functional residual capacity, vital capacity, and total lung capacity are reduced, due to lower respiratory compliance.[36] Residual volume remains unchanged, and a lower expiratory reserve volume is the primary cause of the reduction in functional residual capacity. Closing capacity, the lung volume at which small airways begin to close, is unchanged; thus, the reduction in functional residual capacity can lead, during normal breathing, to lung volumes below

I. Given the diversity of published opinions and cultures within our society, an essential element of preoperative preparation and perioperative care for patients with Do Not Resuscitate (DNR) orders or other directives that limit treatment is communication among involved parties. It is necessary to document relevant aspects of this communication.

II. Policies automatically suspending DNR orders or other directives that limit treatment prior to procedures involving anesthetic care may not sufficiently address a patient's rights to self-determination in a responsible and ethical manner. Such policies, if they exist, should be reviewed and revised, as necessary, to reflect the content of these guidelines.

III. Prior to procedures requiring anesthetic care, any changes in existing directives that limit treatment should be documented in the medical record. These include absolute injunctions as desired by the patient (or the patient's legal representative). When appropriate, the items that should be considered are:
   A. Blood product transfusion
   B. Tracheal intubation or instrumentation
   C. Chest compressions and direct cardiac massage
   D. Defibrillation
   E. Cardiac pacing, internal or external
   F. Invasive monitoring
   G. Postoperative ventilatory support
   H. Vasoactive drug administration

IV. When relevant, the anesthesiologist should describe and discuss the appropriate use of therapeutic modalities to correct deviations of hemodynamic and respiratory variables predictably resulting from anesthetic agents and techniques.

V. Additional issues that may be relevant to discuss are perioperative placement of naso/orogastric tubes or urinary catheters, administration of antibiotics, establishment of intravenous access, maintenance of intravascular volume with nonblood products and treatment with supplemental oxygen.

VI. It is important to discuss and document whether there are to be any exceptions to the injunction(s) against intervention should there occur a specific recognized complication of the surgery or anesthesia.

VII. Concurrence on these issues by the primary physician (if not the surgeon of record), the surgeon and the anesthesiologist is desirable. If possible, these physicians should meet together with the patient (or the patient's legal representative) when these issues are discussed. This duty of the patient's physicians is deemed to be of such importance that it should not be delegated. Other members of the health care team who are (or will be) directly involved with the patient's care during the planned procedure should, if feasible, be included in this process.

VIII. Should conflicts arise, the following resolution processes are recommended:
   A. When an anesthesiologist finds the patient's or surgeon's limitations of intervention decisions to be irreconcilable with one's own moral views, then the anesthesiologist should withdraw in a nonjudgmental fashion, providing an alternative for care in a timely fashion.

Fig. 15-1. Ethical guidelines for the anesthesia care of patients with do not resuscitate orders or other directives that limit treatment (approved by the House of Delegates on October 13, 1993). These guidelines apply to competent patients and also to incompetent patients who have previously expressed their preferences. (Reprinted with permission of the American Society of Anesthesiologists, 520 N. Northwest Highway, Park Ridge, IL 60068.)

B. When an anesthesiologist finds the patient's or surgeon's limitation of intervention decisions to be in conflict with generally accepted standards of care, ethical practice or institutional policies, then the anesthesiologist should voice such concerns and present the situation to the appropriate institutional body.

C. If these alternatives are not feasible within the time frame necessary to prevent further morbidity or suffering, then in accordance with the American Medical Associations's Principles of Medical Ethics, care should proceed with reasonable adherence to the patient's directives, being mindful of the patient's goals and values.

IX. A representative from the hospital's anesthesiology service should establish a liaison with surgical and nursing services for presentation, discussion and procedural application of these guidelines. Hospital staff should be made aware of the proceedings of these discussions and the motivations for them.

X. Modification of these guidelines may be appropriate when they conflict with local standards or policies, and in those emergency situations involving incompetent patients whose intentions have not been previously expressed.

Fig. 15-1. *Continued*

closing capacity with resulting small airway collapse. Ventilation-to-perfusion mismatch occurs and thus reduction in arterial oxygenation (PaO_2). The supine and Trendelenburg's positions worsen these changes.[37] The work of breathing is increased. Oxygen consumption and carbon dioxide production increase with increasing weight, although basal metabolic rate, because it is related to body weight, remains normal. Thus, the morbidly obese patient is at risk of hypoxia during anesthesia and postoperatively, especially when in the supine position. Weight loss can increase functional residual capacity and increase PaO_2.

Cardiovascular System

The changes in the cardiovascular system are complex. An association exists between obesity and coronary artery disease, myocardial infarction, and sudden death, especially in patients older than 50 years.[38] The risk exists of CHF, particularly in men, and of atherothrombotic stroke in women. An association is seen between obesity and hypertension, but the pathophysiology is poorly understood. Systemic vascular resistance is normal, but blood volume is expanded, distending both the right and left ventricles at end diastole. There is an associated increase in stroke volume, increased cardiac output, and thus increased left ventricular stroke work. The increased total body oxygen consumption has already been noted. The elevated preload leads to dilation and eccentric hypertrophy of the left ventricle and reduced compliance of the chamber. This reduced compliance and the increased left ventricular end diastolic volume directly cause an increase in left ventricular end diastolic pressure and pulmonary artery occlusion pressure. CHF can occur from diastolic or systolic dysfunction if the dilated left ventricle fails to hypertrophy sufficiently. Pulmonary hypertension is common and can lead to right ventricular problems. Ventricular arrhythmias are more common than in the nonobese population and could possibly con-

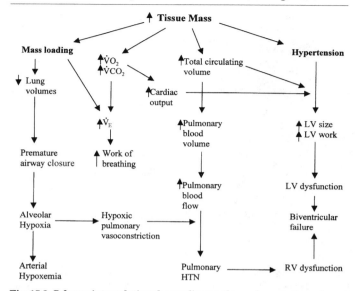

Fig. 15-2. Schema interrelating the cardiovascular and respiratory abnormalities in morbidly obese patients with the pathophysiologic changes found in such patients. (HTN, hypertension; LV, left ventricular; RV, right ventricular; $\dot{V}_E$, minute volume of ventilation; $\dot{V}CO_2$, carbon dioxide production per unit time; $\dot{V}O_2$, oxygen consumption per unit time.) (Reprinted with permission from Buckley FP. Anesthesia and obesity and gastrointestinal disorders. In: Barash PG, Cullen BF, Stoelting RK, eds. *Clinical anesthesia*, 3rd ed. Philadelphia: Lippincott–Raven Publishers, 1996:976.)

tribute to sudden death in this group of patients. The cardiopulmonary changes are summarized in Fig. 15-2.

Gastrointestinal System and Metabolism

A classic paper by Vaughan et al.[39] demonstrated an increase in gastric juice volume and decrease in pH in obese patients; since that time, such patients have been considered at increased risk of regurgitation and aspiration. Increased intraabdominal pressure and an increased incidence of hiatus hernia magnify this risk. In a more recent study,[40] in otherwise healthy, nondiabetic, fasted patients, a lower incidence of combined high-volume, low-pH stomach contents was found in obese surgical patients than in lean patients. One difference between the two studies is that, in the earlier study, intramuscular diphenhydramine hydrochloride and a mixture of fentanyl and droperidol were given preoperatively to the obese group but not to the control group, whereas in the latter study midazolam hydrochloride was given to some patients immediately before transfer to the operating room. Although further study is needed, opinions on the resting gastric contents of obese patients may need to be revised.

An association is seen between obesity and fatty liver, although no causal mechanism is known. Drug metabolism may be altered in obese patients. A higher level of free fluoride ion is found after exposure to methoxyflurane, enflurane and, in some studies, halothane. Conflicting reports are found of free fluoride ion formation with sevoflurane. Obesity is a risk factor for halothane-induced hepatotoxicity. The volume of distribution of some lipid-soluble drugs is increased in obese patients. Because the serum concentration from a given dose is thus lower, the rate of elimination is slower. This applies to thiopental sodium, midazolam hydrochloride, and sufentanil citrate. Fentanyl and propofol seem to behave similarly in obese and nonobese patients. Some muscle relaxants, but not atracurium besylate or cisatracurium besylate, have a slower offset in the obese patient. The physician must realize that drugs may behave unpredictably in the obese patient.

Certain antiobesity drugs have been shown to have effects on the heart and pulmonary vasculature. In the late 1960s and early 1970s, a small epidemic of pulmonary hypertension occurred in Europe, with some deaths, due to the use of aminorex for weight reduction. Fenfluramine hydrochloride and dexfenfluramine hydrochloride are known to be associated with pulmonary hypertension, and the combination of fenfluramine hydrochloride and phentermine hydrochloride (fen-phen) has been associated with fatal pulmonary hypertension after only a brief course of the drugs.[41] In the second half of 1997, reports emerged of an association of valvular heart disease and the combination of fenfluramine hydrochloride and phentermine hydrochloride for weight loss.[42] Several more similar cases were identified, and fenfluramine hydrochloride and dexfenfluramine hydrochloride were removed from the market. However, phentermine hydrochloride remains available. Other reports of the association of appetite suppressants and valvular disease[43-45] showed the wisdom of withdrawing the drugs. The valves involved were mostly left-sided, although right-sided ones were not exempt, and the lesion led to regurgitation in all cases. Although many patients were symptomatic, some valvular lesions have been found in asymptomatic people. It is too early to judge the extent of this association or the natural history of the disease (although one case report has shown a regression of multivalvular regurgitation over a 2-year period).[46] However, in November 1997, the U.S. Department of Health and Human Services (DHSS) issued interim public health recommendations.[47] The DHSS recommended that all persons exposed to either drug for any period should have a medical history taken and should undergo cardiovascular examination. Any person with a history or examination suggestive of valvular disease should undergo an echocardiogram. Practitioners should strongly consider performing echocardiography on all persons who have been exposed to fenfluramine or dexfenfluramine for any period, either alone or in combination with other agents—regardless of whether such patients have cardiopulmonary signs or symptoms—before they undergo any invasive procedure for which antimicrobial endocarditis prophylaxis is recommended by American Heart Association guidelines[48] (see Chapter 16). Patients with significant valvular lesions should have antibiotic prophylaxis when indicated. Because of the prevalence of minimal degrees of regurgitation in the general population, the current case definition of drug-associated valvulopathy should include echocardiographically demonstrated aortic regurgitation of mild or greater severity or mitral regurgitation of moderate or greater severity in exposed patients. For emergency procedures or at other times when cardiac evaluation cannot be performed, empiric antibiotic prophylaxis should be administered.

Preoperative Assessment

In addition to performing a routine evaluation, the physician should focus on issues that are peculiar to the morbidly obese. Questions should be directed at assessing the cardiovascular and respiratory systems (see Chapters 3–5), and the patient's tolerance of exercise and ability to lie flat, especially while sleeping, should be noted. Symptoms of sleep apnea (see below) should be sought. A correctly sized blood pressure cuff should be used; the width of the cuff should be approximately two-thirds the width of the arm, and the cuff should be long enough to encircle the arm. The patient's airway should be carefully assessed because a number of abnormalities may exist, including limitation of flexion and extension of the cervical spine, restricted mouth opening from submental fat, large tongue, and redundant intraoral tissue. The thyromental distance should be assessed. Although many obese patients are normal in this respect, some may have an infantile-type anterior laryngeal opening.

Specific questions should be asked about the recent use of diet tablets and, if any have been taken—particularly fenfluramine hydrochloride, dexfenfluramine hydrochloride, and even phentermine hydrochloride—suspicion of valvular regurgitation or pulmonary hypertension should be entertained. The cardiovascular system should be reviewed carefully. If the history is suggestive of a valvular problem or pulmonary hypertension, or if any murmur is present, echocardiography is indicated, as noted previously. Until more is known of this phenomenon, the DHSS recommendations should be strongly considered.

Preoperative tests should be chosen carefully. The healthy obese patient is likely to have normal pulmonary function tests, but these tests might provide useful information for the extremely obese patient and the patient with a history of lung problems or smoking. ECG, CXR, hematocrit, and measurement of blood glucose level may be advisable for the morbidly obese patient. Preoperative measurement of oxygen saturation while the patient breathes room air may be useful if the patient has an abnormal respiratory history.

Obesity Hypoventilation Syndrome

Five percent to 8% of morbidly obese patients have what is called *obesity hypoventilation syndrome* or *pickwickian syndrome*. The latter term was originally coined by Osler[49] and used by Burwell et al.[50] in their classic description of patients with obesity, excessive daytime sleepiness, snoring, and cor pulmonale. Patients are reminiscent of Joe the Fat Boy from Dickens' *The Posthumous Papers of the Pickwick Club*. The patients may exhibit hypercapnia, severe hypoxemia, periodic breathing, biventricular enlargement (especially of the right ventricle), dependent edema, polycythemia, and pulmonary edema. Compared with patients with simple obesity, pulmonary compliance is dramatically reduced in such individuals and the work of breathing greatly elevated. The cause of the hypercapnia is still not completely known, but an intrinsic problem with the central respiratory center is likely.

These patients have very high anesthetic risk, and even lying flat can be dangerous. The physician must identify these patients, assess their cardiopulmonary systems thoroughly, and emphasize weight reduction before elective surgery because even a relatively minor weight loss can drastically improve their physiologic status.

PATIENTS WITH SLEEP APNEA SYNDROME

Sleep apnea syndrome is characterized by periods of apnea lasting longer than 10 seconds and recurring at least 11 times per hour during sleep.[51] The three subtypes are (a) obstructive, in which airflow is interrupted but respiratory muscle activity continues—that is, upper airway obstruction; (b) central, in which no respiratory muscle activity occurs during periods of apnea; and (c) mixed, in which both patterns occur in the same patient.

More apneic episodes occur during rapid eye movement (REM) sleep than during deep non-REM sleep. Each apneic period is associated with arterial desaturation, which is worse in the obstructive pattern. Sleep is disrupted and daytime somnolence and performance decrement occur. Daytime naps are common.[52] Snoring is a common complaint. The repeated hypoxic episodes can lead to pulmonary hypertension, and cardiac arrhythmias frequently occur when hypoxia develops.

The obstructive pattern occurs because of increased pharyngeal compliance caused by relative hypotonia of the genioglossus and geniohyoid muscles, as suggested by electromyographic findings.[53] This devlopment allows the tongue to fall or be sucked back into the pharynx. The pharyngeal lumen is smaller in these patients. Central sleep apnea syndrome presumably has a central origin but can be associated with myopathic conditions or neurologic or brainstem disorders.

Treatments include the use of continuous positive airway pressure, the use of various tongue-retaining devices, uvulopalatopharyngoplasty (which has good results for snoring and equivocal results for sleep apnea syndrome) and, in severe cases, tracheotomy. Intraoperatively, problems may exist with the airway;[54] postoperatively, nocturnal desaturations may occur.[55] Cases of sudden respiratory arrests associated with epidural opioids have been reported.[56]

Preoperative Assessment

The diagnosis must be sought from the history. Typical are snoring, gasping, choking during sleep, impaired daytime performance, intellectual deterioration, personality changes, or nonrefreshing daytime naps. The airway must be examined carefully. Any related systemic effects should be treated before elective surgery. Administration of preoperative sedatives should be avoided. Patients who use nasal continuous positive airway pressure should be asked to bring the system to the hospital so they can use it while hospitalized.

PATIENTS WITH CANCER

The first thought on meeting a patient with cancer for preoperative assessment is often to concentrate on the anticancer drugs the patient has taken and their possible effects for anesthesia and surgery. This is an important aspect of the assessment of these patients, but one must not forget that cancer has effects that go beyond the drugs involved. This section considers the effects of the various chemotherapeutic agents but also discusses the physiologic disturbances that can occur with some cancers and the problems that can arise from the anatomic location of the tumors.

Chemotherapy

Many patients are taking, or have taken, various chemotherapeutic drugs. The range is increasing, and finding patients who are on novel study regimens is not unusual in academic centers. A detailed history of the drugs involved and the dosages should be elicited. Communication with the oncologist or other physician who is administrating the drugs may be necessary. A number of reviews have been published on the effects of these drugs,[57–60] but a brief outline is given here.

The alkylating agents are used to treat a wide variety of tumors. Rapid destruction of tumor mass can lead to an increase in the breakdown of pyramidine and purine and can give rise to uric acid nephropathy. Bone marrow suppression is common and can be severe. Nitrogen mustard can cause severe local tissue damage. This agent has been delivered into the pleural space in cases of malignant pleural effusion and has been given as an arterial infusion in a technique used for metastatic melanoma called *isolated limb perfusion*. Cyclophosphamide can cause hemorrhagic cystitis and inappropriate water retention. Pulmonary fibrosis is rare. Plasma cholinesterase synthesis is inhibited, and care should be taken when using succinylcholine chloride. The antimetabolites (methotrexate sodium, 5-fluorouracil) cause bone marrow suppression, nausea, vomiting, and diarrhea. Methotrexate sodium can cause renal toxicity because of its effects on renal tubules, and liver damage has occurred. Renal and hepatic function should be evaluated in patients taking these medications.

The major toxic effect of vincristine sulfate is neurologic, and the drug can lead to muscle weakness and wasting. When this occurs, hyperkalemia may arise with the use of succinylcholine chloride. Vinblastine sulfate causes suppression of the bone marrow. *Cis*-platinum has a high incidence of renal toxicity, with a reduction in renal blood flow, reduction in glomerular filtration rate, and loss of magnesium and potassium. Renal function should be optimized perioperatively with administration of fluids and mannitol (see Chapter 8). Other potential nephrotoxic drugs should be avoided. Use of interferon may lead to immune deficiency states, hypotension, sepsis, and hyperthermia during treatment, which resolves on discontinuing the drug. Taxol is derived from the bark of a particular yew tree. It requires Cremophor El for its formulation because it is insoluble. Hypersensitivity reactions can occur that may be due to the Cremophor. Peripheral neuropathies and myelosuppression can limit the dose. Conduction defects, such as second- and third-degree heart block, have been described.

The chemotherapeutic antibiotics have toxic effects of great interest to anesthesiologists. Anthracyclines, of which doxorubicin hydrochloride (Adriamycin) is the best known, causes a dose-dependent cardiotoxicity that manifests chronically as a cardiomyopathy. Daunorubicin has similar actions. An acute cardiac toxicity occurs that can manifest as arrhythmias or, in extreme cases, pump failure. Long-term cardiac changes are more likely if the dose is higher than 550 mg per m^2, the patient has a prior history of heart disease, and cyclophosphamide also has been used. It is more common in patients older than 65 years. The mechanism is thought to occur through oxygen free radicals that damage the sarcoplasmic reticulum and allow calcium build-up in the myocytes. Cardiac muscle has a low amount of the enzyme catalase, which neutralizes oxygen free radicals.

Patients who are on these drugs must be carefully evaluated to determine the degree of cardiac involvement. As always, the history is most important, not just to determine the dosage and other risk factors as indicated above but also to evaluate the degree of the patient's cardiovascular reserve by obtaining details regarding exercise tolerance and cardiac symptoms (see Chapters 3 and 4). Signs of CHF, such as basal crackles, edema, elevated jugular venous pressure, and S_3 gallop, should be sought. A CXR and ECG should be taken and, if the history and physical examination indicates it, an echocardiogram should be arranged to determine ventricular function. The patient's cardiovascular status should be optimized preoperatively, and specialized cardiac monitoring may be indicated intraoperatively.

Bleomycin sulfate, another drug in this group, has a dose-related pulmonary toxicity that occurs in 10% of patients taking the drug. Bleomycin sulfate binds to DNA intracellularly, and a ferrous to ferric conversion liberates electrons, which then form oxygen free radicals and superoxide. The lungs are low in a bleomycin sulfate deactivator, bleomycin hydrolase, and naturally high in concentrations of oxygen. Experimentally, two phases of damage are seen. The first, which occurs soon after treatment, consists of pulmonary edema and hyaline membrane formation. The second phase is a proliferative process, with inflammatory cell infiltration and eventually pulmonary fibrosis.[61] Risk factors are associated with the development of bleomycin sulfate toxicity. These include a total cumulative dose of more than 200 mg, concomitant radiotherapy to the lungs, age older than 65 years, and possibly breathing increased oxygen concentrations. The symptoms include cough, fever, and shortness of breath. A CXR shows progressive basilar infiltrates, pulmonary function tests show a restrictive pattern, and early decrease in the diffusing capacity of carbon monoxide is seen. If the history and physical examination suggest bleomycin sulfate toxicity, then investigation is worthwhile.

Controversy exists as to whether increased inspired oxygen is safe for patients who have taken bleomycin sulfate. Early reports suggested that the incidence of bleomycin sulfate toxicity and death was increased if the inspired oxygen was higher than 28%,[62] but more recently published studies have shown no increase in postoperative pulmonary problems in bleomycin sulfate–treated patients who received 40% oxygen.[63] Despite this finding, many centers still limit the amount of oxygen to 28%.[64] Because pulse oximetry is now available, restricting the inspired oxygen level to the lowest amount compatible with maintenance of satisfactory oxygen saturation would seem prudent.

Mitomycin C causes myelosuppression, and pulmonary toxicity similar to that seen with bleomycin sulfate has been reported. Administration of high-dose corticosteroids at the onset of pulmonary symptoms may be helpful, but the mortality rate is high. Whether increased oxygen concentration is harmful for patients who have received mitomycin C is uncertain.

Pathophysiology

Cancer may be associated with paraneoplastic syndromes.[65] The main syndromes are listed in Table 15-10.

The most common problem is anemia (see Chapter 7), which has a number of causes. These include the anemia of chronic disease, bone marrow suppression by radiotherapy or chemotherapy, direct invasion of the bone marrow, hypersplenism, blood loss from bleeding, autoimmune hemolysis, and deficiency of iron and vitamins. The degree of anemia may approach levels at which preoperative blood transfusion should be considered. In deciding if a transfusion is indicated, a number of factors must be taken into account. These include the likelihood of intraoperative and postoperative bleeding and the general condition of the patient. The old practice of performing a transfusion if the hematocrit reached 30% has been shown to be unnecessary. If coronary artery disease is present, however, maintaining the hematocrit at approximately 30% reduces the incidence of perioperative ischemia. If the patient is otherwise healthy, a hematocrit of 20% might be acceptable for bloodless surgery and anesthesia. Blood transfusion seems to have an immunosuppressive action, which has the risk of enhancing the spread of tumor, although this effect is by no means proven. This same action is useful for renal transplant patients. The suggestion exists that infection risk is increased. The use of a cell-saving procedure intraoperatively may increase the risk of metastases if tumor cells are in the blood. This may be unlikely, but each case should be considered individually.

Thrombocytopenia may be caused by chemotherapy, radiotherapy, or disseminated intravascular coagulation. A platelet transfusion may be necessary if the platelet count is less than 50,000 to 60,000 per cubic millimeter (see Chapter 7). Coagulopathies may be associated with oncologic disease. They may be due to decreased production of coagulation factors, liver dysfunction, vitamin K deficiency, or chemotherapy, or caused by the direct effects of the cancer itself. Immunologic causes and disseminated intravascular coagulation are possible. The causes should be sought and treated if possible before replacement therapy is instituted. In many patients, a hypercoagulable state is present. Occurrence of the Eaton-Lambert syndrome is unusual and is associated primarily with cancer of the lung. Also known as *myasthenic syndrome*, it mimics myasthenia gravis (see Chapter 11A). Limb girdle weakness is the most common symptom,

Table 15-10. Paraneoplastic syndromes

Neuromuscular disorders
   Dermatomyositis and polymyositis
   Myasthenic syndrome (Eaton-Lambert syndrome)
Hematologic disorders
   Anemia associated with cancer
   Granulocytosis
   Thrombocytopenia and thrombocytosis
   Coagulation abnormalities
Endocrinologic disorders
   Pheochromocytoma
   Carcinoid syndrome
   Thyrotoxicosis
   Hypercalcemia and parathyroid disease
Fever, anorexia

Reprinted with permission from Desiderio DP, Kross RA, Bedford RF. Evaluation of the patient with oncologic disease. In: Longnecker DE, Tinker JH, Morgan GE Jr, eds. *Principles and practice of anesthesiology*, 2nd ed. St. Louis: Mosby–Year Book, 1998:386.

although the weakness is not helped by anticholinesterases and, in contrast to myasthenia, the weakness improves with continued exercise. These patients are very sensitive to both depolarizing and nondepolarizing muscle relaxants. Pheochromocytoma and carcinoid are described in Chapter 6.

Anatomic Problems

Patients with cancer may present with problems due to the physical location of the tumor or anatomic problems resulting from the tumor. One anatomic problem may occur when the tumor involves the airway. The upper airway may become obstructed from tumors of the pharynx, larynx, thyroid, or base of the tongue. Tumors involving the jaw may restrict mouth opening. Symptomatically, the patient may complain of dysphagia, hoarseness, or speech disturbance. Wheezing is a late and ominous symptom. Physical examination should determine whether the patient's airway is intrinsically difficult to intubate and the extent of tumor spread. Radiographs, computed tomographic (CT) scans, and flow-volume loops may be necessary to delineate the problem. Fiberoptic intubation may be required, and in advanced cases preoperative tracheotomy may need to be performed under local anesthesia.

Tumors involving the heart and pericardium may produce a pericardial effusion that can lead to cardiac tamponade. The speed of accumulation is important; the heart can adapt to a slow buildup of fluid (up to 300 mL in extreme cases), but rapid accumulation of much smaller volumes can lead to decompensation. The pathophysiology is that of impaired diastolic filling and reduction in cardiac output. The varying rates of accumulation of fluid in different patients lead to great variation in the presentation. Symptoms include cough, dyspnea, chest pain, weakness, and fatigue. The classic triad of quiet heart sounds, increased venous pressure, and decreased arterial pressure is by no means constant. On physical examination the pulse is rapid and jugular venous distension is usually present. Pulsus paradoxicus (an exaggeration of the normal change of approximately 6 mm Hg systemic blood pressure during breathing) may be present. Filling pressures gradually equalize. Although an ECG and CXR may be helpful, the definitive diagnosis can be made with echocardiography. For such patients, anesthesia is fraught with hazards. Invasive monitoring is needed. Maintenance of systemic blood pressure is important, and positive-pressure ventilation may reduce cardiac filling even more.

Secondary involvement of the peritoneum may lead to massive ascites. This can be so severe as to compress the inferior vena cava, decreasing venous return and impinging on the diaphragm.

Anterior mediastinal tumors may be primary or secondary, and they can lead to one of the greatest challenges in anesthesia. The mass may obstruct any of the structures in the mediastinum, including the airway, the heart, and the superior vena cava. The symptoms are syncope, orthopnea, stridor, and even cyanosis. If the superior vena cava is obstructed, facial swelling occurs that can include the neck, resulting in difficult intubation. Raised intracranial pressure is a possibility. Despite all this, very large mediastinal masses may be relatively asymptomatic. The main concerns during induction of anesthesia are loss of the airway and death.[66] The patient should be questioned to determine if a particular body position improves the respiratory symptoms. During anesthesia, placement of the patient in that favored position may allow ventilation when other positions make ventilation impossible. A CT scan may be helpful. Flow-volume loops help to determine how much obstruction exists and whether the obstruction is intrathoracic (limitations on the expiratory limb of the loop) or extrathoracic (limitations on the inspiratory limb). Stridor (inspiratory and extrathoracic) and wheezing (expiratory and intrathoracic), if present, give the same information as the flow-volume loops.

Tumors may be metastatic or primary. Primary tumors are thymomas, lymphomas, or germ cell tumors. Preoperative radiotherapy alters the histology and may make a definitive diagnosis impossible. Thus, preoperative radiotherapy to shrink the tumor may not be advisable. Also, it may initially cause swelling and worsen symptoms. Performing a biopsy (the most common reason for surgery) under local anesthesia may not be feasible for all patients. A general anesthetic may be necessary. The main issue is the airway, especially in cases of superior vena cava obstruction. Fiber-optic intubation may be required. Spontaneous ventilation, or at least the avoidance of positive-pressure ventilation and paralysis, is recommended. The position of the patient may be very important and, as already mentioned, the optimal position should be determined preoperatively. One approach to evaluating these patients is shown in Fig. 15-3 from Neuman et al.[67]

PATIENTS WITH HUMAN IMMUNODEFICIENCY VIRUS

Human immunodeficiency virus (HIV) is the etiologic agent for acquired immunodeficiency syndrome (AIDS). This disease

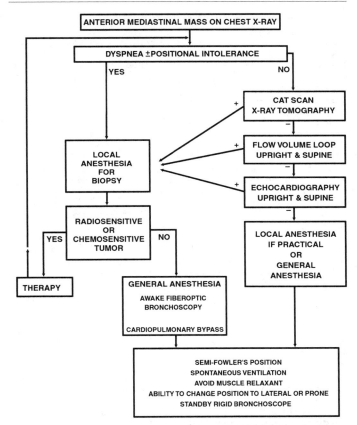

Fig. 15-3. Flow chart describing the preoperative evaluation of the patient with an anterior mediastinal mass. (+ indicates positive finding; − indicates negative workup; CAT, computed axial tomography.) (Reprinted with permission from Neuman GG, Weingarten AE, Abramowitz RM, et al. The anesthetic management of the patient with an anterior mediastinal mass. *Anesthesiology* 1984;60:144–147.)

was first described in 1981, and since then a worldwide epidemic has ensued. Because of this, and because of the risk that health care providers may acquire the disease, clinicians would do well to understand the disease. HIV is a retrovirus in the Lentivirus group of viruses. Diploid RNA strands are surrounded by distinctive proteins to form a core particle. A viral envelope of proteins and glycoproteins allows the virus to attach to the CD4 receptor on the host cell. After attachment, the core is injected into the host cell's cytoplasm and reverse transcriptase forms a double-stranded DNA molecule from the RNA template that enters the host cell's nucleus. Infection is permanent. The virus can remain dormant for long periods, but for unknown reasons rapid virus replication can occur, leading to cell death.

When the virus first came to medical attention, a number of high-risk groups were identified: male homosexuals, bisexuals, intravenous drug abusers, and hemophiliacs. Later, people who had received multiple blood products, prostitutes, and babies of high-risk mothers were found to be infected. Now the virus is known to be transmitted heterosexually, and an increasing number of women are infected. In Africa, the virus is acting as a heterosexually transmitted venereal disease.

The clinical spectrum ranges from asymptomatic but infective patients to those with frank AIDS and life-threatening infection. The Centers for Disease Control and Prevention expanded its classifications of AIDS in 1993 and recognized the prognostic importance of CD4 counts.[68] Three stages of progression are seen. Immediately after infection, a minority of patients show signs of an infection that mimics mononucleosis in some respects. These signs gradually resolve. The virus then remains latent for possibly many years, even though it may continue to replicate. The patient feels well but is infective. The next stage is characterized by chronic lymphadenopathy, which after 3 to 5 years gradually worsens to the third stage, a cell-mediated immune deficiency. This stage is characterized by a large variety of opportunistic infections, as well as by the appearance of tumors such as Kaposi's sarcoma and non-Hodgkin's lymphoma.

The diagnosis can be made by a number of blood tests. The primary screening test is the enzyme-linked immunosorbent assay, which detects the antibody to an extract of a tissue culture growth of HIV. The test is greater than 99% sensitive but generates a number of false-positive results. Confirmation is usually by the Western blot technique, in which viral protein antigens, separated by electrophoresis and blotted onto nitrocellulose strips, are incubated with the patient's serum. If specific antibodies to virus proteins are present, they are detected by a labeled anti-human globulin to the protein bands. Other confirmatory tests include the cytoplasmic immunofluorescent assay and the polymerase chain reaction.

During the preoperative evaluation, the multisystem nature of the disease should be kept in mind.[69] In addition, some high-risk patients, particularly intravenous drug abusers, may have significant illnesses. Questions should be asked to define the involvement of the various organ systems, and although the questions may not be different from those in a normal preoperative evaluation, the likely pathology should be borne in mind.

The pulmonary system in AIDS patients can be affected in a number of ways. Opportunistic infections are common. The most frequently seen is infection with *Pneumocystis carinii*. This can be an insidious and protracted infection in these patients, in contrast to the acute illness usually seen in the immunologically intact patient. History taking may need to be supplemented with pulmonary function tests, but the diagnosis is often difficult, and pulmonary lavage or even lung biopsy may be required for microbiological and histologic confirmation. Kaposi's sarcoma and lymphoid interstitial pneumonitis can affect the lung, and non-Hodgkin's lymphoma can cause mediastinal masses that can compromise large airways. The cardiovascular system can be involved, with pericarditis and pericardial effusion, infective endocarditis, and cardiomyopathy. CHF and arrhythmias that lead to sudden death have been well described. Children with AIDS can develop cardiomyopathy and CHF. In any AIDS patient with suggestive symptoms, a CXR and ECG should be performed and an echocardiogram should be considered.

AIDS patients have a number of neurologic diseases ranging from peripheral neuropathy to the development of central nervous system tumors, such as metastatic Kaposi's sarcoma or primary lymphomas. A subacute encephalopathy is invariably fatal. Atypical septic meningitis is possible, as is AIDS dementia complex and various opportunistic infections. Patients with central nervous system involvement may have raised intracranial pressure and may need CT scanning as part of their workup. Many hematologic problems are seen in AIDS patients, either from the disease itself or due to various treatments, such as zidovudine (AZT) therapy, chemotherapy, or radiotherapy. These may range from simple anemia to coagulation problems (see Chapter 7). Manifestations in the gastrointestinal tract are common, either from direct infection with the HIV virus or from opportunistic infections. Chronic diarrhea, dysphagia, and esophagitis are the usual ones. These can lead to malnourishment (see Chapter 16), dehydration, or electrolyte imbalance. Electrolyte problems, especially hyponatremia, can result from renal involvement, which is common. Acute tubular necrosis, glomerular nephritis, renovascular disease, and a HIV-associated nephropathy may be present. Renal function should be carefully assessed in these patients (see Chapter 8).

Precautions against transmission of the virus to health care workers are important. Logistic problems, cost, and ethical considerations make it impractical to test all patients preoperatively for HIV. Instead, the Centers for Disease Control and Prevention recommends that every patient be assumed to have a communicable disease and that health care workers institute "universal precautions."[70] Any health care worker who is stuck by a contaminated needle or who has extensive areas of broken skin that come into contact with body fluids should immediately contact the employee health department. HIV testing may be appropriate, and the need for prophylactic treatment with AZT should be discussed. The effectiveness of this therapy is controversial, but it may be indicated.

SUMMARY

A number of disparate topics have been discussed in this chapter. A common theme is the need to understand something of the basic pathophysiology and then logically to apply that knowledge to the preoperative assessment. The most effective way of eliciting the necessary information from each patient is by an adequate history taking and physical examination, supplemented by tests specific for each patient and condition.

REFERENCES

1. Lewis L, Robinson RF, Yee Y, et al. Fatal adrenal cortical insufficiency precipitated by surgery during prolonged continuous cortisone infusion. *Ann Intern Med* 1953;39:116–125.
2. Salem M, Tainsh R Jr, Bromberg J, et al. Perioperative glucocorticoid coverage: a reassessment 42 years after emergence of a problem. *Ann Surg* 1994;219:416–425.
3. Lamberts SWJ, Bruining HA, de Jong FH. Corticosteroid therapy in severe illness. *N Engl J Med* 1997;337:1285–1292.

4. Kehlet H. *Clinical course on hypothalamic-pituitary-adrenal cortical function in glucocorticoid-treated surgical patients.* Copenhagen: FADL's Forlag, 1976.
5. Holzman RS, Hirshman CA. Anaphylactic reactions and anesthesia. In: Longnecker DE, Tucker JL, Morgan GE, eds. *Principles and practice of anesthesiology,* 2nd ed. St. Louis: Mosby, 1998:2400.
6. Holzman RS. Latex allergy: an emerging operating room problem. *Anesth Analg* 1993;76:635–641.
7. Dailland P. Analgesia and anaesthesia and breast feeding. In: Reynolds F, ed. *Effects on the baby of maternal analgesia and anaesthesia.* London: WB Saunders, 1993:252–270.
8. Wilson JT. Determinants and consequences of drug excretion in breast milk. *Drug Metab Rev* 1983;14:619–652.
9. O'Brien T. Excretion of drugs in human milk. *Am J Hosp Pharmacol* 1974;31:844–854.
10. Rathwell JP, Visconti CM, Ashburn MA. Management of non-obstetric pain during pregnancy and lactation. *Anesth Analg* 1997;85:1075–1087.
11. Committee on Drugs. The transfer of drugs and the chemicals into human milk. *Pediatrics* 1994;93:137–150.
12. *Jehovah's Witness and the question of blood.* New York: Watchtower Bible and Tract Society, 1977:38–49.
13. *Cruzan v Missouri,* 497 US 261 (1990).
14. *Superintendent of Balchortown State School v Spikewicz,* 373 MA 728, 370 NE2d 117 (1977).
15. *Public Health Trust of Dade County v Wons* 541 S2d 96, 14 FL L Weekly 112 (1989).
16. *Application of President and Directors of Georgetown College Inc.* 3 31 F2d 1000, (DC Cir 1964); cert. denied at 84 SCt 1883.
17. Spence RK. Management of surgical patients with specific problems. In: Petz LS, Swisher SM, Kleinman S, et al., eds. *Clinical practice of transfusion medicine,* 3rd ed. New York: Churchill Livingstone, 1966:600–606.
18. Rothenberg D. Jehovah's Witnesses and transfusion. In: Lake GL, Rice LJ, Sperry RJ, eds. *Advances in anesthesia.* St. Louis: Mosby, 1996:14:238–241.
19. In re EG, No. 66089 Illinois Supreme Court, November 13, 1989.
20. Glaser RB. Morbidity and mortality from major vascular surgery. In: Roizen MF, ed. *Anesthesia for vascular surgery.* New York: Churchill Livingstone, 1990:1–27.
21. Moore LE, Stiff JL. Evaluation of the geriatric patient. In: Longnecker DE, Tinker JH, Morgan GE Jr, eds. *Principles and practice of anesthesiology,* 2nd ed. St. Louis: Mosby–Year Book, 1998:473–486.
22. Lubin MF. Is age a risk factor for surgery? *Med Clin North Am* 1993;77:327–333.
23. Marx GH, Matteo CV, Orkin LR. Computer analysis of post anesthetic death. *Anesthesia* 1973;39:54–58.
24. Goldman L, Caldera DC, Nussbaum SR, et al. Multifactorial index of cardiac risk in noncardiac surgical procedures. *N Engl J Med* 1977;297:845–850.
25. Tiret L, N'Doye P, Hatton F. Complications associated with anaesthesia—a prospective survey in France. *Can Anaesth Soc J* 1986;33:336–344.
26. Variakojis RJ, Roizen MF, McLeskey CH, ed. *Geriatric anesthesiology.* Baltimore: Williams & Wilkins, 1997:165–185.
27. Roizen MF. Preoperative evaluation. In: Miller RD, ed. *Anesthesia,* 4th ed. New York: Churchill Livingstone, 1994:827–882.
28. Quigley HA. Mortality associated with ophthalmic surgery: a twenty-year experience. *Am J Ophthalmol* 1974;77:517–524.
29. Backer CL, Tinker JH, Robertson DM. Myocardial reinfarction following local anesthesia for ophthalmic surgery. *Anesth Analg* 1980;59:257–262.

30. *Code of medical ethics: current opinions with annotation*. Chicago: American Medical Association, 1997:59–61.
31. Truog RD. "Do-Not-Resuscitate" orders during anesthesia and surgery. *Anesthesiology* 1991;74:606–608.
32. Cohen CB, Cohen PJ. Do-Not-Resuscitate orders in the operating room. *N Engl J Med* 1991;325:1879–1882.
33. Quill TE, Brody H. Physician recommendations and patient autonomy: finding a balance between physician power and patient choice. *Ann Intern Med* 1996;125:763–769.
34. Margolis JO, McGrath BJ, Kussin PS, Schwinn DA. Do not resuscitate (DNR) orders during surgery: ethical foundations for institutional policies in the United States. *Anesth Analg* 1995;80:806–809.
35. Ethical guidelines for the anesthesia care of patients with "do-not-resuscitate" orders or other directions that limit treatment. In: *American Society of Anesthesiologists Directory of Members*. Park Ridge, IL: American Society of Anesthesiologists, 1998:448.
36. Snyder DS. Evaluation of the obese patient. In: Longnecker DE, Tinker JH, Morgan GE Jr, eds. *Principles and practice of anesthesiology*, 2nd ed. St. Louis: Mosby, 1998:507–527.
37. Vaughan RW. *Pulmonary and cardiovascular derangements in the obese patient*. Contemporary Anesthesia Practice Series, vol 5. Philadelphia: FA Davis Co, 1982:19–39.
38. Hubert HB, Feinlieb M, McNamera PM, et al. Obesity as an independent risk factor for cardiovascular disease: a 26-year follow-up of participants in the Framingham heart study. *Circulation* 1983;67:968–977.
39. Vaughan RW, Bauer S, Wise L. Volume and pH of gastric juice in obese patients. *Anesthesiology* 1975;43:686–689.
40. Harter RL, Kelly WB, Kramer MG, et al. A comparison of the volume and pH of gastric contents of obese and lean surgical patients. *Anesth Analg* 1998;86:147–152.
41. Mark EJ, Patalas ED, Chang HT, et al. Fatal pulmonary hypertension associated with the short-term use of fenfluramine and phentermine. *N Engl J Med* 1997;337:602–606.
42. Connolly HM, Crary JL, McGoon MD, et al. Valvular heart disease associated with fenfluramine-phentermine. *N Engl J Med* 1997;337:581–588.
43. Kahn MA, Herzog CA, St. Peter JV, et al. The prevalence of cardiac valvular insufficiency assessed by transthoracic echocardiography in obese patients treated with appetite-suppressant drugs. *N Engl J Med* 1998;339:713–718.
44. Jick H, Vasilakis C, Weinrauch LA, et al. A population-based study of appetite-suppressant drugs and the risk of cardiac-valve regurgitation. *N Engl J Med* 1998;339:719–724.
45. Weissman NJ, Tighe JF Jr, Gottdiener JS, Gwynne JT. An assessment of the heart-valve abnormalities in obese patients taking dexfenfluramine, sustained-release dexfenfluramine, or placebo. *N Engl J Med* 1998;339:725–732.
46. Cannistra LB, Cannistra AJ. Regression of multivalvular regurgitation after the cessation of fenfluramine and phentermine treatment [Letter]. *N Engl J Med* 1998;339:771.
47. U.S. Department of Health and Human Services. Cardiac valvulopathy associated with exposure to fenfluramine or dexfenfluramine: U.S. Department of Health and Human Services interim public health recommendations, November 1997. *JAMA* 1997;278:1729–1731.
48. Dajani AS, Taubert KA, Wilson W, et al. Prevention of bacterial endocarditis. Recommendations of the American Heart Association. *JAMA* 1997;277:1794–1801.
49. Osler W. *The principles and practice of medicine*, 8th ed. New York: Appleton, 1919:190.
50. Burwell C, Robin E, Whaley R, Bickellmann A. Extreme obesity associated with alveolar hypoventilation: a Pickwickian syndrome. *Am J Med* 1956;21:811–818.

51. Nunn JF. *Nunn's applied respiratory physiology*, 4th ed. Oxford: Butterworth–Heinemann, 1993:333–337.
52. Guilleminault C, Tilkian A, Dement WC. The sleep apnea syndrome. *Ann Rev Med* 1976;27:465–484.
53. Brown IG, Bradley TD, Phillipson EA, et al. Pharyngeal compliance in snoring subjects with and without obstructive sleep apnea. *Am Rev Respir Dis* 1985;132:211–215.
54. Rafferty TD, Ruskis A, Sasaki C, Gee JB. Perioperative considerations in the management of tracheotomy for the obstructive sleep apnea patient: three illustrative case reports. *Br J Anaesth* 1980;52:619–621.
55. Isono S, Sha M, Suzukawa M, et al. Preoperative nocturnal desaturations as a risk factor for late postoperative nocturnal desaturations. *Br J Anaesth* 1998;80:602–605.
56. Ostermeier AM, Roizen MF, Hautkappe M, et al. Three sudden postoperative respiratory arrests associated with epidural opioids in patients with sleep apnea. *Anesth Analg* 1997;85:452–460.
57. Chung F. Cancer, chemotherapy and anesthesia. *Can Anaesth Soc J* 1982;29:364–371.
58. Desiderio DP. Cancer chemotherapy: complications and interactions with anesthesia. *Hosp Formulary* 1990;25:176.
59. Selvin BL. Cancer chemotherapy: implications for the anesthesiologist. *Anesth Analg* 1981;60:425–434.
60. Perry MC. Toxicity: ten years later. *Semin Oncol* 1992;19:453–457.
61. Sikic BI. Biochemical and cellular determinants of bleomycin cytotoxicity. *Cancer Surv* 1986;5:81–91.
62. Goldiner PL, Carlon GC, Cvitkovic E, et al. Factors influencing postoperative morbidity and mortality in patients treated with bleomycin. *BMJ* 1978;1:1664–1667.
63. LaMantia KR, Glick JH, Marshall BE. Supplemental oxygen does not cause respiratory failure in bleomycin-treated surgical patients. *Anesthesiology* 1984;60:65–67.
64. Desiderio DP, Kross RA, Bedford RF. Evaluation of the patient with oncologic disease. In: Longnecker DE, Tinker JH, Morgan GE Jr, eds. *Principles and practice of anesthesiology*, 2nd ed. St. Louis: Mosby–Year Book, 1998:379–396.
65. Bunn PA, Ridgeway EC. Paraneoplastic syndromes. In: DeVita VT, Hellman S, Rosenberg SA, eds. *Cancer principles and practice of oncology*, 3rd ed. Philadelphia: JB Lippincott, 1989.
66. Mackie AM, Watson CB. Anaesthesia and mediastinal masses. *Anaesthesia* 1984;39:899–903.
67. Neuman GG, Weingarten AE, Abramowitz RM, et al. The anesthetic management of the patient with an anterior mediastinal mass. *Anesthesiology* 1984;60:144–147.
68. Centers for Disease Control. 1993 revised classification system for HIV infection and expanded surveillance case definition for AIDS among adolescents and adults. *MMWR Morb Mortal Wkly Rep* 1992;41(RR17):1–19.
69. Berkowitz ID, Fehr JJ. Evaluation of the patient with acquired immunodeficiency syndrome and other serious infections. In: Longnecker DE, Tinker JH, Morgan GE Jr, eds. *Principles and practice of anesthesiology*, 2nd ed. St. Louis: Mosby, 1998:410–425.
70. Centers for Disease Control and Prevention. Leads from the *MMWR*. Update: universal precautions for prevention of transmission of human immunodeficiency virus, hepatitis B virus and other bloodborne pathogens in health-care settings. *JAMA* 1988; 260:462–465.

Perioperative Management Issues

Mary Kraft

Because increasing numbers of patients are being interviewed and educated about anesthesia and surgery in times and places more remote than their hospital beds the night before surgery, the anesthesiologist is advised to be familiar with changing concepts in **fasting guidelines**, **deep venous thrombosis prophylaxis**, **endocarditis prophylaxis**, and **nutritional evaluation and management**.

FASTING GUIDELINES

Although pulmonary aspiration of gastric contents is a rare event (occurring in approximately 1 in 3,000 cases of general anesthesia), it is associated with significant morbidity and a mortality rate of 1 in 71,000 general anesthesia cases.[1] Patients with conditions predisposing them to an increased risk of aspiration, such as a history of incompetence of the lower esophageal sphincter with reflux, hiatal hernia, diabetes mellitus, gastric motility disorders, intraabdominal masses (including the gravid uterus), and bowel obstruction, are specifically excluded from the following discussion on liberalized nil per os (NPO) guidelines for elective surgery. A thorough preoperative screening history reveals such conditions and should be obtained for every patient presenting for anesthesia.

Obesity was once thought to increase a patient's risk of aspiration because of increased volume and low pH of gastric contents. Harter et al.[1] have disproved this idea by demonstrating that these patients, if otherwise healthy (and fasting for 10 to 12 hours), actually had a lower incidence of combined high-volume, low-pH stomach contents than did lean patients.

The most current guidelines for preoperative fasting for the adult patient (see Chapter 13 for pediatric fasting guidelines) recommend that "fasting from solids (and) nonhuman milk should exceed a period of 6 hours before procedures requiring general anesthesia, regional anesthesia, or sedation/analgesia."[2] Some published data support the offering of clear liquids (including black coffee or tea, excluding any containing fat, oil, or alcohol) up to 2 hours before the procedure.[3]

The American Society of Anesthesiologists Task Force on Preoperative Fasting[2] has not recommended the routine use of gastrointestinal stimulants (in patients who have no apparent increased risk) to decrease the risk of pulmonary aspiration because of insufficient published evidence that examines the relationship between these drugs and the frequency of pulmonary aspiration. Likewise, because of insufficient evidence demonstrating effectiveness in preventing the consequences of aspiration in low-

Table 16-1. Risk factors for pulmonary aspiration

History of incompetence of the lower esophageal sphincter with reflux
Symptomatic hiatal hernia
Diabetes mellitus
Gastric motility disorders
Intraabdominal masses (including the gravid uterus)
Bowel obstruction

risk patients, histamine$_2$ receptor antagonists and proton pump inhibitors are not recommended for routine use in patients with no apparent increased risk for aspiration. Those patients who are at risk (Table 16-1) should not be given particulate antacids.[2]

PREVENTION OF DEEP VENOUS THROMBOSIS

Although relatively rare in the general population, deep venous thrombosis (DVT) and pulmonary embolism (PE) are significant causes of morbidity and mortality in the population hospitalized for serious illness or major surgery. Yearly, pulmonary emboli are responsible for the mortality of 50,000 to 100,000 hospitalized patients with an otherwise favorable prognosis and account for 5% to 10% of all deaths in U.S. hospitals.[4]

Determining figures for the total incidence and fatality rates for venous thromboembolism is difficult because typical signs and symptoms (leg pain and swelling, shortness of breath, chest pain) are absent in more than 50% of affected patients, including a majority of those who die of PE.[4] Estimates are that the prevalence of clinically significant venous thromboembolism is 600,000 cases per year in the United States.

Risk factors for developing DVT are outlined in Table 16-2. The predisposing factors in thrombogenesis were proposed by Rudolph Virchow in 1856. Virchow's triad, consisting of blood

Table 16-2. Risk factors for deep venous thrombosis

Prior thromboembolism
Age older than 40 yr
Major surgery
Malignancy
Obesity
Multiple trauma
Varicose veins
Myocardial infarction
Congestive heart failure
Paralytic stroke
Fracture (hip or leg)
Total hip or knee replacement
Estrogen use
Prolonged immobilization
Parturition

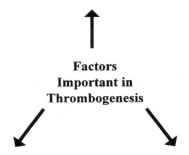

Stasis
Prolonged immobility or bedrest

**Factors
Important in
Thrombogenesis**

Vessel wall injury
Surgical procedure or vessel trauma
Indwelling catheters
Injection of irritating substances
Thromboangiitis obliterans

Hypercoagulable states
Malignant tumors
Oral contraceptives
Blood dyscrasias
Idiopathic thrombophlebitis

Fig. 16-1. Virchow's triad of predisposing factors in thrombogenesis. (Reprinted with permission from Sculco TP, Establishing a universal protocol for deep vein venous thrombosis following orthopedic surgery: total knee arthroplasty. *Orthopedics* 1996;19:6–8.)

flow stasis, vessel wall injury, and hypercoagulable states, is illustrated in Fig. 16-1.[5]

Of the several risk factors illustrated in Table 16-2, the anesthesiologist should be aware of three important factors in particular: a prior history of DVT, a prior history of PE, and impending surgery for total hip replacement or total knee replacement. Patients with DVT are at a greater risk for recurrence, especially if they are exposed to a new risk factor within 6 months of the first occurrence. Patients undergoing lower extremity orthopedic operations are also at much greater risk for developing DVT. Anderson and Wheeler cite three studies suggesting that 50% of patients undergoing elective total hip replacement develop DVT, and the incidence is even higher for those undergoing total knee replacement.[4]

Because the morbidity and mortality from DVT and PE are significant in high-risk populations, prophylaxis should be undertaken in this patient group. No method of prophylaxis is completely effective. Several methods provide some measure of protection. These modalities can be divided into mechanical and pharmacologic methods. Mechanical methods, such as the use of graduated compression stockings and intermittent pneumatic compression, are designed to reduce venous stasis, one of the three components of Virchow's triad. Graduated compression stockings are low cost, low risk, and have been shown to be reasonably effective in reducing the incidence of DVT in general surgery patients. They can easily be combined with other methods of prophylaxis in high-risk surgical patients. Intermittent pneumatic compression appears to be effective in reducing calf DVT, but whether it prevents PE is uncertain. It is useful, however, in patients in whom anticoagulant therapy is contraindicated (e.g., neurosurgical patients) or less effective (patients undergoing total knee replacement).[4]

Pharmacologic methods for prophylaxis commonly include administration of low-dose heparin sodium, low-molecular-weight heparins (LMWHs), warfarin sodium, and antiplatelet agents. Although customarily the surgeon orders these drugs and monitors the patient taking them, the anesthesiologist must be aware of their use and pharmacokinetics. Knowledge of when to withhold therapy in anticipation of anesthesia is important in considering a regional anesthetic technique without concern for additional risk from bleeding. Of course, the appropriate coagulation parameter should be measured in a timely fashion before the start of anesthesia or surgery.

The standard dosage of low-dose heparin sodium is 5,000 units 2 hours before surgery as a subcutaneous injection and then every 8 or 12 hours postoperatively. In general surgery patients, the use of low-dose heparin sodium reduces PE deaths by 50%. However, it is less effective after hip surgery and ineffective in patients undergoing knee surgery.[4] In this dosing regimen, the risk of major bleeding is small; but even so, the regimen should not be used in patients undergoing brain, eye, or spine surgery. Patients receiving this regimen usually do not have a prolonged partial thromboplastin time, and a time limit need not be set for performance of regional anesthesia.

LMWHs (enoxaparin sodium, dalteparin sodium, ardeparin sodium, danaparoid sodium) have a longer half-life than low-dose heparin sodium. Trials seem to indicate that LMWHs may be more effective than low-dose heparin sodium in preventing thromboembolic complications in patients undergoing lower extremity orthopedic surgery. However promising these drugs are in the prevention of PE in these patients, clearly an associated high risk exists of patients' developing epidural or spinal hematomas when LMWH is used concurrently with spinal or epidural anesthesia, or spinal puncture.[6]

Reasons for the increased risk of spinal hematoma with the use of LMWH and spinal or epidural anesthesia include (a) the lack of a convenient assay to monitor coagulation (anti–factor Xa levels cannot readily be measured in most institutions), (b) the fact that LMWH dosage is not adjusted for weight, (c) the fact that the anticoagulant effect of LMWH is only partially reversed by protamine, and (d) the marked differences in the pharmacokinetics and pharmacodynamics of LMWH and standard heparin. Specifically, LMWH has a plasma half-life two to four times that of standard heparin (longer in patients with renal failure). Peak activity occurs 3 to 4 hours after subcutaneous administration of LMWH and has fallen by only 50% 12 hours after injection.[7]

Therefore, Horlocker and Wedel make the following recommendations:

- The smallest effective dose of LMWH should be administered perioperatively. The U.S. Food and Drug Administration (FDA) has approved the use of enoxaparin sodium, 40 mg once daily, as an alternative dosage regimen for thromboprophylaxis after total hip replacement. Single daily dosing results in a true trough in anticoagulant activity, during which time needle placement and catheter removal can occur.
- LMWH therapy should be delayed as long as possible: a minimum of 12 hours and ideally 24 hours postoperatively. This is within the FDA-approved dosage schedule and is particularly relevant for patients with indwelling catheters.

- Administration of antiplatelet or oral anticoagulant medications in combination with LMWH may increase the risk of spinal hematoma. Education of the entire patient care team is necessary to avoid potentiation of the anticoagulant effects.
- The risk of spinal hematoma is almost certainly increased in patients with indwelling catheters who receive LMWH. Removal of the catheter before initiation of LMWH therapy may be a compromise that provides superior analgesia for 24 hours but eliminates the risk of concomitant epidural hematoma and LMWH therapy.
- Catheter removal should occur when anticoagulant activity is low. Twice daily dosing of LMWH results in two peaks and no trough of anti–factor Xa activity. Skipping the evening dose of LMWH before an anticipated morning removal of the epidural catheter is unlikely to significantly increase the risk of thromboembolic events, but it should provide safe conditions for catheter removal.[7]

Oral anticoagulants such as warfarin sodium are highly effective in preventing thromboembolic phenomena when they are administered in dosages that prolong the prothrombin time to an international normalized ratio of 2.0 to 3.0.[4] Because these drugs do not become effective for several days after initiation of treatment, they leave patients vulnerable to the formation of DVT in the acute postoperative period. In addition, they carry a risk of bleeding, and their use must be carefully monitored. The recommendation is that their use be limited to very high risk patients, such as those who have sustained hip fractures and those undergoing total hip replacements.[4]

Although the literature suggests that decreasing platelet activation by the use of drugs such as aspirin may decrease the incidence of DVT and PE, no definitive evidence exists that these drugs are as effective as the others previously discussed.[4]

Because the incidence of DVT after total knee replacement is reportedly as high as 84% of all unprotected patients and may be as high as 68% of patients who receive prophylaxis, ensuring that these patients are on the best prophylactic regimen possible is important.[5] The anticoagulant therapy considered to be most effective by the American College of Chest Physicians Consensus Conference on Antithrombotic Therapy is postoperative unmonitored subcutaneous administration of fixed-dose LMWH twice daily. Intermittent pneumatic compression was identified as the most effective nonpharmacologic prophylaxis. A combination of these two preventive measures should be considered for patients having risk factors in addition to total knee replacement itself.[5]

PREVENTION OF BACTERIAL ENDOCARDITIS

Anesthesiologists must be acquainted with conditions and operations requiring antibiotic prophylaxis for subacute bacterial endocarditis. According to the recommendations of the American Heart Association,[8] prophylaxis for subacute bacterial endocarditis is recommended for patients with high-risk cardiac conditions (prosthetic valves, previous occurrence of subacute bacterial endocarditis, complex cyanotic congenital heart disease, and surgically constructed systemic pulmonary shunts or conduits). Prophylaxis is also recommended for those in a moderate risk category: those with other congenital cardiac malformations (except isolated secundum, atrial

Table 16-3. Procedures for which subacute bacterial endocarditis prophylaxis is and is not recommended

Endocarditis prophylaxis recommended

Respiratory tract
   Tonsillectomy and/or adenoidectomy
   Surgical operations that involve respiratory mucosa
   Bronchoscopy with a rigid bronchoscope
Gastrointestinal tract[a]
   Sclerotherapy for esophageal varices
   Esophageal stricture dilation
   Endoscopic retrograde cholangiography with biliary obstruction
   Biliary tract surgery
   Surgical operations that involve intestinal mucosa
Genitourinary tract
   Prostatic surgery
   Cystoscopy
   Urethral dilation

Endocarditis prophylaxis not recommended

Respiratory tract
   Endotracheal intubation
   Bronchoscopy with a flexible bronchoscope, with or without biopsy[b]
Tympanostomy tube insertion
Gastrointestinal tract
Transesophageal echocardiography[b]
   Endoscopy with or without gastrointestinal biopsy[b]
Genitourinary tract
   Vaginal hysterectomy[b]
   Vaginal delivery[b]
   Cesarean section
   In uninfected tissue:
      Urethral catheterization
      Uterine dilatation and curettage
      Therapeutic abortion
      Sterilization procedures
Insertion or removal of intrauterine devices
Other
   Cardiac catheterization, including balloon angioplasty
   Implantation of cardiac pacemakers, implantation of defibrillators, insertion of coronary stents
   Incision or biopsy of surgically scrubbed skin
   Circumcision

---

[a]Prophylaxis is recommended for high-risk patients; optional for medium-risk patients.

[b]Prophylaxis is optional for high-risk patients.

Reprinted with permission from Dajani AS, Taubert KA, Wilson W, et al. Prevention of bacterial endocarditis, recommendations by the American Heart Association. *JAMA* 1997;277:1794–1801.

Table 16-4. Prophylactic regimens for dental, oral, respiratory tract, and esophageal procedures

Situation	Agent	Regimen[a]
Standard general prophylaxis	Amoxicillin	Adults: 2.0 g; children: 50 mg/kg orally 1 h before procedure
Unable to take oral medications	Ampicillin	Adults: 2.0 g i.m. or i.v.; children: 50 mg/kg i.m. or i.v. within 30 min before procedure
Allergic to penicillin	Clindamycin _or_	Adults: 600 mg; children: 20 mg/kg orally 1 h before procedure
	Cephalexin[b] or cefadroxil[b] _or_	Adults: 2.0 g; children: 50 mg/kg orally 1 h before procedure
	Azithromycin or clarithromycin	Adults: 500 mg; children: 15 mg/kg orally 1 h before procedure
Allergic to penicillin and unable to take oral medications	Clindamycin _or_	Adults: 600 mg; children: 20 mg/kg i.v. within 30 min before procedure
	Cefazolin sodium[b]	Adults: 1.0 g; children: 25 mg/kg i.m. or i.v. within 30 min before procedure

[a]Total children's dose should not exceed adult dose.
[b]Cephalosporins should not be used in individuals with immediate-type hypersensitivity reaction to penicillins (urticaria, angioedema, or anaphylaxis).
Reprinted with permission from Dajani AS, Taubert KA, Wilson W, et al. Prevention of bacterial endocarditis, recommendations by the American Heart Association. _JAMA_ 1997;277:1794–1801.

septal defect, surgical repair of atrial septal defect, ventricular septal defect, or patent ductus arteriosus without residual beyond 6 months), acquired valvular dysfunction (e.g., rheumatic heart disease), hypertrophic cardiomyopathy, and mitral valve prolapse with valvular regurgitation or thickened leaflets (as evidenced by audible clicks _and_ murmurs of mitral regurgitation or by mitral insufficiency demonstrated by Doppler ultrasonography).

Although bacteremias occur during normal daily events such as chewing and tooth brushing, significant bacteremias associated with subacute bacterial endocarditis are attributable to certain procedures. Invasive oral or dental procedures, such as odontectomies and tonsillectomies, fall into this category, as does the use of a rigid bronchoscope. Endotracheal intubation itself does not require antibiotic prophylaxis. For a more inclusive list of those procedures for which prophylaxis is and is not recommended, see Table 16-3.

Tables 16-4 and 16-5 present antibiotic prophylactic regimens. Antibiotic administration should be timed to ensure adequate concentrations in the serum during and after the procedure. This can be readily achieved by giving the antibiotic intravenously at the time of induction. Antibiotic administration should not be continued for more than 6 to 8 hours after the procedure to minimize the risks of microbial resistance.

Table 16-5. Prophylactic regimens for genitourinary and gastrointestinal (excluding esophageal) procedures

Situation	Agents[a]	Regimen[b]
High-risk patients	Ampicillin plus gentamicin	Adults: ampicillin 2.0 g i.m. or i.v. plus gentamicin 1.5 mg/kg (not to exceed 120 mg) within 30 min of starting procedure; 6 h later, ampicillin 1 g i.m./i.v. or amoxicillin 1 g orally
		Children: ampicillin 50 mg/kg i.m. or i.v. (not to exceed 2.0 g) plus gentamicin 1.5 mg/kg within 30 min of starting procedure; 6 h later, ampicillin 25 mg/kg i.m./i.v. or amoxicillin 25 mg/kg orally
High-risk patients allergic to ampicillin/ amoxicillin	Vancomycin plus gentamicin	Adults: vancomycin 1.0 g i.v. over 1–2 h plus gentamicin 1.5 mg/kg i.m./i.v. (not to exceed 120 mg); complete injection/infusion within 30 min of starting procedure
		Children: vancomycin 20 mg/ kg i.v. over 1–2 h plus gentamicin 1.5 mg/kg i.m./ i.v.; complete injection/ infusion within 30 min of starting procedure
Moderate-risk patients	Amoxicillin or ampicillin	Adults: amoxicillin 2.0 g orally 1 h before procedure, or ampicillin 2.0 g i.m./i.v. within 30 min of starting procedure
		Children: amoxicillin 50 mg/ kg orally 1 h before procedure, or ampicillin 50 mg/ kg i.m./i.v. within 30 min of starting procedure
Moderate-risk patients allergic to ampicillin/ amoxicillin	Vancomycin	Adults: vancomycin 1.0 g i.v. over 1–2 h; complete infusion within 30 min of starting procedure
		Children: vancomycin 20 mg/ kg i.v. over 1–2 h; complete infusion within 30 min of starting procedure

[a]Total children's dose should not exceed adult dose.

[b]No second dose of vancomycin or gentamicin is recommended.

Reprinted with permission from Dajani AS, Taubert KA, Wilson W, et al. Prevention of bacterial endocarditis, recommendations by the American Heart Association. *JAMA* 1997;277:1794–1801.

Patients already taking antibiotics when presenting for a procedure should be given a drug from another class rather than an increased dose of the antibiotic the patient has been taking. Manipulation of infected tissues (such as incision and drainage of an abscess) may result in a bacteremia. Patients who are at high or moderate risk for endocarditis should receive antimicrobial prophylaxis before the procedure. The prophylaxis should be directed at the organism most likely to cause the infection. Clindamycin is an acceptable alternative for those allergic to penicillins; vancomycin is the drug of choice for those who are unable to take oral antibiotics or who are known to have methicillin-resistant *Staphylococcus aureus* bacteremia.[8]

NUTRITIONAL EVALUATION AND MANAGEMENT

Patients presenting for anesthesia and surgery may be malnourished, either because of a chronic disease process (e.g., cancer or difficulty swallowing after a stroke) or because of a relatively more acute one, such as intermittent bowel obstruction. Recognition of malnutrition is important because of the associated postoperative complications, which range from prolonged hospital stay for patients undergoing total hip replacement,[9] to more major morbidity, such as wound breakdown, abscesses, infections, anastomotic breakdowns, respiratory failure, and death.[10]

Therefore, the preoperative patient's nutritional status should be evaluated, with an eye to improving the nutrition of a severely malnourished patient before surgery, when possible. Although authors differ in their opinions as to what is most important in assessing nutritional status, reasonable agreement exists about the importance of factors such as weight change over a 6-month period before surgery (weight loss greater than 10% is considered significant), change in dietary intake (relative to normal), gastrointestinal symptoms (that persisted for longer than 2 weeks), decreased functional capacity (from lethargic to bedridden), and physical factors (loss of subcutaneous fat, muscle wasting, ankle edema, sacral edema, ascites). Detsky et al. have incorporated these factors into a short scale, called the Subjective Global Assessment, presented as Fig. 16-2.

Detsky et al.[11] rate these physical factors as normal (0), mild (1+), moderate (2+), or severe (3+). They suggest that the best places to look for loss of subcutaneous fat are the triceps region of the arms, the midaxillary line at the costal margin, the interosseous and palmar areas of the hand, and the deltoid region of the shoulder. Muscle wasting is best examined in the quadriceps femoris and deltoid region. They classify the nutritional status of patients as well nourished (class A), moderately malnourished (class B, weight loss of at least 5% without stabilization or weight gain, poor dietary intake, and mild loss of subcutaneous tissue), or severely malnourished (class C, ongoing weight loss of at least 10%, severe subcutaneous tissue loss, muscle wasting, and edema).

A number of laboratory tests have been suggested by various authors to document malnutrition; the only consistency among them, however, is that a serum albumin level of 3.5 g/dL or less in the general surgical population and 3.9 g/dL or less in those undergoing total hip replacement was found to be an accurate

History

1. Weight change
   Overall loss in past 6 months: amount + _____ kg; _____ %
   Change in past 2 weeks: _____ increase
                                _____ no change
                                _____ decrease

2. Dietary intake change (relative to normal)
   _____ no change
   _____ change _____ duration = _____ weeks
                   _____ type: _____ suboptimal   _____ full liquid
                                            solid diet   diet
                                    _____ hypocaloric _____ starvation
                                            liquid diet

3. Gastrointestinal symptoms (that persisted for >2 weeks)
   _____ none   _____ nausea   _____ vomiting
   _____ diarrhea   _____ anorexia

4. Functional capacity
   _____ no dysfunction (e.g., full capacity)
   _____ dysfunction _____ duration = _____ weeks
                       _____ type: _____ working suboptimally
                                        _____ ambulatory
                                        _____ bedridden

**Physical (for each trait specify: 0 = normal, 1+ = mild,
2+ = moderate, 3+ = severe)**
   _____ loss of subcutaneous fat (triceps, chest)
   _____ muscle wasting (quadriceps, deltoids)
   _____ ankle edema
   _____ sacral edema
   _____ ascites

Subjective Global Assessment rating (select one)*
   _____ A = well nourished
   _____ B = moderately (or suspected of being) malnourished
   _____ C = severely malnourished

**Fig. 16-2. Features of the Subjective Global Assessment scale. *Class A
indicates those with <5% weight loss or >5% total weight loss but
recent gain and improvement in appetite; class B indicates those with
5% to 10% weight loss without recent stabilization or gain, poor
dietary intake, and mild (1+) loss of subcutaneous tissue; class C indicates ongoing weight loss of >10% with severe subcutaneous tissue
loss and muscle wasting, often with edema. (Derived from Detsky AS,
Smalley PS, Chang J. Is this patient malnourished? *JAMA* 1994;271:
54–58.)**

predictor of malnutrition.[9] The combination of history and
physical examination as suggested here and serum albumin
level provide slightly improved accuracy than either indicator
alone.

When possible, nutritional status should be improved preoperatively in those patients found to be severely malnourished.
Enteral nutrition is the preferred means of obtaining the desired
results. If the gut cannot be used (e.g., in cases of enterocutane-
ous fistulas, severe pancreatitis), total parenteral nutrition,
although not without its own risks, is acceptable. A large study

published in 1991[11] demonstrated that severely malnourished patients who received total parenteral nutrition had fewer noninfectious complications than controls (5% versus 43%), with no concomitant increase in infectious complications.

REFERENCES

1. Harter RL, Kelly WB, Kramer MG, et al. A comparison of the volume and pH of gastric contents of obese and lean surgical patients. *Anesth Analg* 1998;86:147–152.
2. Practice guidelines for preoperative fasting and the use of pharmacologic agents to reduce the risk of pulmonary aspiration: application to healthy patients undergoing elective procedures. A Report by the American Society of Anesthesiologists Task Force on Preoperative Fasting. *Anesthesiology* 1999;90:896–905.
3. Phillips S, Hutchinson S, Davidson T. Preoperative drinking does not affect gastric contents. *Br J Anaesth* 1993;70:6–9.
4. Anderson FA, Wheeler HB. Venous thromboembolism. *Clin Chest Med* 1995;16:235–251.
5. Sculco TP. Establishing a universal protocol for deep vein venous thrombosis following orthopedic surgery: total knee arthroplasty. *Orthopedics* 1996;19:6–8.
6. Reports of epidural or spinal hematomas with the concurrent use of low molecular weight heparin and spinal/epidural anesthesia or spinal puncture. FDA Public Health Advisory. December 15, 1997.
7. Horlocker TT, Wedel DJ. Spinal and epidural blockade and preoperative low molecular weight heparin: smooth sailing on the Titanic. *Anesth Analg* 1998;86:1153–1156.
8. Dajani AS, Taubert KA, Wilson W, et al. Prevention of bacterial endocarditis, recommendations by the American Heart Association. *JAMA* 1997;277:1794–1801.
9. Del Savio GC, Zelicof SB, Wexler LM, et al. Preoperative nutritional status and outcome of elective total hip replacement. *Clin Orthop* 1996;326:153–161.
10. The Veterans Affairs Total Parenteral Nutrition Cooperative Study Group. Perioperative total parenteral nutrition in surgical patients. *N Engl J Med* 1991;325:525–532.
11. Detsky AS, Smalley PS, Chang J. Is this patient malnourished? *JAMA* 1994;271:54–58.

Organizational Infrastructure of a Preoperative Evaluation Center

Stephen P. Fischer

The successful development and implementation of an anesthesia preoperative evaluation center (APEC) program require financial commitment, adjustment of support resources, focused leadership, and a hospital and departmental dedication to change.[1] The anesthesiologist is the specialist most knowledgeable and experienced in evaluating perioperative medical complexities as they relate to anesthesia and surgery. As such, the anesthesiologist is best qualified to determine the preoperative patient preparation needed for optimal anesthesia care.

Increasing numbers of surgical patients are entering the hospital on an outpatient basis or as same-day admissions.[2] This trend is expected only to increase and reflects a national environment of cost consciousness and the growing managed care market.[4–6] It presents the anesthesiologist with additional clinical challenges and a decreased amount of time to evaluate patients who are often medically complex. Approximately 28 million patients undergo surgery annually in the United States. With the rising age of patients, complex surgical procedures are being performed, often frequently, on patients with serious coexisting conditions.[3]

Establishment of a centralized APEC is a positive investment for the anesthesia group and the hospital.[1,7–12] Increasingly, anesthesiologists direct the preoperative assessment and preparation of patients for surgery with the aim of ensuring safe and efficient care while controlling costs by reducing unnecessary testing and preventable cancellations on the day of surgery.[13] The APEC can become a recognized center for establishing a standard of efficient clinical services, decreased costs, and increased patient/surgeon satisfaction.[14]

CONCERNS AND PROBLEMS

Many medical centers, hospitals, and anesthesia groups have adopted some method of anesthesia preoperative screening or evaluation before the day of surgery in response to the increasing volume of patients admitted on the day of surgery. Nationally, estimates are that 70% to 80% of surgical patients enter the hospital for immediate admission.[2]

Preoperative programs are often informal with limited hours of operation. The majority of patients are evaluated at the end of the day when anesthesiologists are available outside the operating room (OR). This can result in significant patient waits of up to 2 or 3 hours for assessment when patient volume is high and creates an environment of frustration and dissatisfaction.

Overcrowded and uncomfortable patient waiting areas, inadequate patient examination facilities and equipment, lack of medical records or consultant reports, and unavailability of phlebotomy and technical and registration support contribute to staff and patient discontent. These problems will continue to increase as the American health care system actively transforms to a system of outpatient medicine coupled with limited resources and decreasing financial support.

OPERATIONAL GOALS

The conceptual goal of the APEC program is to provide cost-effective patient management in a centralized, integrated clinic for patients about to undergo surgery and anesthesia. The primary focus of the APEC program is to determine if the patient is sufficiently prepared and if proceeding with anesthesia is appropriate.

Provision of a dedicated, centralized location is the best framework for increasing efficiency and decreasing the logistic shuffling of patients, medical charts, test results, and other pertinent information throughout the hospital. Integration and coordination of services, including on-site registration and insurance authorization, together with on-site laboratory and diagnostic facilities, are imperative to establishing clinical integration and service value. Additional operational goals of an APEC are reviewed in Table 17-1.

Table 17-1. Summary of operational goals adopted for anesthesia preoperative evaluation center (APEC) of Stanford University Hospital

To improve the patient's, surgeon's, and insurance company's perception of the preoperative evaluation experience by increasing personalized patient care, comfort, and convenience.

To institute an anesthesia scheduling system to ensure timely patient access and flow.

To ensure the presence of an anesthesiologist on site when patients are present.

To appoint a medical director of the APEC to coordinate all activities.

To ensure the availability of medical records and surgical notes at the time of the preoperative evaluation.

To decrease logistical shuffling of patients to multiple hospital service areas.

To improve education of patients and families about the elements of their surgical procedure and the proposed anesthesia, including postoperative pain control options.

To ensure and coordinate cost-effective ordering of preoperative laboratory and diagnostic studies.

To provide a medical consultation service for evaluation of medically complex inpatients and outpatients.

To decrease cancellations and delays of operative procedures on the day of surgery.

To enlist the skills of a registered nurse practitioner to assist in preoperative evaluations and patient and family education.

To develop protocols, policies, and clinical pathways.

To perform quality assurance reviews.

To maximize efficiency in operating room function and turnover time by coordinating all preoperative information into one location (the APEC).

To enhance patient and surgeon satisfaction.

Table 17-2. Business plan outline for an anesthesia preoperative evaluation center (APEC)

Executive summary (four sentences summarizing the APEC program content)

Description of an APEC

    APEC objective or mission

    Names of proposed APEC medical director, department chair

    Location within the hospital (define an area even if currently occupied)

    Development stage (Does a preoperative program currently exist?)

    Services of the APEC (see operational goals in Table 17-1)

    Anesthesiology specialty information [i.e., anesthesiologists are the experts in operating room (OR) medicine and preoperative evaluation]

Preoperative program analysis

    Preoperative patient volume and acuity (present a graph for past years)

    Anticipated growth trends

    Vulnerability to economic factors (decreasing fee-for-service and increasing managed care focus, hospital needs to decrease costs)

    Technological factors (anesthesia and surgical procedures are increasingly more advanced; anesthesiologists are uniquely qualified to determine optimal preoperative and OR patient management)

    Regulatory issues (APEC conforms to local, state, and federal policies)

    Financial considerations

Target market

    All outpatients and same-day admissions

    Medically complex patients undergoing anesthesia and surgery

Competition

    Competitive position (the anesthesiologist is the OR and preoperative medicine expert)

    Barriers to entry (primary care physicians and consultants believe they have specialty knowledge to clear patients for anesthesia and surgery)

    Future competition (see above)

Marketing strategies

    Increased visibility is viability

    Hospital news media (who anesthesiologists are and what they do)

    Strategic partnerships (with department of nursing and hospital administration)

    Informal assurance that cases will not be canceled or delayed by anesthesia

    Presentations at surgical grand rounds and conferences

APEC operations

    Facilities (e.g., examination rooms, phlebotomy and electrocardiography room)

    Equipment and supplies

    Variable labor requirements (e.g., nurse practitioner, anesthesiologist)

    Daily anticipated operations and flow

    Quality assurance and utilization review

    Management information systems

APEC management and organization

    Clinical and administrative director

continued

Table 17-2. *Continued*

Inclusion of department of nursing and hospital administration
Organizational management flow chart
APEC developmental goals
  Short term (clinical practice changes)
  Long term (e.g., facility renovations)
  Time line (demonstrates a development plan)
  Growth strategy (project 6-month, 1-year, 5-year goals)
  Risk evaluation (as long as patients have surgical needs, risk is
    minimal)
Financial matters
  Income statement (consider a facility fee, anesthesia medical
    consultation charge; project hospital cost savings)
  Variable expenditures (APEC personnel and resources, 90% of
    expenditures; facility housekeeping and supplies)
  Balance sheet

IMPLEMENTATION STRATEGIES

The development of an APEC program requires, foremost, the commitment of the anesthesia departmental chair to support necessary changes. A written business plan should be developed and presented to the hospital administration to obtain financial and political support. Table 17-2 suggests sequential elements of an APEC business plan that details APEC program development and strategies in terms familiar to hospital administrators.

Anesthesia faculty support and consensus regarding evaluation guidelines are imperative to the success of the APEC. The anesthesia group must define and review practice policies and clinical guidelines to avoid day-of-surgery conflicts, delays, and cancellations.

An alliance with the department of nursing can provide shared financial support for nursing staff resources, such as a registered nurse practitioner (RNP) to assist in the evaluations and nurse educators for patient and family education. These resources usually are based in nursing administration, and this strategic alliance creates a financial and strategic link to hospital administration.

Cancellations and delays on the day of surgery can be a prominent source of aggravation and frustration for a surgeon and the patient. The surgeon's hesitation to send patients to the APEC can be reduced by identifying the clinical advantages of the APEC. One example is the structuring of an informal assurance that, if a patient is evaluated and deemed medically stable and appropriate for anesthesia by the APEC, the case will proceed to surgery without cancellation or delay by the anesthesiologist. The only exception would be a case in which the patient experiences an adverse medical event or illness between the time of evaluation and the time of the planned surgery.

FACILITY DEVELOPMENT

Development of a centralized facility together with capital equipment expenditures is important to coordinate services and

Table 17-3. Facilities of the anesthesia preoperative evaluation clinic at Stanford University Hospital

Six combination office and examination rooms.
A patient and family education room (for preoperative teaching).
A patient-centered media and video room.
A phlebotomy and electrocardiography room.
An on-site office for the anesthesia preoperative medical director.
A registration and reception area.
On-site restroom facilities.
A large, comfortable patient lounge.
An area for admissions and financial services.
Facilities are approximately 2,200 square feet.

to increase efficiency. The facilities of the APEC at Stanford University Hospital are listed in Table 17-3. Not all of the concepts and changes seen at Stanford need to be implemented to improve the overall system and cost effectiveness of preoperative evaluation; however, certain advantages accrue to the anesthesiologist and department of anesthesiology when such an APEC program is established.

STRUCTURE AND DAILY OPERATIONS

The concept of an APEC program is illustrated in Fig. 17-1. Patients from all surgical services are evaluated through the APEC before proceeding to the OR or out-of-OR locations.

Figure 17-2 illustrates a typical flow pattern in the APEC program. During periods of increased patient volume into one area, the flow pattern can be changed to promote timeliness and efficiency. For example, patient education can precede the anesthesiology evaluation. Laboratory test requirements can often be

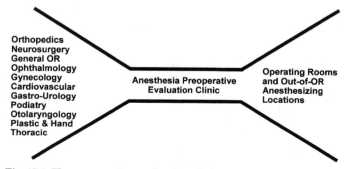

Orthopedics
Neurosurgery
General OR
Ophthalmology
Gynecology
Cardiovascular
Gastro-Urology
Podiatry
Otolaryngology
Plastic & Hand
Thoracic

Anesthesia Preoperative Evaluation Clinic

Operating Rooms and Out-of-OR Anesthesizing Locations

Fig. 17-1. The preoperative evaluation clinic conceptually is the final pathway that determines a patient's stability and appropriate preparation for anesthesia and surgery. (OR, operating room.)

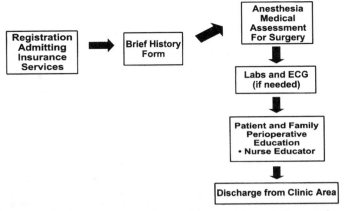

Fig. 17-2. Basic flow diagram of patient progress through the anesthesia preoperative evaluation clinic. (ECG, electrocardiogram; labs, laboratory tests.)

determined when the patient arrives in the APEC by the anesthesiologist's review of the patient's medical history and anesthesia questionnaire. Thus, laboratory testing can be obtained before the formal patient evaluation when adjustment of the patient flow pattern is required. Direct involvement and awareness of APEC operations are primary responsibilities of the anesthesiology medical director.

Patient Appointments with the Anesthesia Preoperative Evaluation Program

To decrease long patient waits (of up to several hours) when anesthesiologists are not available or when high patient volume occurs in the late afternoon, an anesthesia scheduling appointment system becomes mandatory. At Stanford, patients are given appointments (as with any other medical specialty) between the hours of 8:30 a.m. and 5:30 p.m., Monday through Friday. Twenty minutes is allocated for patients categorized as class 1 or 2 according to the American Society of Anesthesiologists Physical Status (ASA-PS) scale, and 30 minutes for patients categorized as ASA-PS class 3 or 4.

To maintain compliance with the preoperative anesthesia appointment system, the surgeon is required to book an anesthesia appointment before obtaining an OR reservation for an elective case. Because of this method of gentle leverage, virtually all patients are scheduled into the APEC, and several daytime slots are available for drop-in, nonappointment, urgent surgical cases.

A list of patients scheduled for anesthesia preoperative evaluation is faxed to the medical records department 24 hours in advance of appointments. Under this practice, 95% of medical records are present at the time of patient assessment.

Staff Resources

An on-site anesthesia preoperative medical director provides immediate clinical consultation, supervision of staff, and evaluation of concerns or problems that can result in OR cancellations and delays. Personal communication between the anesthesia medical director and the assigned anesthesiologist on the day before surgery is important in certain medically complex cases. This communication allows discussion of concerns, avoidance of delays, and optimal intraoperative planning.

Staff requirements in the APEC program are specific to the institution, patient demographics, and anesthesia group. A facility such as Stanford University Hospital, which evaluates 50 to 60 patients per day, requires the following staff resources to maintain consistency of flow as well as efficiency of services: one RNP per 12 to 15 patients, one phlebotomy and electrocardiography technician per 25 patients, one nurse educator per 25 patients, and one admission and insurance clerk per 20 to 25 patients during an 8-hour APEC day.

Staff resource figures assume that at least 75% of patients are scheduled and arrive on time. In addition, a patient-clinic coordinator such as an office manager or nurse can be used to supervise various APEC services and flow management. This individual is responsible for completion of the final preoperative patient chart, including physician orders, consents, surgical history and physical documentation, consultant reports, the anesthesia preoperative evaluation, the historical medical record, diagnostic and laboratory results, and any vital information that provides a smooth transition to the OR without delay or mismanagement on the day of surgery.

Patient preoperative charts are completed and available for the assigned anesthesiologist to review throughout the day before surgery. The efficiency of the APEC at Stanford University Hospital and the completed chart preparation has resulted in a significant decrease in OR delays for first cases of the day. Currently at Stanford University Hospital, 90% of all patients scheduled for a 7:30 a.m. start time enter the OR by 7:10 a.m.

Admission and Insurance Authorization

A satellite area for patient insurance confirmation and admission registration is physically within the APEC. This area provides increased access for patients, service efficiency, and enhanced patient satisfaction. Patients are hospital registered and insurance authorized before entering the APEC system, to avoid inadvertent processing of patients who are potentially ineligible for their surgical procedure. Cross-trained staff provide patient reception in the APEC as well as coordination of insurance authorization.

TEAMWORK ALLIANCE

The APEC is a constructive partnership between the departments of anesthesiology and nursing and the hospital administration to achieve the common goals of decreased costs, delivery of efficient quality services, enhanced clinical productivity, and patient and staff satisfaction. It has a necessary focus on team-work, problem solving, and cooperation.

The RNP has had an evolving role in the APEC. With the increasing volume of patients requiring preoperative assessment and the staffing requirements of anesthesiologists in the OR, using the clinical skills of RNPs is practical.

Clinical supervision is provided by the anesthesia medical director. Standardized clinical procedures are developed for assessment and management of patients within the APEC. The RNP is recognized as an integral member of the preoperative team by the physicians, staff, and patients.

Anesthesia education is provided for the RNPs through intra-operative observation of the various anesthetic techniques. This observation allows a visual understanding and practical interpretation of regional anesthetic protocols, general anesthesia, and monitored anesthesia care so that the RNP can better inform the patient and family during the APEC evaluation. Complex clinical cases and preoperative topics of interest are presented at the weekly APEC staff meeting for review and discussion.

PATIENT AND FAMILY PREOPERATIVE EDUCATION

The goal of preoperative education is to increase the perisurgical knowledge and comfort of the patient by decreasing anxiety and fear. The preoperative teaching center is located in the APEC and provides individualized perioperative education for patients and families. In this personal interaction between a nurse educator, patient, and family, standardized teaching care plans developed by each surgical specialty and the departments of anesthesiology and nursing are used.

The APEC's preoperative education program has eliminated the need for multiple surgical teaching resources by coordinating the education of all surgical patients. Patients have an opportunity, if they choose, to view and handle various anesthetic and surgical equipment such as epidural catheters, oxygen masks, surgical drains, and catheters, and to inspect anatomic models and other materials to increase understanding and decrease anxiety.

A private media/video room has modular stations in which patients can view tapes specific to their surgery and proposed anesthesia. A patient-oriented tape tours the procedures of hospital registration, preoperative assessment, the OR and recovery room, and rehabilitation, and discusses other perioperative topics such as options for postoperative pain management.

All patients are contacted by telephone by cross-trained staff from the preoperative, admitting, and postoperative recovery units the evening before surgery to assure compliance with preoperative instructions, medication regimens, and specific hospital arrival times. All laboratory and diagnostic studies are reviewed at 6 p.m. The anesthesia medical director is available to resolve any concerns of patients, surgeons, or anesthesiologists.

RESIDENT EDUCATION AND RESEARCH

Significant opportunity is available in the APEC for resident and staff education in preoperative medical assessment of patients. Resident training in perioperative medicine has become an issue of great importance during the 1990s. It not only provides increased recognition and visibility of anesthesiologists among colleagues and patients but, more important, confirms the primary expertise of the anesthesiologist in perioperative medicine.

Multiple academic reprints and textbooks have been published on preoperative medical complexities as they relate to intraoperative management. Most studies have not captured the necessary protocols, data, and statistics required to measure clinical, medical, and financial outcomes. This area of research remains available.

At Stanford University Hospital, the anesthesia residents participate in a 1-week rotation in the APEC with no on-call or OR assignments. At the request of the Department of Internal Medicine and the Department of Surgery, both a medical and surgical resident participate in educational sessions and preoperative patient evaluations in the APEC under the direction of the anesthesiology medical director. The purpose is to provide an interdisciplinary approach and teaching of perioperative medicine. Clinical issues and perspectives on patients' medical complexities as they relate to anesthetic, medical, and surgical management are reviewed. Residents are encouraged to participate in preoperative clinical research and attend the monthly APEC journal club.

CONCLUSION

The anesthesia preoperative assessment is a medical evaluation of the patient's current condition integrated with the anesthesiologist's knowledge of the operative events that potentially may occur. The presurgical patient presents the anesthesiologist with significant clinical challenges in providing the most appropriate care and the best outcome possible.

The APEC can become a strategic framework for the expansion of the anesthesiologist's practice beyond the OR. It provides the anesthesiologist with increased hospital visibility and leadership in the changing health care system.

Anesthesiologists have the ability to redefine their specialty by assuming responsibility as perioperative managers of the surgical patient. Anesthesiologists can contribute to the goals of cost-effective, enhanced quality of patient care. The foundation of this challenge begins with the anesthesia preoperative evaluation.

REFERENCES

1. Fischer SP. Development and effectiveness of an anesthesia preoperative evaluation clinic in a teaching hospital [Special article]. *Anesthesiology* 1996;85:196–206.
2. Roizen MF. Preoperative evaluation. In: Miller RD, ed. *Anesthesia*, 4th ed. New York: Churchill Livingstone, 1994:827–882.
3. Mangano DT. Preoperative risk assessment: many studies, few solutions: is a cardiac risk assessment paradigm possible? *Anesthesiology* 1995;83:897–901.
4. Macario A, Vitez TS, Dunn B, et al. Where are the costs in perioperative care? Analysis of hospital costs and charges for inpatient surgical care. *Anesthesiology* 1995;83:1138–1144.

5. Vitez TS. Principles of cost analysis. *J Clin Anesth* 1994;6:357–363.
6. Johnstone RE, Martinec CL. Costs of anesthesia. *Anesth Analg* 1993;76:840–848.
7. Pollard JB, Zboray AL, Mazze RI. Economic benefits attributed to opening a preoperative evaluation clinic for outpatients. *Anesth Analg* 1996;82:407–410.
8. Starsnic MA, Guarnieri DM, Norris MC. Efficacy and financial benefit of an anesthesiologist-directed university preadmission evaluation clinic. *J Clin Anesth* 1997;9:299–305.
9. Boothe P. Changing the admission process for elective surgery: an economic analysis. *Can J Anaesth* 1995;42:391–394.
10. Hand R, Levin P, Stanziola A. The causes of canceled elective surgery. *Qual Assur Utiliz Rev* 1990;5:2–6.
11. Conway JB, Goldberg J, Chung F. Preadmission anaesthesia consultation clinic. *Can J Anaesth* 1992;39:1051–1057.
12. Rinegan BA. Preadmission and outpatient consultation clinics [Editorial]. *Can J Anaesth* 1992;39:1009–1011.
13. Wiklund RA, Rosenbaum SH. Medical progress: anesthesiology [Review article]. *N Engl J Med* 1997;337:1132–1141.
14. Deutschman CS, Traber KB. Evolution of anesthesiology [Editorial]. *Anesthesiology* 1996;85:1–3.

Development of Practice Guidelines

L. Reuven Pasternak

The development of guidelines for the preoperative evaluation of the surgical patient has posed a formidable challenge for anesthesiologists. The challenges and current state of the art in guideline development are presented in this chapter. Methodologies and a recommended algorithm for timing of the evaluation and its content are provided. The reader should understand that this is a dynamic process and is subject to variations depending on the nature of the practice and the practice environment. Nonetheless, the fundamentals presented here are the basis on which these variations may be developed.

IMPERATIVE FOR DEVELOPMENT

Guideline development has progressed rapidly during the 1990s as a means for health care providers to seek an organized method of evaluating a large amount of information from an increasing diversity of print and electronic sources. The explosion of medical knowledge has made it impossible for practitioners to rely on a few specialty journals or experts to address all issues within their specialties. The pressures to formulate guidelines go beyond a desire to distill the clinical data and include attempts to address the regulatory, economic, and practice organization issues facing clinicians on a daily basis.

The preoperative assessment of the surgical patient is a classic example of a case in which these pressures are felt. Preoperative evaluation provides one of the most formidable challenges for anesthesiologists from both a clinical and an organizational perspective. Although the relative merits of alternative surgical and anesthetic techniques have been extensively reviewed in the literature and other forums, the issue of appropriate preoperative preparation has remained ambiguous and, in many instances, frustrating. The importance of this issue is demonstrated by the fact that preoperative care affects 26 million surgical cases in the United States each year at a cost in excess of $10 billion in a patient population with increasing medical and surgical acuity. Other contributing issues in this area include the following:

- Although the surgeon has retained the opportunity to examine and assess the patient before the scheduling of surgery, the anesthesiologist no longer has guaranteed access to the patient, as previously existed with routine preoperative admissions. The anesthesiologist has lost a uniform way of obtaining appropriate laboratory and clinical information in a timely fashion.
- The designation by third-party payers of procedures to be performed on an outpatient and same-day admission basis is

generally determined by the presumed complexity of the procedure and not by the patient's underlying medical problems or potential issues associated with anesthesia. Consequently, the anesthesiologist often must manage patients with complex medical conditions undergoing complex surgery with little prior information.

• Organized health plans often seek to retain control of the process as much as possible, including determination of when and where tests and consultations are to be performed.

• Many hospitals and surgical units have yet to organize and develop preoperative evaluation units because of the expense of providing staff and space at a time when financial constraints are increasingly severe.

• Anesthesiologists often provide care at several institutions whose clinical and administrative staffs are seeking a consistent approach to clinical management, especially in the context of clinical paths.

• No consistent system has existed for risk assessment to determine appropriate preoperative management.

The aggregation of health care into contractual units of multispecialty providers has caused all health care providers to carefully review the rationale for their activities and to insist that activities be performed on a value-added basis.

Although anesthesiologists have been approaching this issue with considerable caution, others have already disseminated information on preoperative evaluation based on their own specialty society of initiatives and guidelines. Hence, anesthesia-directed efforts in this area are needed.

PROMISE AND PERILS

The attraction of guidelines is to provide direction to the clinician. Guidelines are intended to serve as a resource that allows for individual interpretation. Unlike protocols, which are based on definitive clinical evidence that mandates adherence to specific recommendations, guidelines can be interpreted by the clinician on a case-by-case basis. Nonetheless, several prerequisites must be met before guidelines can be formulated for preoperative evaluation, or for any clinical activity. Among these is a systematic approach to the available scientific data and an adequate number of well-designed studies or data that establishes a clear trend. Equally important, and often overlooked, is a target audience of clinicians who accept the prior two tenets and are receptive to a critical evaluation of their practice, based on scientific evidence rather than custom.

The systematic approach to guideline development has shown considerable improvement and sophistication over time. In the past, guidelines were based on everything from formal literature analysis to consensus development and, on occasion, represented ad hoc statements lacking any critical analysis. Guidelines often were viewed as a rapid response to clinical dilemmas subject to resolution by a simple vote of interested parties. This approach, although providing the comfort of an answer to a perceived problem, tended to reinforce the ongoing predisposition of the interested parties rather than advancing the cause of scientific evaluation. Although simple in its approach, it reminds one of the observation attributed to the journalist H. L. Mencken that "every problem has a simple solution; unfortunately, it is always wrong." Hunt and McKibbon[1] note the methodologic difficulties associated with the retrieval and analysis of the information required for developing guidelines, and provide insight into the challenge of conducting a comprehensive literature review. Of great concern is the need to rely on retrospective studies whose design, execution, and interpretation may not have addressed the issues raised or may not stand up to scientific scrutiny. Cook et al.[2] present an excellent summary of the relationship between these reviews and the development of guidelines, and note in their algorithm the great complexities inherent in this effort, including the importance of recognizing the different practice considerations beyond those of science, such as geographic variation and practice organization. The evidence-based guideline is the seminal development that has served to provide structure in this area. Guyatt et al.[3] assert that evidence-based practice, when applied to clinical practice, "de-emphasizes intuition, [and] unsystematic clinical experience . . . and stresses the examination of evidence from clinical research." When applied to the broader area of guideline formulation, the evidence-based model provides a rigorous format for guideline development that has been adopted by numerous professional, academic, and governmental bodies. When the algorithm of guideline development devised by Cook et al.[2] is merged with appropriate scientific evidence, the result is a truly scientific guideline. The level of the scientific evidence required in establishing the guideline then becomes the limiting factor in the guideline development process. The American College of Cardiology and American Heart Association (ACC/AHA) guidelines[4] (see Chapter 3) for cardiovascular evaluation of the cardiac patient undergoing noncardiac surgery represent an analysis based in large part on a consensus approach and a reasonableness doctrine.

Other organizations, such as the American Society of Anesthesiologists (ASA), have used a very rigorous approach based on an evidence and outcomes model. Such a model sets a very high criterion for the inclusion of studies in guideline development and requires that a specific linkage exist between a defined intervention, such as a specific test or the timing of the performance of the preoperative evaluation, and a specific outcome, such as mortality or morbidity. Failure to provide a specific linkage in a manner that is supported by data from studies showing consistent trends in a rigorous scientific manner results in exclusion of the guideline from consideration. Under the algorithm of the ASA (Fig. 18-1), a search of the literature regarding a given issue results in three potential outcomes: *definitive findings* with firm and consistent scientific data; *marginal findings*, in which a limited number of appropriate studies show trends that agree with consensus opinion; and *no guidance,* when the literature does not contain an adequate number of studies meeting methodological standards. In its Task Force on Preoperative Evaluation, the ASA panel found that, of the initial 901 articles reviewed, only 163 qualified as original studies and, of these, only 11 satisfied the criteria for inclusion. As a result, insufficient scientific evidence was available to establish guidelines, and the ASA task force had to defer the proposal of guidelines.

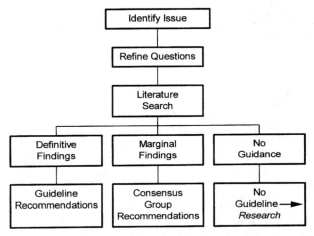

Fig. 18-1. American Society of Anesthesiologists algorithm for guideline development.

This experience illustrates one of the pitfalls of guideline development. Reliance on the existing literature can be a disappointing process, and the result points to the need for more directed research in the area of interest. One always runs the risk of having to advise colleagues that insufficient information exists for guidance and that individual judgment must be the guiding principle.

PHILOSOPHY OF THE PROCESS

Although an adequate number of studies were lacking, several distinct trends and statements have emerged from the work of the ASA task force that are recognized as guiding principles for preoperative evaluation. Although not scientific in their formulation, these precepts are based on clinical issues regarding the nature of the preoperative process and the role of the anesthesiologist.

Philosophy of the Preoperative Evaluation

The preoperative evaluation of the patient undergoing surgery is carried out to address issues concerning the safety and efficiency of the perioperative process. As such, it is designed to reduce the risk to patients and to the system in which they are receiving their care. The *preanesthesia evaluation* is the portion of the assessment that is designed to address issues related to the perioperative management of the surgical patient by anesthesiologists. It is a focused assessment designed to deal with issues of relevance to anesthesia. Although anesthesiologists should be concerned about primary care issues such as health screening and maintenance, preanesthesia evaluation systems are not expected to be responsible for these activities if they are not related to the safety and efficiency of the perioperative process.

In those circumstances in which these activities are undertaken, they should be performed in association with the appropriate primary and specialty care services.

Role of the Primary Care Provider and Specialist

Primary care providers and associated specialists furnish information that is used by anesthesia staff to evaluate the appropriateness of patients for surgery. Other providers do not clear patients for anesthesia but address issues of the medical stability of the patient. Specifically, the items to be resolved are the medical issues of the patient, how they are being managed, and whether they are being managed as optimally as is reasonably possible. Requests by anesthesia staff for consultations or elaboration on existing information should be raised in this manner, rather than in a fashion that implies a request for guidance on appropriate anesthetic management. The expectation is that before surgery the patient is in as optimal a condition as can be expected, with new exacerbations or chronic existing conditions addressed before the patient undergoes elective surgical procedures.

Value-Added Approach to the Preanesthesia Process

All preanesthesia activities, including evaluation before the day of surgery, testing, and consultation, should be undertaken on the reasonable expectation that they will enhance the safety, comfort, and efficiency of the process for the patient and the clinical staff. Decisions concerning preanesthesia management should consider how the evaluation will affect the management and outcome of the process. Evaluations and interventions that have no demonstrated beneficial effect have no value to the clinician, patient, or manager and should not be undertaken out of custom or convenience. The preanesthesia process is concerned with issues of physiologic morbidity, patient satisfaction, and operational efficiency and integrity of the surgical system.

CURRENT STATE

As noted earlier, the ASA Task Force on Preoperative Evaluation identified fewer than 11 original research articles that met the most stringent criteria of outcome- and evidence-based information. This number was deemed insufficient to allow specific recommendations to be made. Despite the inability of the literature to provide a basis for definitive guidelines, some preliminary data provide assistance in this area. Fischer's article[5] on the value of a preoperative screening clinic at Stanford University Hospital established the usefulness of an anesthesia-based and anesthesia-organized screening and evaluation system in enhancing patient care and operational efficiency (see Chapter 17). Through application of the value-added approach in an anesthesia-directed unit, the preoperative screening clinic was able to effect major reductions in testing (18% to 90%; depending on the test), consultation (70% to 98%, depending on specialty), and surgery cancellations (from 2% to 0.2%). Unpublished data from the

Johns Hopkins Bayview Medical Center have demonstrated a reduction in surgery cancellations from 15% to 2% and an improvement in morning on-time starts from less than 30% to more than 80% through the use of a preoperative system.

The optimal timing of the preanesthesia evaluation and the staff who should perform it have yet to be established. Assertions by some that all patients should have a preanesthesia visit before the day of surgery are not supported by evidence. Many successful units have reported that evaluations accomplished by actual visit rather than by data acquisition may be performed in as few as one-fourth to one-third of cases without compromising patient safety, convenience, or anxiety reduction. Timing and specifics of the evaluation should consider parochial issues of the practice environment, geography, and other factors that call for a carefully considered local solution rather than a broad mandate.

Nonetheless, ASA task force participants determined that an algorithm could be used for the timing of the preanesthesia evaluation that might fit most situations (Fig. 18-2). The determining factors in this enterprise are the risks to the patient. The risk associated with the performance of surgery and anesthesia is generally recognized to be related to two principal factors. These are the nature of the patient's medical condition before undergoing surgery and the nature of the surgical procedure itself. Although outcome studies in this area are few, those that exist clearly establish the interactive nature of these forces. The most significant of these is the confidential investigation of perioperative deaths conducted in Great Britain,[6] which demonstrated that one-half of all morbidity was attributable at least in part to a combination of these factors. The current system for risk classifi-

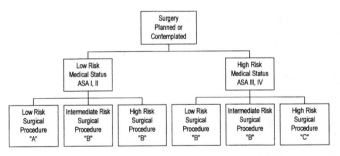

Fig. 18-2. Illustrative algorithm for preanesthesia evaluation adapted from that developed by the American Society of Anesthesiologists Task Force on Preanesthesia Evaluation. Low-risk procedure poses minimal physiologic stress and risk to the patient independent of medical condition (e.g., office-based, minor surgery); intermediate-risk procedure poses moderate physiologic stress and risk with minimal blood loss, fluid shift, or postoperative change in normal physiology; high-risk procedure poses significant perioperative and postoperative physiologic stress. A, patient may have preanesthesia assessment on day of surgery, based on available preoperative data; B, patient may require preanesthesia consultation, based on the nature of the patient's medical condition and planned procedure; C, patient should have preanesthesia consultation with anesthesia staff before the day of surgery.

Table 18-1. American Society of Anesthesiologists' medical classification system

Class	Description
1	No physiologic, biochemical, or psychiatric disturbance
	Example: healthy without any concurrent medical problems
2	Mild to moderate physiologic disturbance under good control
	No significant compromise of normal activity
	Condition may potentially affect safety of surgery and anesthesia
	Examples: well-controlled hypertension, well-controlled asthma, mild obesity, tobacco abuse
3	Major systemic disturbance, difficult to control
	Significant compromise of normal activity
	Significant impact on surgery and anesthesia
	Examples: stable angina, chronic obstructive pulmonary disease
4	Severe, potentially lethal systemic disorder
	Major impact on surgery and anesthesia
	Examples: congestive heart failure, respiratory failure
5	Moribund patient, surgery as last effort to save life

cation used by the ASA (Table 18-1) is based on an analysis of mortality; and the system has not been assessed with regard to patient morbidity or administrative problems. Although this system remains to be tested in this format, it still serves as the basis for medical risk classification. Surgical classification systems have not used a standardized format. However, general consensus is seen across specialties in delineating procedures as low risk, medium risk, or high risk. This format has been adopted by the ACC/AHA guidelines and is part of the model adopted by the ASA Task Force on Preoperative Evaluation (see Fig. 18-2).

REFERENCES

1. Hunt DL, McKibbon A. Locating and appraising systematic reviews. *Ann Intern Med* 1997;126:532–538.
2. Cook DJ, Greengold NL, Ellrodt G, Weingarten SR. The relation between systematic reviews and practice guidelines. *Ann Intern Med* 1997;127:210–215.
3. Guyatt GH. Evidence based medicine. *JAMA* 1992;2420–2425.
4. Eagle K, Brundage B, Chaitman B, et al. Guidelines for perioperative cardiovascular evaluation for noncardiac surgery. A report of the American College of Cardiology/American Heart Association Task Force on Assessment of Diagnostic and Therapeutic Cardiovascular Procedures. *Circulation* 1996;93:1278–1317.
5. Fischer SP. Development and effectiveness of an anesthesia preoperative evaluation clinic in a teaching hospital. *Anesthesiology* 1996;85:196–206.
6. Buck N, Devlin HB, Lunn JL. *Report of a confidential enquiry into perioperative deaths.* London: The King's Fund Publishing House, 1987.

Preoperative Data Management

Michael S. Higgins

GOALS OF PREOPERATIVE DATA COLLECTION

In practical terms, the primary goal of preoperative data collection is to inform care providers about the medical history and current condition of the patient. This information assists in the process of risk assessment and modification, and the selection of an appropriate anesthetic plan. In addition, preoperative documentation must meet specific requirements of hospitals, insurance organizations, the federal government (Health Care Financing Administration), and professional organizations such as the American Society of Anesthesiologists. By creating a common record, the data collection process may serve part of the documentation needs of nursing and surgical teams in addition to those of the anesthesiologist (Table 19-1).

Tracking of the important descriptors of each patient's medical condition allows reasonable comparisons to be made between sentinel outcomes. Such analyses will be required by the Health Care Financing Administration's Health Care Quality Improvement Program, which addresses the quality of health care provided to federal beneficiaries.[1] Outside pressures from health care management progressively demand justification of outcomes and cost, which necessarily requires an "apples-to-apples" comparison of patients that only electronic systems can readily provide. If practitioners do not take the lead in defining quality outcomes and the relevance of preoperative predictors, then physician performance will be left to others with far less knowledge.[2,3]

The advent of relatively inexpensive information systems has made it possible to consistently and accurately assess medical details for large numbers of patients. With these new sources of information, preoperative evaluation can improve both individual patient management and entire processes of perioperative care. With the heightened emphasis on these new goals of preoperative data collection, focusing on issues relating to the evolution of preoperative data collection systems is essential.

SOURCES OF PREOPERATIVE INFORMATION

A wide range of sources may provide valuable patient information (Table 19-2). One vital source is the patient's verbal history and examination. Other sources may include hospital and clinic medical records. Important components of the medical record are prior inpatient evaluations, preoperative and intraoperative anesthetic records, and testing reports. Records of particular interest are those of the surgeon, primary care provider, and

Table 19-1. Goals of preoperative data collection

Succinctly describe past medical history
Accurately determine the current medical status
Meet legal documentation requirements
Support perioperative quality improvement efforts
Form foundation for outcome analysis
Support institutional information integration

other specialists. Critically important information may reside in records outside of the current institution, such as primary care provider notes and laboratory information. With the advent of contractual limitations in health systems, these access-related inconveniences are likely to increase.

Traditional systems providing data for the majority of preanesthetic care are largely paper based, except for laboratory and other testing information, which may be obtained through enterprise-wide data retrieval systems. When possible, these systems can take advantage of institutional data. Usually, ADT (admission/discharge/transfer) and laboratory information are available for electronic uploading (Fig. 19-1). Because this is an important resource for clinicians, access to hospital information resources should be a high priority in system design and development.[4] Paper-based medical records systems are extremely expensive to maintain and are fraught with inefficiencies arising from misplaced or incomplete records. Information systems of the future can overcome the limitations of paper-based systems by allowing simultaneous access by multiple caregivers. If data quality, security, and ownership issues are properly addressed, future preoperative electronic record (PER) systems conceivably will allow universal information access independent even of the system to which the patient "belongs."

SYSTEMS FOR RECORDING AND REPORTING PREOPERATIVE INFORMATION

The traditional system for recording and reporting data is handwritten documentation on paper. This documentation has consisted of either a handwritten annotation in the progress

Table 19-2. Sources of preoperative information

The patient
Previous anesthetic records
Inpatient hospitalization summaries*
Surgical notes regarding current problem
Recent internist/subspecialist notes*
Laboratory and other testing reports*

*Both internal and external.

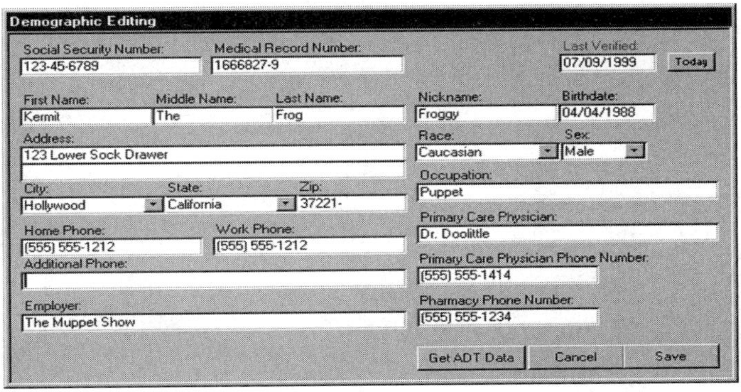

Fig. 19-1. Networked systems can access information in hospital database systems such as admission, discharge, and transfer (*ADT*) data. (Courtesy of Department of Anesthesiology, Vanderbilt University.)

notes of the medical record or a combination of handwritten notes and marked check boxes (listing medical conditions) on a preprinted form. Paper-based preoperative record systems offer several advantages: they are inexpensive, completely portable, require little training to use, and are relatively fast. Nevertheless, they are woefully inadequate to meet the current health care information requirements.

Compared with paper systems, the use of a PER system should meet the information needs that are evolving with the dramatic changes in health care management and delivery. Information systems are used to improve efficiency, increase flexibility, inform the care process, and actually implement changes in care. To improve efficiency, the PER must address problems of information availability, content, and format. Flexibility is required by health care restructuring, orientation to goals of managed care, and the need to serve physician, administrator, and patient.

By addressing these needs, the PER serves as the starting point of any information system designed to improve the perioperative process. The PER can improve the clarity of the preoperative information by using a standard vocabulary and reporting method. It can improve consistency and accuracy of the preoperative evaluation by providing a template for the evaluation and requiring the entry of specific items with specific terms. Error detection can be implemented by setting value limits for fields (e.g., vital signs) and incorporating spelling and grammar analysis tools.

Decision-support algorithms can suggest testing and consultation requirements by applying anesthesiologist-specific guidelines. Profiling testing practices can identify unnecessary costs and potentially reduce those costs.[5] The use of information systems in preoperative evaluation can track surgeon-ordered testing and compare it to internal algorithms or to requirements selected by the anesthesiologist (Fig. 19-2). This tool can demonstrate the magnitude of unindicated testing to focus cost-reduction efforts on specific tests or specific surgical departments (Fig. 19-3).

Process improvement can be achieved by reporting evaluation times, visit lengths, and cancellations. Credentialing support

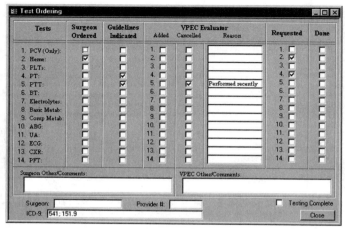

Fig. 19-2. The preoperative electronic record can be used to track testing practices and suggest areas for cost reduction. (Courtesy of Department of Anesthesiology, Vanderbilt University.)

can be achieved by examining user-specific evaluation times, evaluation correction, and consultation and testing rates. By reviewing individual anesthesiologists, evaluation critiques can be related to the practitioner to achieve maximal learning benefit (Fig. 19-4). Information availability can be universal and simultaneous, meeting the needs of multiple users.

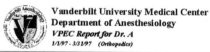

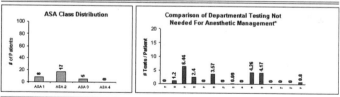

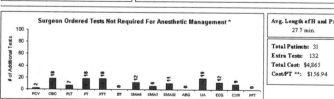

Fig. 19-3. Reports can be generated to supply feedback to surgical teams. *Tests not required for anesthetic management. **Patient charges. ASA, American Society of Anesthesiologists; Cost/PT, cost per patient; Xa–Xo, physician A through physician O. (Courtesy of Department of Anesthesiology, Vanderbilt University.)

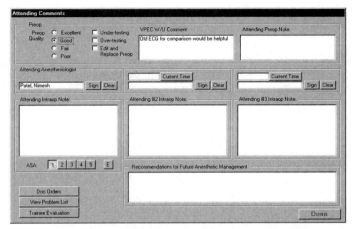

Fig. 19-4. Evaluation critiques can efficiently provide teaching to other members of the evaluation team. (Courtesy of Department of Anesthesiology, Vanderbilt University.)

Guideline Support, Outcomes Monitoring, and Quality Improvement

National emphasis is given to the development of clinical practice guidelines to ensure that patient care is provided in a consistent, cost-effective manner (see Chapter 18). Variability in outcomes has been demonstrated to result largely from the high variability in information delivery, combined with human cognitive and memory constraints.[6] The electronic medical record could provide a powerful tool to minimize the variability by collecting the required information and applying a programmed algorithm to suggest an appropriate care plan. For example, an algorithm for reduction of aspiration risk could identify a patient with risk factors (diabetes mellitus, neuropathy, pregnancy, hiatal hernia) and suggest the appropriate precaution (histamine blockers, motility agent, rapid-sequence induction technique) (Fig. 19-5). Unfortunately, a great deal of effort is required to input the data required to design and update guideline algorithms, as was shown in a case study analyzing a guideline for acute postoperative pain management.[7]

Analysis of aggregate data of perioperative outcomes (administrative, economic, clinical) and costs has become important.[3] Traditionally monitored outcomes have been broadened from morbidity and mortality statistics to include patient satisfaction and quality-of-life measures. Adjusting for risk factors, care complexity, and severity of illness is absolutely essential when interpreting or comparing outcomes. The American Society of Anesthesiologists Physical Status score is a commonly used severity-of-illness indicator that has demonstrated correlation with postoperative mortality,[8] but it has been shown to be a poor predictor of hospitalization costs.[9] To identify specific pre-

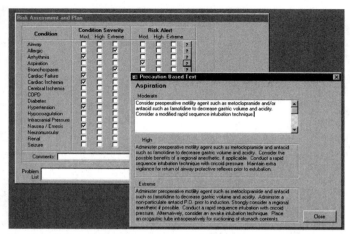

Fig. 19-5. Internal algorithms can assess patient severity of illness based on entered evaluation elements and suggest a possible course of action to reduce perioperative risk. (Courtesy of Department of Anesthesiology, Vanderbilt University.)

operative predictors that can be modified to affect specific postoperative outcomes, a significantly higher level of detail is required. The PER, based on codified medical language, can deliver the level of granularity required.

Clinical Research, Knowledge Discovery, and Decision Analysis

With the burgeoning of evidence-based medicine, much of quality improvement and knowledge discovery blend seamlessly into clinical research.[10] Although the PER generally contained observational data, the valid contributions of this data type have now been recognized.[11] At the very least, information from observational analysis can be used to generate hypotheses for subsequent clinical trials and provide reliable data for sample-size calculations. The PER can become a tool for data collection that simplifies this onerous aspect of investigation. Database applications can be designed or modified to add special dictionary or vocabulary tables and unique data indexing strategies for research support.[12]

That large preoperative databases can provide important information to support clinical decision making and knowledge discovery seems logical. Unfortunately, providing easy access to data and supplying simple tools to manage complex medical databases are difficult tasks. A precursor to developing such tools is an understanding of clinician knowledge-seeking behavior so that ideal retrieval methods can be designed. Combined with knowledge discovery tools, the PER may be able to identify new predictors of outcomes and suggest new care algorithms to reduce untoward events. Knowledge discovery tools support explorations of large, incomplete data sets such as medical databases that are difficult to approach using standard statistical methodologies. These tools have utility for the practitioner who wants to answer the questions, "What complications is my patient at risk of experiencing?" and "What strategies can reduce these risks in this patient, at my institution, at this time?"[13] By helping health care providers answer practical management questions, the PER, in conjunction with these techniques, promises to advance patient care and research.

Preoperative Electronic Record Design

If a demand for information exists that can be supplied only by a PER, why have computer-based record systems not been widely adopted? Significant problems exist with the data, which often reside on isolated systems, and the capture of data from clinicians in a coded and structured form has proven to be extremely difficult. Both problems must be solved before the PER can be implemented widely.

International standards for exchanging data between systems are necessary for efficient and accurate sharing of data. Health Level 7 (HL7)[14] is an international standards group formed to focus on the interface requirements of the health care system. The group has developed standards for exchanging medical record content such as patient registry, orders, and test results. HL7 message content is used by more than 2,000 hospitals and health system vendors in North America, Asia, and Europe. Nevertheless, the HL7 standard has yet to be fully adopted by many manufacturers because of the expensive retooling required, and it has not fully permeated the market.

The lack of code standards has been identified as the most important barrier to the development of electronic medical records systems, outcomes management, and quality assurance.[15] To achieve its full utility in providing for "apples-to-apples" comparisons among institutions, the data contained in the PER at each institution must be in the same codified form or in a form that can be linked to similar elements in other systems. This task has been extremely difficult to accomplish because of the relatively inefficient interfaces required to perform medical documentation. Use of coding schemes requires significant programming expertise and development cost. For these reasons, use of coding in the PER has largely been absent and remains to be developed.

In contrast to the easy coding of information such as laboratory values, the coding of physician-entered data is a complex task. Physicians usually record observations as free text. Some notes may be problem oriented, some structured, and others just free-floating text associated with figures and idiosyncratic abbreviations and acronyms. Coding requires menu selection, which takes longer than free text entry, because it does not conform to clinicians' thought processes. Rather, users must find the best code from the available choices, which may be limited. This limitation requires time for reorientation and degrades the precision of the system when the "best fit" remains imperfect. This effect on accuracy is difficult to quantify but requires further investigation.

If the ultimate solution to designing the PER is to combine codified text with free-form entry, then the data subset that is important for coding must be selected. This depends on the inter-

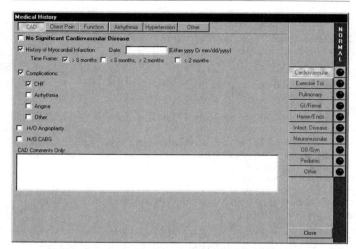

Fig. 19-6. To achieve efficient and accurate data entry, a combination of check boxes and free text entry is optimal. (Courtesy of Department of Anesthesiology, Vanderbilt University.)

ests and goals of the user. For the purposes of preoperative evaluation, this task can best be achieved by asking the questions, "What does our experience and the literature suggest are predictors of perioperative complications?" "What are important elements that determine the need for preoperative testing, additional evaluation, and treatment?" "What elements influence the selection of a specific plan of perioperative anesthetic care and postoperative management?"

For example, the literature suggests that surgery performed after a recent myocardial infarction is associated with a higher incidence of perioperative death.[16] This finding would suggest that codifying the occurrence of prior myocardial infarction should include the date or at least indicate if it occurred more than 3 to 6 months earlier. Other information related to the myocardial infarction could be collected in a free-text form. This method provides for the collection of information using check boxes as well as free text for information that would be difficult to code (Fig. 19-6).

Selecting essential elements is a difficult but important task. The tendency is to seek too many variables when only a fraction are important for decision making. The participation of consensus panels should be pursued when supportive data are lacking. Although selecting critical data elements can be time consuming, doing so not only produces an efficient data collection tool but often can also improve the care process.

Security Issues

The importance of trust and confidentiality in the preoperative interaction is critical. Significant economic, psychological, and social harm can occur when data security is violated, especially in the risk-based health care system in the United States. Maintenance of security is difficult because of the need for many individuals to access the information from many sites at the same time. The goals of information security are (a) to ensure patient privacy and confidentiality (prevent unauthorized disclosure of information), (b) to ensure the integrity of health care data (prevent unauthorized modification of data), and (c) to ensure the availability of data for authorized persons (prevent withholding of information).

Paper-based systems carry high risks of small violations (parts of individual records). Paper records abound in many unsecured and unsupervised areas such as patient rooms, nursing stations, medical records hubs, and even waste systems. Nevertheless, paper systems carry a low probability of large breeches, given the physical limitation of acquiring large numbers of records. This is dramatically different from electronic systems, which allow access to massive data sets of entire populations. Because of this risk, the relatively cavalier approach to security found in paper-based systems cannot be tolerated in the electronic environment.[17]

Security concerns raise issues of access control (user authentication and authorization), and data integrity concerns create the need for data authentication and error detection protocols. Data availability problems suggest the need for access control, data encryption, system reliability, and data backup methods. Because most environments using electronic systems also depend on a paper record, the security risks of both systems must be considered.

Although federal and state laws are inconsistent with regard to the protection of private electronic health data, the Medical Records Confidentiality Act of 1995 (SB 1360) proposes measures to ensure confidentiality. Debate still remains as to whether this measure might actually increase security risks by creating a national database and allowing the release of information without patient or physician consent. Institutional policies will be a major determinant of local security measures, although widespread implementation is highly sensitive to cost constraints.

Partial answers to security concerns include the use of passwords with expiration time limits, user authentication cards, or other identification systems. Techniques such as differential access rights according to user group (i.e., physician, nurse) offers a minor degree of control. Audit systems that trace all inquiries and transactions at first seem like a perfect solution, but detecting which of thousands of daily transactions actually constitutes a security violation is problematic.

Protecting data from interception is a security matter of great debate with the advent of the Internet.[18] Eliminating outside violations by eliminating Internet access would seem desirable. Unfortunately, remote access services are highly desired by users. In reality, most incursions occur within network systems, not from without. Thus, these precautions may unnecessarily limit user productivity while accomplishing little in terms of security.

The weakest link in data security systems is the human link. An essential element of any security policy is the application of penalties for violations. Equally important is appropriate education regarding the need for privacy and confidentiality. Explicit examples of what constitutes a violation and the methods to prevent and detect violations must be understood by all users. Because most violations are the result of seemingly innocent curiosity, simple measures can deter these activities, such as login screens that remind users of the confidential nature of the information and special reminders when information is requested about hospital employees, public figures, or celebrities.

Informed consent should be considered because patients normally must release their medical records for use by others. The availability of information in electronic systems and the detached manner by which it can be accessed often neglect this important issue of patient control. Disclosure of information requires that the patient (a) be told what information is to be disclosed, (b) understands what is being disclosed, (c) is competent to provide consent, and (d) consents willingly. Most research can be conducted using aggregates of data without patient identifiers.

The U.S. Food and Drug Administration has issued regulations that provide criteria for acceptance of electronic signatures and records as equivalent to signatures and records executed on paper.[19] These guidelines elaborate simple security measures that are essential for electronic signature modules and should be incorporated in cases in which this feature is applied.

System down time and software failures can result in significant loss of vital data for PER users, and the reliability of these systems is a security concern. Continuous transmission of data to a central server can eliminate the loss of data due to isolated system failure. Evolving technologies and system management procedures should address redundancy and backup issues to prevent potential violation of data integrity.

In summary, although a breach of security in a PER system risks access to data for a large population of patients, acceptable security can be provided if the proper policies and best available technologies are used. In fact, electronic security measures can be superior to those for paper record systems, which cannot offer security features such as providing an audit trail of who reviewed or edited what part of what record at what time.

Transition to a Preoperative Electronic Record

The decision as to whether to purchase an off-the-shelf system or design or develop a homegrown solution can be difficult. Although turnkey solutions are the result of extensive development by software experts, they may lack many of the essential features for health care. These products can be exceedingly expensive to purchase and often require extensive modification (if it is even possible) for a specific environment. Homegrown solutions can generally deliver a tailored product for a specific environment (which can continuously evolve) but may require significant programming expenses and prolonged development time. Whatever the ultimate solution, developing a plan for electronic documentation is an essential step that ensures that the final product addresses the needs of the documentation environment. A documentation plan can form the foundation for a request for proposal, which can be used to compare software companies (Table 19-3).

Several anesthesiology organizations have successfully developed and implemented components of perioperative information systems, although few have produced robust PER modules.[20–24] Most anesthesiology-based systems have focused on the collection of intraoperative data, emphasizing physiologic variables, drug

Table 19-3. Items to include in software request for proposal

Company information
  Mission statement
  Years in business
  Financial statements
  Organization structure and size
  Technical support provisions
General software information
  Years current program in use
  Clients with software in clinical use (describe)
  Detailed description of software features (flow oriented)
  Standard, optional, and custom features (costs)
  Patient privacy features
  Documentation and help systems
  Error minimization features
  Standard reports
  Clinical and administrative report customization
Technical software information
  Software-developing environment
  Source code ownership
  Licensing requirements (client-server)
  Communication standards
  Security features (authentication, encryption, audit)
  Data protection and backup features
  Routine maintenance requirements

use, and time flow. Most anesthesiology quality-tracking systems have included few preoperative predictors and rather have focused on the intraoperative correlates of postoperative outcomes.[21] The CAPE (Computer Assisted Patient Evaluation) system has been used to identify patients at high risk of postoperative respiratory complications.[22] This and other systems have linked some preoperative evaluation elements to postoperative outcomes but are limited because of a lack of a coding scheme and restricted linking to other data sources. Most data entry in these systems has been redundant to the charting process, which has significant time and cost implications.[23–25] Collection of important predictor and outcome data as part of the routine documentation process, storage in coded format, and linkage to other databases would be ideal.

As programming tools become more available and the need for data collection expands, additional attempts at local system development will be made. Such systems must be developed according to evolving guidelines for health care software to ensure their success.[26] To advance communication and compatibility, now is the time to develop a minimal anesthesiology data set consisting of a common core of data elements to be collected for every anesthetic encounter and common among all anesthetizing locations worldwide. Such a concept has been promoted in other professional groups with some success[27] and would provide extensive patient care and knowledge discovery benefits.

Preoperative Electronic Record Implementation

The task of translating physician thoughts into a codified data structure is the greatest challenge to the success of the PER system. When software requires large amounts of text entry, a keyboard may be optimal; when all data are entered by list or item selection, a pointing device may be optimal. The task of data entry can be time consuming and tedious.

One hopes that the evolution of data entry technology can minimize this problem. In addition to standard keyboard and mouse/trackball entry modalities, more user-friendly modes of data entry are available, including touch screen and pen-pad devices. Voice-recognition systems have greatly improved in speed and accuracy but are still difficult to use in active and noisy environments, and they remain processor dependent, with significant implications for hardware expenditures.

Scan-form technologies are relatively inexpensive and require limited hardware resources. Unfortunately, they involve redundant data entry, which decreases chances of completion and degrades quality of information as the number of items increases. Translation of text entries is limited if it exists at all. Still, these systems can provide access to aggregates of selected data and serve as a bridge to the PER system.

Processor systems range from computer workstations and notebook computers to handheld devices. With the advent of reliable radiofrequency spread spectrum (2.4 GHz) network systems, point-of-care data entry for the mobile care provider has become possible. Portable devices raise issues regarding device security and maintenance. Cost can vary widely; the general principle is that the newest, most attractive hardware is likely to be the most expensive and potentially least tested.

Unlike individual computers, networked systems can take advantage of instantaneous data storage and sharing among users and other information systems. This provides tremendous benefits in data security and access. Processing may be handled at the end-user site (local processing), the server (terminal emulation), or a combination of the two, which provides for a wide range of possible hardware solutions. Future anesthesiology information systems will likely be composed of an assortment of hardware configurations, data entry methods, and processing configurations.

Many preoperative centers gather medical information from patients in the form of a written questionnaire to help focus the interview and obtain an accurate medical history in less time. Early work demonstrated the ability of systems using data generated from computer questionnaires to detect findings missed by anesthesiologist interview.[28] Subsequent work with HealthQuiz has shown an inconsistent ability to reduce the interview time or add new information compared with written patient questionnares.[29,30]

The training of system users is often inappropriately underemphasized in the implementation of electronic systems. The most well-designed software can fail if the users are not familiar with it. Training can also be a valuable step in software development (alpha and beta testing). Significant user "buy-in" can be achieved before full system implementation with this approach, and it is helpful for groups developing systems or modifying turnkey solutions. Survey instruments are being developed for use in medical information science that may be useful in determining design and implementation issues (such as user skills, attitudes, and expectations).[31]

SUMMARY: "PAPER OR PLASTIC?"

Information access has become more critical in the current rapid-paced health care environment. The paper record can be in only one place at a time, whereas the electronic record is available at numerous sites simultaneously. The content of electronic medical records can be presented clearly and consistently, which may result in more effective communication of medical issues and reduce errors. Paper records cannot take advantage of real-time rule-based warnings and suggestions, which can reduce error rate and ensure the application of clinical practice guidelines that have become essential in a resource-limited environment. The costs of PER systems may actually be less than those of paper-based systems when the inefficiencies and delays of a paper system, along with the armies of personnel required to care for these mammoth documents, are taken into account. Provided that the necessary guidelines are followed, moving forward prudently to ensure the development of a completely functional, reliable, and secure PER system is essential.

REFERENCES

1. Grant JB, Hayes RP, Pates RD, et al. HCFA's health care quality improvement program: the medical informatics challenge. *J Am Med Inform Assoc* 1996;3:16–26.
2. Roizen MF. Preoperative evaluation: a shared vision for change. *J Clin Anesth* 1997;9:435–436.
3. Fisher DM, Macario A. Economics of anesthesia care: a call to arms! *Anesthesiology* 1997;86:1018–1019.
4. Gibby DL, Lemeer G, Jackson K. Use of data from a hospital online medical records system by physicians during preanesthetic evaluation. *J Clin Monit Comput* 1996;12:405–408.
5. Vogt AW, Henson LC. Unindicated preoperative testing: ASA physical status and financial implications. *J Clin Anesth* 1997;9:437–441.
6. Elson RB, Faughnan JG, Connelly DP. An industrial process view of information delivery to support clinical decision making: implications for systems design and process measures. *J Am Med Inform Assoc* 1997;4:266–278.
7. Miller PL, Frawley SJ. Trade-offs in producing patient-specific recommendations from a computer-based clinical guideline: a case study. *J Am Med Inform Assoc* 1995;4:238–242.
8. Vacanti CJ, Van Houten RJ, Hill RC. A statistical analysis of the relationship of physical status to postoperative mortality in 68,388 cases. *Anesth Analg* 1970;49:564–566.
9. Macario A, Vitez TS, Dunn B, et al. Hospital costs and severity of illness in three types of elective surgery. *Anesthesiology* 1997;86:92–100.
10. Haynes RB, Hayward RA, Lomas J. Bridges between health care research evidence and clinical practice. *J Am Med Inform Assoc* 1995;6:342–350.
11. Duncan PG. That was then, this is now! The value of observing change. *Anesth Analg* 1998;86:225–227.
12. Nadkarni PM, Brandt C, Frawley S, et al. Managing attribute-value clinical trials data using the ACT/DB client-server database system. *J Am Med Inform Assoc* 1998;5:139–151.

13. Tsai YS, King PH, Higgins MS, et al. An expert-guided decision tree construction strategy: an application in knowledge discovery with medical databases. Paper presented at American Medical Information Association Fall Symposium, Nashville, TN, October 1997.

14. *Health Level Seven. An application protocol for electronic data exchange in healthcare environments, with special emphasis on inpatient acute care facilities.* Version 2.3 (1996). Health Level Seven, Inc., 900 Victors Way, Suite 122, Ann Arbor, MI 48108.

15. McDonald CJ. The barriers to electronic medical record systems and how to overcome them. *J Am Med Inform Assoc* 1997;4:213–221.

16. Steen PA, Tinker JH, Tarhan S. Myocardial reinfarction after anesthesia and surgery. *JAMA* 1978;239:2566–2570.

17. Cushman R. Serious technology assessment for health care information technology. *J Am Med Inform Assoc* 1997;4:259–265.

18. Siwicki B. Applying the Internet in health care. *Health Data Manag* 1998;6:38–48.

19. *Electronic signatures.* 21 CFR part 11. Rockville, MD: Food and Drug Administration, Department of Health and Human Services.

20. Weiss YG, Cotev S, Drenger V. Patient data management systems in anaesthesia: an emerging technology. *Can J Anaesth* 1995;42:914–921.

21. Edsall DW. Quality assessment with a computerized anesthesia information management system (AIMS). *QRB Qual Rev Bull* 1991;17:182–193.

22. Chase CR, Merz BA, Mazuzan JE. Computer assisted patient evaluation (CAPE): a multi-purpose computer system for an anesthesia service. *Anesth Analg* 1983;62:198–206.

23. Strauss PL, Turndorf H. A computerized anesthesia database. *Anesth Analg* 1989;68:340–343.

24. Bashein G, Barna CR. A comprehensive computer system for anesthetic record retrieval. *Anesth Analg* 1985;64:425–431.

25. Rose DK, Cohen MM, Wigglesworth DF, Yee DA. Development of a computerized database for the study of anesthesia care. *Can J Anaesth* 1992;39:716–723.

26. Miller RA, Gardner RM. Recommendations for responsible monitoring and regulation of clinical software systems. *J Am Med Inform Assoc* 1997;4:442–457.

27. Goossen WT, Epping PJ, Feuth T, et al. A comparison of nursing minimal data sets. *J Am Med Inform Assoc* 1998;5:152–163.

28. Tompkins BM, Tompkins WJ, Loder E, Noonan AF. A computer-assisted preanesthesia interview: value of a computer-generated summary of patient's historical information in the preanesthesia visit. *Anesth Analg* 1980;59:3–10.

29. Lutner RE, Roizen MF, Stocking CV, et al. The automated interview versus the personal interview: do patient responses to preoperative health questions differ? *Anesthesiology* 1991;75:394–400.

30. Beers RA, O'Leary CE, Franklin PD. Comparing the history-taking methods used during a preanesthesia visit: the HealthQuiz versus the written questionnaire. *Anesth Analg* 1998;86:134–137.

31. Cork RD, Detmer WM, Friedman CP. Development and initial validation of an instrument to measure physicians' use of, knowledge about, and attitudes toward computers. *J Am Med Inform Assoc* 1998;5:164–176.

Case Studies in Preoperative Evaluation

Francisco DeLaCruz and BobbieJean Sweitzer

Preoperative assessment frequently involves the evaluation of surgical patients with multiple, complex disease processes. Limited by time constraints, the perioperative physician is presented with a challenging and often difficult task. All patients, particularly those with comorbid conditions, warrant careful and thoughtful preoperative evaluations. A routine assessment and particular attention to specific aspects of an individual's illnesses are necessary. Obtaining a focused history, performing a physical examination, ordering and analyzing laboratory tests, assessing operative risk, and planning for the perioperative period are important.

In this chapter, several cases in preoperative assessment are presented and discussed. In these cases, the patients present to the perioperative physician with multiple medical problems. The integrative process of preoperative preparation is investigated as an exercise in medical management of the surgical patient.

CASE 1

A 54-year-old woman with type 2 diabetes mellitus (DM) presents to the preoperative clinic for evaluation 3 days before a right total knee replacement. She has rheumatoid arthritis (RA) and began taking steroids in the last year. She had one previous general anesthetic and was told by her anesthesiologist that it was "difficult to put a breathing tube in."

Medical History

A complete history should be obtained, with the focus on her significant problems, including DM, RA, steroid use, and possible difficult airway management.

Diabetes Mellitus (see Chapter 6)

To evaluate the impact of the patient's DM, the history should focus on the duration of disease, therapy, adequacy of blood glucose control, and associated complications.

The patient was diagnosed with DM 12 years ago. She is taking 40 mg of glipizide per day and has difficulty following her recommended diet. She walks 1 mile daily. By history, her blood glucose level has been difficult to control, and chart review, with documentation of elevated hemoglobin A_{1C} levels, confirms this.

This patient's long history of DM increases the risk of complications such as cerebrovascular and coronary artery disease, peripheral vascular disease, nephropathy, and autonomic and peripheral neuropathy. Control of her disease may delay the onset of end organ dysfunction.[1]

Further history should attempt to elicit information indicating dysfunction of her cardiovascular, autonomic, renal, neurologic, and ophthalmologic systems.

She has no history of myocardial infarction and denies angina or dyspnea, even with her daily walks. She complains of dizziness on standing and has frequent heartburn associated with a bitter taste in her mouth, especially while recumbent. She complains of numbness in her fingers and toes that developed over the last 3 years. Chart review reveals a history of bilateral laser retinal photocoagulation and a baseline creatinine level of 2.7 mg per dL (Table 20-1).

Although "silent" ischemia can occur with DM and should be considered,[2] the patient has good exercise tolerance and no symp-

Table 20-1. Normal values for common diagnostic test results

Variable	Value
Sodium (mmol/L)	135–145
Potassium (mmol/L)	3.3–4.9
Chloride (mmol/L)	97–110
Carbon dioxide (mmol/L)	22–31
Blood urea nitrogen (mg/dL)	8–25
Creatinine (mg/dL)	0.5–1.7
Hemoglobin A_{1C} (%)	4.4–6.3
Phosphate (mg/dL)	2.5–4.5
Magnesium (mEq/L)	1.3–2.2
Protein (g/dL)	6.2–8.2
Albumin (g/dL)	3.6–5.0
Bilirubin (mg/dL)	0.2–1.3
Alanine/SGPT (IU/L)	7–53
Aspartate/SGOT (IU/L)	11–47
Amylase (IU/L)	35–118
GGT (IU/L)	20–76 (males)
	12–54 (females)
Lactate dehydrogenase (IU/L)	90–280
Serum ethanol (mg/dL)	0
White blood cell count (mm^3)	3,800–9,800
Hematocrit (%)	40–50 (males)
	36–44 (females)
Platelet count (mm^3)	140,000–440,000
Prothrombin time (sec)	10.7–13.0
Partial thromboplastin time (sec)	25–33
Calcium (mg/dL)	8.9–10.3
Serum myoglobin (ng/mL)	0–85
Urine myoglobin (+ or –)	Negative

GGT, γ-glutamyltransferase; hemoglobin A_{1C}, glycated hemoglobin; SGOT, serum glutamic oxalacetic transaminase; SGPT, serum glutamic pyruvic transaminase.

toms of cardiac disease. She has symptoms of reflux and possibly postural hypotension, which suggest autonomic dysfunction.[3] The patient has evidence of peripheral neuropathy, retinopathy, and moderate nephropathy.

Rheumatoid Arthritis (see Chapter 10)

So that the severity of the patient's RA can be assessed, information should be obtained on the duration of the disease, extent of joint involvement, and therapy.

The patient has stiffness and pain in her neck, hands, and knees, especially in the morning. She has pain with swallowing and mouth opening, which limits her jaw movement. She denies any neurologic symptoms with neck movement.

The patient had taken large doses of ibuprofen, but since starting prednisone she lowered the dosage of ibuprofen to 200 mg three times per day. She has never taken cytotoxic drugs. She is taking ranitidine hydrochloride for ulcer prophylaxis and for her heartburn.

Despite her medications, she has significant temporomandibular joint, cricoarytenoid, and atlanto-occipital symptoms, as suggested by painful mouth opening, odynophagia, and neck pain, respectively. This raises concerns about potential airway difficulties.

The degree of cardiac and pulmonary involvement of RA should be sought.

The patient denies dyspnea, chest pain, fatigue, orthopnea, or peripheral edema, even during her walks.

The lack of dyspnea or exercise intolerance argues against RA-associated pericarditis or pulmonary fibrosis.

Steroid Use (see Chapter 15)

Does this patient need perioperative steroid administration because of hypothalamic-pituitary-adrenal axis suppression?[4] The steroid dose as well as the duration and extent of the surgery are important in determining the need for perioperative steroids.

Her dosage of prednisone has been 10 mg per day for the last 3 months. Before that, it was 5 mg per day for 4 months.

Given the patient's high dose (more than 5 mg of prednisone per day) and long duration of treatment (longer than 1 week), she should be given perioperative steroids.[4]

Difficult Airway (see Chapter 14)

Review of the patient's previous anesthetic record is important.

Chart review shows that with her previous anesthesia she had poor neck extension and mouth opening, which led to a grade III laryngoscopic view with a MacIntosh 3 blade.[5] This improved to a grade II view with cricoid pressure. Three intubation attempts were made; intubation was finally successful with a 6.5 styletted tube.

One must consider that, in the 3 years since her last laryngoscopy, her RA may have progressed, and she may have an even more difficult airway.

Physical Examination

The examination should focus on the patient's neurologic, cardiovascular, musculoskeletal, and endocrinologic systems through examination of the central and peripheral nervous systems, heart, joints, and body habitus. The examination of the airway, particularly with the patient's history of difficult airway, should be thorough.

The patient is 5 ft 5 in. and 186 lb. Her temperature is 36.6°C, pulse is 73 beats per minute (bpm) while sitting and 94 bpm while standing, and respiration rate is 16 breaths per minute. The blood pressure is 125/82 mm Hg while sitting and 104/71 mm Hg while standing.

Several retinal hemorrhages and old laser scars are seen with funduscopy. She has a Mallampati class III airway, thyromental distance of 6 cm, and no macroglossia.[6] The patient has significant limitation of neck flexion and extension but denies pain with neck movements. Her mouth opens 2 cm and she has no loose teeth, prosthetic devices, hoarseness, or stridor. Her face is rounded.

Her lung examination is normal with good expansion and excursion, and bilateral clarity of breath sounds. She has tenderness at the costochondral junctions.

The cardiovascular examination is notable for normal, regular heart sounds without murmurs or heart rate variability with inspiration and expiration. She has strong pulses in all extremities. She has no peripheral bruits or edema.

Her abdomen is obese with reddish striae. Her upper back has a slight prominence consistent with a "buffalo hump."

She has mild ulnar deviation of all fingers. She has good strength in all muscle groups but decreased sensitivity to pinprick and vibration diffusely in her fingertips. The right hand numbness worsens slightly with neck extension.

Several manifestations of DM are confirmed. She has orthostatic hypotension and absence of heart rate variability, consistent with autonomic neuropathy.[3] She has evidence of peripheral neuropathy. The decreased mobility seen in the atlanto-occipital joint may occur with DM.[7] She has no signs of cardiac or peripheral vascular disease.

Evidence of RA is present, including hand deformities, painful costochondral joints, and limitation of the temporomandibular and cervical joints. Heart valve fibrosis and aortitis may occur in RA,[8] but the absence of murmurs argues against both.

The patient has signs of Cushing's syndrome from chronic steroid use, including a posterior neck fat pad, truncal obesity, abdominal striae, and rounded face. However, she lacks hypertension and proximal muscle weakness.

A potentially difficult airway is suggested by poor neck mobility, a possibly unstable cervical spine, and limited mouth opening. The lack of hoarseness or stridor suggests a normal cricoarytenoid joint.

Diagnostic Testing (see Chapter 2)

Because of her DM, an electrocardiogram (ECG) and measurement of electrolytes, glucose, blood urea nitrogen (BUN), creatinine, and hemoglobin A_{1C} are warranted. Her history of RA calls for a chest radiograph (CXR), cervical neck films, ECG, and hematocrit. Steroid use warrants measurement of electrolyte and glucose levels. Investigating the degree of hypothalamic-pituitary-adrenal axis suppression is probably not beneficial.

A CXR is normal. Lateral neck films with flexion reveal a 3.2-mm anterior separation of the odontoid from the atlas arch. The ECG is notable for nonspecific ST and T wave changes.

The sodium, potassium, chloride, and carbon dioxide levels are normal. The glucose level is 284 mg per dL, BUN level is 30 mg per dL, and creatinine level is 1.3 mg per dL. The level of hemoglobin A_{1C} is 8.5%. The hematocrit is 34%, white blood cell count is 9,900 per mm^3, and platelet count is 150,000 per mm^3.

An adrenocorticotropic hormone stimulation test, which can assess adrenal function, was not performed because the decision to give perioperative steroids is based on the dosage and duration of her steroid treatment[4] (see Chapter 15).

These tests confirm poor diabetic control and moderate renal dysfunction. Nonspecific ST changes on the ECG are not strongly suggestive of significant coronary artery disease. The neck film, with more than 3 mm of odontoid-atlas separation, shows atlanto-occipital instability.

Assessment

This 54-year-old woman, categorized as American Society of Anesthesiologists Physical Status (ASA-PS) class 3, has type II DM, poorly controlled with an oral hypoglycemic agent.[9] Autonomic neuropathy with neurogenic gastroparesis and reflux, peripheral neuropathy, moderate nephropathy, and retinopathy are present. She has RA with diffuse joint pain, atlanto-occipital instability, limited neck and temporomandibular joint motion, and probably carpal tunnel syndrome. She has neurologic symptoms with neck extension. She has a history of being a difficult intubation. She has been taking a moderate dose of steroids for several months.

Management

The patient should discontinue her oral hypoglycemic the evening before surgery because the long half-life puts her at risk for perioperative hypoglycemia while fasting. Its absence, however, may lead to hyperglycemia. Therefore, scheduling her case as the first of the day and controlling her perioperative blood glucose with administration of regular insulin would be ideal.

Perioperative glucocorticoid administration should be based on the patient's preoperative glucocorticoid dosage and duration and the anticipated surgical stress. In addition to her regular prednisone dose, she should receive a supplementary dose of hydrocortisone equivalent of 50 to 75 mg per day (50 mg given intraoperatively) for 1 to 2 days, because she is about to undergo a moderate surgical stress[4] (see Chapter 15).

The patient is a candidate for regional or general anesthesia. Use of a regional technique may prevent the need for airway manipulation. Awake fiberoptic intubation should be discussed with the patient if general anesthesia is preferred.

Given the patient's significant reflux symptoms, preoperative administration of metoclopramide to promote gastric emptying and oral sodium citrate to raise gastric pH with continuation of her ranitidine hydrochloride are indicated. Because of her reflux symptoms, history of difficult intubation, evidence of cervical spine subluxation, limited mouth opening, and neck movement, a rapid-sequence induction of general anesthesia is contraindicated (see Chapter 14).

CASE 2

A 57-year-old man, accompanied by his wife, presents for evaluation before an inguinal hernia repair. He has a long history of alcoholism complicated by cirrhosis. A new right carotid bruit was noted recently.

Medical History

Alcoholism (see Chapter 12)

Before surgery, an assessment of the severity, duration, treatment, and systemic manifestations of alcoholism is important.

The patient has drunk heavily for the past 15 years. He underwent a 12-step treatment program 2 years ago, abstaining for 2 months. He had several episodes of severe diarrhea, memory loss, and "the shakes" during that time. He did not take disulfiram. Thereafter, he continued drinking a fifth of hard alcohol per day. His last drink, 3 oz of whiskey, was 4 hours earlier.

The long history of alcoholism increases the risk of perioperative withdrawal and delirium tremens as well as systemic complications such as nutritional deficiency, gastritis, esophagitis, cirrhosis, and coagulation disorders.[8] The symptoms he experienced while abstaining suggest physical dependence.

The patient's alcohol tolerance suggests the presence of cross-tolerance to some anesthetic agents such as benzodiazepines, hypnotics, inhalational agents, and opioids. Eliciting a history of disulfiram use is important, because it is a dopamine β-hydroxylase inhibitor that may lead to hypotension under general anesthesia due to inadequate norepinephrine stores.[10]

His recent alcohol intake is significant. If emergency surgery were required, the alcohol would lower anesthetic requirements. Withdrawal symptoms of nausea, vomiting, tremors, autonomic overactivity, and confusion can be anticipated 6 to 8 hours after his last drink.[8] Delirium tremens, manifested as hypotension or hypertension, tachycardia, hyperthermia, seizures, or hallucinations, begins 48 to 72 hours later.

The cardiac, gastrointestinal, pulmonary, and central nervous systems may be adversely affected by alcoholism and should be assessed.

The patient denies chest pain, dyspnea, or palpitations, even with exertion. He denies abdominal pain. The patient and his wife deny memory, walking, or balance difficulties.

The patient has no symptoms of cardiomyopathy or dysrhythmias. The absence of abdominal complaints argues against gastritis, pancreatitis, or hepatitis. He lacks the gait disturbances of

Wernicke's encephalopathy and the memory loss of Korsakoff's psychosis.

Cirrhosis (see Chapter 9)

The diagnosis, cause, and treatment of the patient's cirrhosis should be verified.

The patient's cirrhosis was diagnosed by a liver biopsy 1 year ago after he presented with weight loss, anorexia, fever, and nausea. His wife oversees his medical regimen of lactulose, vitamin supplements, and spironolactone.

Alcoholic hepatitis is the most likely cause of his cirrhosis, although other causes, including viral hepatitis and primary biliary cirrhosis, should be considered.

The patient continues to drink, and his cirrhosis may have progressed. However, the use of lactulose, vitamin K, and spironolactone may reduce the incidence of encephalopathy, coagulopathy, and ascites, respectively.

To assess the severity of the cirrhosis, the history should focus on the neurologic, hematologic, gastrointestinal, immunologic, and nutritional systems.

The patient's wife says that he often becomes confused and agitated for no apparent reason. He bruises easily and bleeds for prolonged periods after small cuts. An endoscopy 3 months earlier showed "big veins" in his esophagus. His abdominal girth has decreased with the use of spironolactone but is still large. He has had two episodes of pneumonia in the last year but no other serious infections. His appetite, poor for years, has worsened, and his wife states that he has lost 40 lb in 3 months.

The patient's mental status changes and bleeding problems suggest encephalopathy and coagulopathy. The endoscopy confirmed esophageal varices secondary to portal hypertension. His history is consistent with ascites, immunologic compromise with recent pneumonia, and poor nutritional status.

Carotid Bruit (see Chapter 4)

Whether the incidental carotid bruit is associated with symptoms should be determined.

The patient recalls several episodes of left-arm "tingling" and weakness. He has had four of these events in the last month, each lasting seconds to minutes. He denies visual, language, or coordination problems.

Temporary focal neurologic symptoms that last less than 24 hours are consistent with transient ischemic attacks. His transient ischemic attacks occur in an area supplied by the right carotid artery, and their presence increases the probability that the stenosis is high grade.[11] Carotid endarterectomies decrease mortality and stroke in patients with symptomatic, high-grade (70% to 99%) stenosis,[12] so further studies are indicated (see Diagnostic Studies, below).

Carotid artery disease is associated with cardiac and peripheral vascular disease, so their presence should be sought.

The patient denies chest pain, dyspnea, or palpitations, even with moderate exercise. He denies claudication and excessive coolness of his extremities.

Physical Examination

The physical examination should assess the complications and severity of this patient's alcoholism, cirrhosis, and cerebrovascular disease.

The patient is cachetic and his breath smells of alcohol. He is 5 ft 11 in. and weighs 137 lb. His temperature is 36.9°C, pulse is 82 bpm, and respiratory rate is 32 breaths per minute. The blood pressure is 131/76 mm Hg and equal in both arms.

The patient's sclera and skin are not jaundiced, but several spider angiomas are present.

Lateral and rotational head movements produce no neurologic symptoms.

The lung examination is normal, with good expansion, excursion, and bilateral clarity.

The cardiovascular examination is notable for normal, regular heart sounds without murmurs, a point of maximal impulse that is not diffuse or lateralized, and strong pulses in all extremities. The patient has a right carotid bruit.

The patient's abdomen is nontender and distended, and a fluid wave is present. He has hepatomegaly and an easily palpable spleen.

The extremities show multiple small bruises and diffuse edema.

Neurologic examination is notable for normal mental status, short-term and long-term memory, and cranial nerves. The patient has generalized weakness of all motor groups but no focal findings or gait abnormalities. He has normal sensation to pinprick, light touch, and proprioception in all extremities. He is hyperreflexive bilaterally with down-going plantar reflexes. He has asterixis.

Evidence exists that the patient is malnourished. The spider angiomas, splenomegaly, and ascites are suggestive of portal hypertension with collateral flow. The normal heart examination argues against alcoholic cardiomyopathy. The patient's normal mental status suggests that acute intoxication, withdrawal, and hepatic encephalopathy are absent. However, the asterixis and increased reflexes are indicative of hepatic encephalopathy.

Bruising, icterus, and edema suggest poor hepatic function.

Aside from the bruit, little evidence exists for diffuse cerebrovascular or peripheral vascular disease.

Diagnostic Testing

The patient's alcoholism warrants measurement of blood alcohol level, ECG, CXR, and complete blood cell count. Measurement of serum glutamic oxalacetic transaminase (SGOT), serum glutamic pyruvic transaminase (SGPT), γ-glutamyltransferase (GGT), and lactate dehydrogenase (LDH) levels; tests of synthetic liver function [albumin level, prothrombin time (PT), partial thromboplastin time (PTT)]; measurement of electrolyte, BUN, creatinine, and magnesium levels; and a CBC are indicated because of his cirrhosis. The presence of a symptomatic carotid bruit warrants Doppler ultrasonographic imaging.

A CXR is normal. Doppler ultrasonography of the carotid arteries shows 30% occlusion of the left and 85% occlusion of the right bifurcation.

The ECG is normal.

The levels of sodium, potassium, chloride, carbon dioxide, BUN, creatinine, and serum glucose are normal. The magnesium level is 1.1 mEq per L. The protein level is 4.6 g per dL, the albumin level is 2.1 g per dL, and the bilirubin level is 2.3 mg per dL. The level of SGPT is 102 IU per L, the SGOT level is 94 IU per L, the amylase level is 73 IU per L, the GGT level is 123 IU per L, and the LDH level is 352 IU per L. The level of serum ethanol is 76 mg per dL. The hematocrit is 37%, the white blood cell count is 10,300 per mm³, and the platelet count is 78,000 per mm³. The PT is 16.1 seconds and the PTT is 54 seconds.

The serum ethanol level confirms recent alcohol intake. The patient has evidence of poor nutrition (low total protein and albumin levels), evidence of compromised hepatic synthetic function (elevated PT and PTT and low albumin level), and hepatocellular damage. With the exception of mild hypomagnesemia, the electrolyte profile is unaffected by his cirrhosis and alcoholism. No evidence is seen of alcohol-induced cardiomyopathy or conduction abnormalities from the CXR and ECG. A moderate anemia with thrombocytopenia is present.

The carotid Doppler ultrasonography indicates a high-grade right carotid lesion.

Assessment

This 57-year-old man categorized as ASA-PS class 3 has cirrhosis secondary to alcoholism, carotid artery disease, and malnutrition. Portal hypertension, ascites, splenomegaly, esophageal varices, hepatocellular damage with synthetic dysfunction, coagulopathy, hypomagnesemia, hypoalbuminemia, and thrombocytopenia complicate his cirrhosis. Because of cirrhosis, elevated PT and bilirubin levels, reduced albumin level, moderate ascites, and poor nutrition,[13] he is classified as a Child's grade C (Pugh modification) (see Chapter 9), and his surgical risk is high.[14]

Management

Because of his high-grade, symptomatic carotid lesion, he should undergo carotid endarterectomy before his inguinal hernia repair.[12]

The pharmacodynamics and pharmacokinetics of many drugs may be changed because of his poor hepatic function, altered volume of distribution, lowered protein binding, and possible encephalopathy. A nasogastric tube may cause variceal bleeding and should be avoided. The patient may benefit from nutritional support[15] through increase in and monitoring of his preoperative caloric intake (see Chapter 16). Vitamins K and B$_{12}$ and thiamine should be given before surgery.

Potential anesthetic techniques for this procedure include regional, general, or monitored anesthesia care. A central neuraxial block (spinal, epidural) is contraindicated given the patient's compromised coagulation and thrombocytopenia. However, administration of vitamin K and a transfusion of 12 to 20 mL per kg of fresh frozen plasma and three units of concentrated platelets may normalize the PT and increase his platelet count to more than 100,000 per cubic millimeter. If general anesthesia is performed, avoidance of hypotension with induction and mechanical ventilation is important because hepatic blood flow in cirrhosis is highly dependent on hepatic artery pressure. Monitored anesthesia care with local anesthesia may be preferable.

CASE 3

A 7-year-old boy with asthma presents to the preoperative clinic 5 days before a scheduled herniorrhaphy. He has a "cold," and it has worsened his asthma. However, his upper respiratory symptoms and asthma are improving.

The patient had a cousin who died under anesthesia from "overheating."

Medical History

The important medical issues for this patient are asthma, a recent upper respiratory tract infection (URI), and a possible family history of malignant hyperthermia.

Asthma (see Chapter 5)

Information regarding onset, medications, hospitalizations, complications, and exacerbating factors[16] is important in assessing the severity of the patient's asthma.

The patient's asthma was diagnosed at age 3 years, and he is taking inhaled albuterol, cromolyn sodium, and beclomethasone dipropionate. He has been to the emergency department several times for exacerbations and is hospitalized one or two times per year. Fourteen months ago, he was intubated for 1 day and placed on a steroid taper for 1 month. Cold weather, cats, dogs, exercise, pollen, and URIs aggravate his symptoms.

Frequent exacerbations, a history of intubation, and use of steroids indicate severe asthma.

The current status of the patient's asthma should be assessed. A history of recent exposure to exacerbating factors and a subjective assessment by the patient and his parent about his current status are important.

The patient had no dyspnea or wheezing until 2 weeks ago, when he "caught a cold." His illness began with sneezing and rhinorrhea and progressed to a dry cough and wheezing. His mother almost brought him to the emergency department 8 days ago, but he improved with more frequent doses of albuterol. He still has a slight cough and wheezing, but the nasal discharge has been clear and he has been afebrile.

URI (see next section) is implicated as the exacerbating factor. Despite improvement, the patient still has acute asthma symptoms.

Upper Respiratory Tract Infection (see Chapter 13)

Unlike allergic rhinitis, a recent URI is more likely to cause intraoperative[17] and postoperative[18] complications in the pediatric patient. Therefore, determining the severity, time course, and characteristics that distinguish the URI (e.g., purulent nasal discharge, fever, cough) from allergic rhinitis is important. In addition, signs and symptoms indicative of a URI (sore throat, sneezing, rhinorrhea, congestion, nonproductive cough, temperature higher than 101°F, laryngitis, malaise)[19] should be sought.

In addition to his other symptoms, the patient had a sore throat, congestion, and malaise. He has not had purulent nasal discharge, laryngitis, fevers, or limitation of activity. He has had allergic rhinitis before, but unlike his current illness, it occurs in summer and lasts only hours.

The patient exhibits several of the criteria for a mild URI. Despite the mildness of the symptoms, which are resolving, his URI is still of concern because it is recent and, most important, is associated with coexisting asthma.

Malignant Hyperthermia (see Chapter 14)

Further history regarding the cousin's anesthetic course, mode of inheritance, possible existence of a malignant hyperthermia–associated condition, and previous anesthetics given to this patient may determine if he is at increased risk for malignant hyperthermia.

A history of specific diseases associated with malignant hyperthermia, including osteogenesis imperfecta, muscular dystrophies, and myotonia, should be sought.

The patient's cousin died at age 5 years. Under anesthesia, he had jaw rigidity, tachycardia, hypercarbia, acidosis, and eventually hyperthermia and arrhythmias that resulted in death. No autopsy was performed. The cousin was the son of the patient's maternal uncle, who had had one general anesthetic without problems. The patient's maternal grandfather, however, died while under anesthesia. The patient's mother denies any "muscle disorders" in the family. At age 4, the patient had no problems during a general anesthesia with halothane but did not receive muscle relaxants. The patient's parents have not had a general anesthetic.

Although malignant hyperthermia is likely in the case of the patient's cousin, one must also consider the differential diagnosis of neuroleptic malignant syndrome in the setting of phenothiazine administration, thyroid storm, sepsis, and pheochromocytoma. A posthumous muscle biopsy with a caffeine-halothane contracture test would have been diagnostic[20] (see Chapter 14).

The inheritance of susceptibility to malignant hyperthermia is probably autosomal dominant with variable penetrance,[21] and this family's pattern is consistent. Neither the patient nor his maternal uncle had reactions under general anesthesia, but this does not rule out susceptibility to malignant hyperthermia in either of them.

Physical Examination

The physical examination should look for signs of acute asthma, URI, and features associated with malignant hyperthermia susceptibility.

The patient's temperature is 37.2°C, pulse is 110 bpm, and respiratory rate is 25 breaths per minute. The blood pressure is 105/55 mm Hg.

The patient is breathing with slight difficulty and at a rapid rate. He is using accessory muscles but is speaking in full sentences. He is congested, has clear nasal discharge, and has a slight cough. His lungs have diffuse, late expiratory wheezes. He has no pulsus paradoxus or cyanosis. No chest wall, back, or extremity deformities, or muscle wasting is seen.

Tachypnea, accessory muscle recruitment, cough, and wheezing are signs of an acute asthma exacerbation. The rhinorrhea and cough are evidence of a URI. The patient lacks several features associated with myopathies linked to malignant hyperthermia,[8] including pectus carinatum, muscle wasting or hypertrophy, kyphosis, or lordosis.

Diagnostic Testing

Indicated tests include a CXR, measurement of peak airway flows (simple spirometry), and creatine phosphokinase level. A muscle biopsy for a caffeine-halothane contracture test is not indicated because avoidance of malignant hyperthermia triggering agents is simple and preferable, regardless of the results of this costly, inconvenient, and potentially inaccurate test. For a patient with known susceptibility to malignant hyperthermia, baseline calcium, potassium, and myoglobin levels are indicated.

A CXR is clear with mild hyperinflation. The patient's current peak flow is 225 L per minute, although his maximum is 300 L per minute. The creatine phosphokinase level is 574 IU per L. The levels of potassium, calcium, and serum and urine myoglobins are normal.

The CXR and decreased peak flows are consistent with an asthma exacerbation. An elevated creatine phosphokinase level is 70% to 80% predictive for malignant hyperthermia if a patient has known susceptibility to malignant hyperthermia,[21] so a presumptive diagnosis is made.

Assessment

This 7-year-old boy categorized as ASA-PS class 3 has moderate asthma as assessed according to the Global Initiative for Asthma (GINA) scale[22] (Table 20-2) with a current exacerbation, resolving URI, and a high likelihood of susceptibility to malignant hyperthermia.

Management

This patient's pulmonary status should be optimized before surgery. His procedure should probably be postponed until 2 weeks or more after the resolution of his symptoms,[23] although this practice has not been examined. He should continue his current medications, and an inhaled β-agonist should be given just before surgery. "Stress-dose" steroids are not required prophaylactically[4] (see Chapter 15). Agents that can trigger malignant hyperthermia should be avoided, but prophylaxis with dantrolene sodium is controversial[24] (see Chapter 14). Consent for muscle biopsy under anesthesia should be discussed with the family.

Table 20-2. Global Initiative for Asthma classification of asthma severity*

Intermittent
  Intermittent symptoms <1 time per wk
  Brief exacerbations (hours to a few days)
  Nighttime asthma symptoms <2 times per mo
  Asymptomatic and normal lung function between exacerbations
  PEF or FEV_1 >80% of predicted; variability <20%
Mild persistent
  Symptoms >1 time per week but <1 time per day
  Exacerbations possibly affecting activity and sleep
  Nighttime asthma symptoms >2 times per mo
  PEF or FEV_1 >80% of predicted; variability 20–30%
Moderate persistent
  Symptoms daily
  Exacerbations affecting activity and sleep
  Nighttime asthma symptoms >1 time per wk
  Daily use of inhaled short acting β_2-agonist
  PEF or FEV_1 >60% to <80% of predicted; variability >30%
Severe persistent
  Continuous symptoms
  Frequent exacerbations
  Frequent nighttime asthma symptoms
  Limitation of physical activities by asthma symptoms
  PEF or FEV_1 <60% of predicted; variability >30%

FEV_1, forced expiratory volume in 1 second; PEF, peak expiratory flow.
*Meeting only one criterion for a given grade qualifies a patient.

CASE 4

A 64-year-old woman with a history of coronary artery disease and angina presents to the preoperative clinic 1 week before a sigmoidectomy for diverticulosis. A nurse notes a new cardiac murmur.

Medical History

Coronary Artery Disease (see Chapter 3)

In 1996, a task force of the American College of Cardiology and American Heart Association released guidelines for perioperative cardiovascular evaluation for noncardiac surgery.[25] In these guidelines, the perioperative risk and need for diagnostic studies are based on the patient's history and the presence of clinical predictors of increased perioperative risk. A history of these clinical predictors, including myocardial infarction, angina, congestive heart failure (CHF), arrhythmias, valvular disease, DM, stroke, hypertension, and low functional capacity should be sought.

The patient had an anterior wall myocardial infarction 3 years ago. She has since been treated with atenolol, aspirin, and nitrates. She has chest pain and shortness of breath after walk-ing up a flight of stairs but never at rest. She denies paroxysmal nocturnal dyspnea, orthopnea, peripheral edema, or a history of CHF. Her heart sometimes "skips a beat," but she denies presyn-copal symptoms. She has hypertension controlled with atenolol. She has no history of a stroke or DM.

The patient's only **major** clinical predictor of perioperative car-diovascular risk is the possibility of valvular disease suggested by a murmur. She has **intermediate** predictors of mild stable angina and prior myocardial infarction. Her **minor** predictor is low func-tional capacity (fewer than four metabolic equivalents), but this must be interpreted carefully because noncardiac causes such as lung pathology and deconditioning may cause this finding.

The history of previous cardiac evaluations and interventions is important.

After her myocardial infarction, the patient had an exercise stress test, but it was nondiagnostic because her "legs were too weak." She had a dipyridamole thallium stress test showing no perfusion to a small anteroseptal area and no areas of reperfu-sion. She has not undergone coronary angiography, percutaneous transluminal coronary angioplasty, or coronary artery bypass grafting.

The patient's previous tests confirm the anterior wall myocardial infarction but show no other areas at risk. However, her disease may have progressed, especially given her exertional chest pain.

New Cardiac Murmur (see Chapter 4)

Valvular abnormalities are associated with various features[26] that should be sought from the history. The patient with aortic stenosis may have a history of hypertension, syncope, angina, or CHF.[26] Rheumatic heart disease, CHF, hoarseness, or hemoptysis may be present in the patient with mitral stenosis. Mitral regur-gitation may be secondary to endocarditis, rheumatic heart dis-ease, or a collagen vascular disease, and may manifest as CHF. Marfan's syndrome, aortic dissection, collagen vascular disease, and syphilis can cause aortic regurgitation.

A chart review shows that the patient has controlled hyperten-sion, an elevated cholesterol level, and angina. She does not have CHF, syncope, or any history suggestive of a particular valvular lesion.

Physical Examination

The physical examination should focus on predictors of cardio-vascular risk, including CHF, arrhythmias, hypertension, and valvular abnormalities. It should also define the cause of the murmur and its significance.

The patient's temperature is 36.9°C, pulse is 65 bpm, and respi-ratory rate is 17 breaths per minute. The blood pressure is 125/85 mm Hg.

Both lungs are clear. The heart rhythm is regular. The patient has a grade II systolic murmur, loudest at the right upper sternal border during midsystole, which radiates to the right carotid artery (see Chapter 4). S_2 is absent. The carotid pulse has a slow *rate of rise, and a delay is seen between the brachial and radial pulses. Valsalva's maneuver decreases the intensity of the murmur. The point of maximal impulse is discrete and not lateralized. Jugular venous pulse is diffuse, biphasic, and 2 cm above the angle of Louis while recumbent at 30 degrees. She has no hepatosplenomegaly or peripheral edema.*

The location, timing, and radiation of the murmur suggest aortic stenosis, and it is the only predictor of cardiovascular risk implied by the physical examination. The slow rate of rise of the carotid pulse, absent second heart sound, and brachial-radial delay also indicate aortic stenosis.[26,27] The patient has no evidence of CHF.

Diagnostic Testing

The need for cardiac diagnostic studies is based on previous studies, current clinical predictors, and the risk of the surgical procedure.[25]

The ECG shows Q waves in leads II, III, aVF, V_2, V_3, and V_4. No ST abnormalities are present. The CXR is normal except for calcification of the aortic valve. Hematocrit is 38% and platelet count is 172,000 per mm^3.

Because a recent stress test is unavailable, the preoperative workup is based on the presence of the two **intermediate** clinical predictors: mild angina and prior myocardial infarction. The patient may have the **major** clinical predictor of severe valvular disease, so its presence should be defined by echocardiography.

A two-dimensional transthoracic echocardiogram shows an aortic valve area of 0.6 cm^2 with an estimated transvalvular gradient of 50 mm Hg. Her left ventricular ejection fraction is 50% with concentric hypertrophy and a moderate area of anteroinferior wall akinesis.

The echocardiogram shows critical aortic stenosis (area less than 0.7 cm^2), which is a major predictor of cardiovascular risk. Because the patient will need aortic valve surgery, she should undergo coronary angiography to evaluate her coronary arteries because of her history of angina and a prior myocardial infarction.

Cardiac angiography shows a 75% left main coronary artery occlusion with mild diffuse distal disease of the left anterior descending and circumflex arteries. Aortic valve area is 0.5 cm^2 with a transvalvular gradient of 57 mm Hg.

Assessment

This 64-year-old woman categorized as ASA-PS class 3 has a significant left main coronary artery lesion with critical aortic stenosis and is scheduled for a high-risk procedure associated with large fluid shifts. She has a high risk of perioperative cardiac morbidity in her current state.

Management

Before the sigmoidectomy, the patient should undergo coronary artery bypass grafting for the left main arterial lesion and replacement or reconstruction of the aortic valve. These procedures are indicated to reduce her long-term morbidity and mortality related to her cardiac disease and not merely because of her scheduled sigmoidectomy.

When this patient returns for her sigmoidectomy, subacute bacterial endocarditis prophylaxis is indicated[28] (see Chapter 16).

REFERENCES

1. Diabetes Control and Complications Trial Research Group. Diabetes control and complications trial. *Diabetes* 1995;44:968–993.
2. Milan Study on Atherosclerosis and Diabetes Group. Prevalence of unrecognized silent myocardial ischemia and its association with atherosclerotic risk factors in noninsulin-dependent diabetes mellitus. *Am J Cardiol* 1997;79:134–139.
3. Watkins PJ. Diabetic autonomic neuropathy. *N Engl J Med* 1990;322:1078–1079.
4. Salem M, Tainsh RE, Bromberg J, et al. Perioperative glucocorticoid coverage: a reassessment 42 years after emergence of a problem. *Ann Surg* 1994;219:416–425.
5. Cormack RS, Lehane J. Difficult tracheal intubation in obstetrics. *Anaesthesia* 1984;39:1105–1111.
6. Mallampati SR, Gatt SP, Gugino LD, et al. A clinical sign to predict difficult tracheal intubation: a prospective study. *Can Anaesth Soc J* 1985;32:429–434.
7. Hogan K, Rusy D, Springman SR. Difficult laryngoscopy and diabetes mellitus. *Anesth Analg* 1988;67:1162–1165.
8. Stoelting RK, Dierdorf SF. *Anesthesia and coexisting disease*, 3rd ed. New York: Churchill Livingstone, 1993:447, 526–527, 613.
9. American Society of Anesthesiologists. New classification of physical status. *Anesthesiology* 1963;24:111–115.
10. Diaz JH, Hill GE. Hypotension with anesthesia in disulfiram treated patients. *Anesthesiology* 1979;51:355–358.
11. Sauvé JS, Laupacis A, Ostbye T, et al. Does this patient have a clinically important carotid bruit? *JAMA* 1993;270:2843–2845.
12. North American Symptomatic Carotid Endarterectomy Trial Collaborators (NASCET). Beneficial effect of carotid endarterectomy in symptomatic patients with high-grade carotid stenosis. *N Engl J Med* 1991;325:445–453.
13. Strunin I. Preoperative assessment of the patient with liver dysfunction. *Br J Anaesth* 1978;50:25–34.
14. Pugh RN, Murray-Lyon IM, Dawson JL, et al. Transection of the oesophagus for bleeding oesophageal varices. *Br J Surg* 1973;60:646–649.
15. Michel L, Serrano A, Malt RA. Nutritional support of hospitalized patients. *N Engl J Med* 1981;304:1147–1152.
16. Larsen LG. Asthma in children. *N Engl J Med* 1992;326:1540–1545.
17. McGill WA, Coveler LA, Epstein BS. Subacute upper respiratory infections in small children. *Anesth Analg* 1979;58:331–333.
18. Cohen MM, Cameron CB. Should you cancel the operation when a child has an upper respiratory tract infection? *Anesth Analg* 1991;72:282–288.
19. Tait AR, Knight PR. Intraoperative respiratory complications in patients with upper respiratory tract infections. *Can J Anaesth* 1987;34:300–303.
20. Larach MG. Standardization of the caffeine halothane contrac-

ture test. North American Malignant Hyperthermia Group. *Anesth Analg* 1989;69:511–515.

21. Rosenberg H, Fletcher JE, Seitman D. Pharmacogenetics. In: Barash PG, Cullen BF, Stoelting RK, eds. *Clinical anesthesia*, 3rd ed. Philadelphia: Lippincott–Raven Publishers, 1996:489–505.

22. Lenfant C, Khaltaev N. Global initiative for asthma. In: *Global strategy for asthma management and prevention*. National Heart, Lung, and Blood Institute/World Health Organization Workshop Report. Bethesda, MD: National Institutes of Health, 1993:1–176.

23. Coté CJ, Ryan JF, Todres ID, Goudsouzian NG. *A practice of anesthesia for infants and children*, 2nd ed. Philadelphia: WB Saunders, 1993:46.

24. Hackl W, Mauritz W, Winkler M, et al. Anaesthesia in malignant hyperthermia susceptible patients without dantrolene prophylaxis: a report of 30 cases. *Acta Anaesthesiol Scand* 1990;34:534–537.

25. Executive summary of the ACC/AHA task force report: guidelines for perioperative cardiovascular evaluation for noncardiac surgery. Report of American College of Cardiology/American Heart Association Task Force on Practice Guidelines (Committee on Perioperative Cardiovascular Evaluation for Noncardiac Surgery) *Anesth Analg* 1996;82:854–860.

26. Carabello BA, Crawford FA. Valvular heart disease. *N Engl J Med* 1997;337:32–39.

27. Etchells E, Bell C, Robb K. Does this patient have an abnormal systolic murmur? *JAMA* 1997;277:564–571.

28. Dajani AS, Taubert KA, Wilson W, et al. Prevention of bacterial endocarditis. Recommendations by the American Heart Association. *JAMA* 1997;227:1794–1801.

Page numbers followed by *f* indicate figures;
those followed by *t* indicate tables.

427